HANDBOOK OF PATHOLOGY AND PATHOPHYSIOLOGY OF CARDIOVASCULAR DISEASE

Developments in Cardiovascular Medicine

Previous volumes are still available

HANDBOOK OF PATHOLOGY AND PATHOPHYSIOLOGY OF CARDIOVASCULAR DISEASE

by

STEPHEN M. FACTOR, MD, FCAP, ACC
Professor of Pathology and Medicine
Albert Einstein College of Medicine
Bronx, New York

MARIA A. LAMBERTI – ABADI, MD
Assistant Professor of Pathology
Albert Einstein College of Medicine
Bronx, New York

and

JACOBO ABADI, MD
Assistant Professor of Pediatrics
Albert Einstein College of Medicine
Bronx, New York

KLUWER ACADEMIC PUBLISHERS
Boston / Dordrecht / London

Distributors for North, Central and South America:
Kluwer Academic Publishers
101 Philip Drive
Assinippi Park
Norwell, Massachusetts 02061 USA
Telephone (781) 871-6600
Fax (781) 681-9045
E-Mail <kluwer@wkap.com>

Distributors for all other countries:
Kluwer Academic Publishers Group
Distribution Centre
Post Office Box 322
3300 AH Dordrecht, THE NETHERLANDS
Telephone 31 78 6392 392
Fax 31 78 6392 254
E-Mail <services@wkap.nl>

 Electronic Services <http://www.wkap.nl>

Library of Congress Cataloging-in-Publication Data

A C.I.P. Catalogue record for this book is available
from the Library of Congress.

Printed on acid-free paper.

Printed in the United States of America

*The Publisher offers discounts on this book for course use and bulk purchases.
For further information, send email to mimi.breed@wkap.com.*

To my darling wife, and my lovely children with deepest appreciation for all your help and encouragement along the way. To my parents, for making me what I am. And, of course, with love to Raja. SMF

With love to my husband Yaco, our children Daniela, Adriana and David, my mom Renee, my brother Victor, and especially to my dad Jose A. (Cucho) Lamberti, MD, whose memory is a driving force in my life. MA

To my wife Lala and our kids, with all my HEART. You are the light of my life. To my parents, sister, and grandmother Sara, with love. JA

TABLE OF CONTENTS

PREFACE

Autopsy derives from the greek word *autopsia*, which means act of seeing with one's own eyes. It remains the most objective and accurate method to understand human.disease. Unfortunately, the volume of autopsies in teaching hospitals has decreased dramatically over the past years. The crucial factors that account for this are the recent progress and development of new technologies, especially in diagnostic imaging, immunology, cell biology and genetics. Additionally, the perpetual fear of legal liability by physicians accounts for its further decline. Consequently, physicians and medical students are engaged in fewer autopsies and are not reaping the rich educational rewards that accompany these examinations. The purpose of the autopsy is not only to establish the cause of death, but also to determine the nature and course of the disease process. Our goal with this book is to emphasize the importance of the post-mortem exam and the correlation between pathologic material and clinical data by analyzing actual cases with problem-based methodology. The focus of this handbook is on cardiovascular disease, and when appropriate, other disease categories are included if they have an impact on cardiovascular function.

The approach is more than the usual clinico-pathological correlation. Rather, we attempt to present the material from the perspective of the autopsy table. We use the clinical data as the initial framework and the autopsy findings to develop a true understanding of the disease and the associated pathophysiology of the condition. This approach is similar to the "gross" autopsy conferences that have been carried out at our institution for over 30 years. The format of the case presentation is logical and uniform with emphasis in teaching current medical concepts. Relevant clinical information is correlated and evaluated in the context of the macroscopic and microscopic findings obtained in the post-mortem exam. All cases are followed by a comprehensive discussion and review of the disease and pertinent literature is cited. We use extensive photographic material to illustrate each case and facilitate learning.

We address the new issue of legal liability by presenting cases that have medico-legal implications. A thorough discussion on the impact of significant discrepancies between the autopsy findings and clinical diagnoses is also included. This is particularly important in an era that demands quality assurance and performance improvement from the medical professionals.

Scientific methodology and common sense are still essential despite the forever growing knowledge of the medical sciences. Hopefully, with this book, we will succeed in guiding physicians and medical students in their continuous search for answers.

Chapter 1

PRACTICAL CARDIAC ANATOMY: FROM A TO Z

Introduction

It may represent a bias of the authors, but it appears to be a truism to state that the heart is the most complex anatomical structure in the body. Yes, the brain has an intricate spatial and electrical anatomy with numerous nuclei and interconnections, but it does not approach the complexity of the heart anatomically or physiologically. No organ other than the heart is divided into pumping chambers dependent on blood flow moving between two separate circulatory circuits, with the timing of blood movement within the chambers occurring within fractions of a second. This movement must be coordinated by a neural network (e.g. conduction system), heart valves, vascular supply, connective tissue and muscle cells. The heart is dependent on maintaining its own nutrition, while at the same time supplying oxygenated blood to the entire body. During the process of pumping, chamber contraction affects the supply of blood to the tissue performing the pumping, sometimes with adverse consequences. There must be an adequate flow of oxygenated blood to the heart cells, because they have very high metabolic requirements. Although myocytes are organized as individual cells and do not form a syncytium, they must 'talk' to each other electrically and functionally. The cells must each contract, but this contraction must then be coordinated so that groups and layers of cells are shortening sequentially within a very short period of time. Otherwise, this would lead to hypokinesia (decreased contraction), dyskinesia (abnormal contraction), or akinesia (absence of contraction).

Many books have been written on cardiac anatomy, both descriptive and illustrated. Detailed descriptions are available of the complex structural and functional anatomy of the heart; but most of such works do not provide adequate explanations for acquired pathophysiology or contractile dysfunction. The rationale for this book is different: we are attempting to correlate actual case material with clinically relevant findings, and to show how clinical manifestations, pathophysiology and pathology interact to produce disease. Furthermore, we want to show how there is a certain logic and analytical process that goes into each case, if one understands clinical findings **and** pathology. Our goal in this book is not to re-teach cardiac anatomy. Those who are interested or stimulated to do so can find any number of adequate books and atlases on the subject. We want to provide a brief outline of some basic features of cardiac anatomy, and by doing so, make pathophysiology and disease manifestations meaningful.

The following provides an alphabetical functional anatomical glossary. It is not proposed as a complete list, but one that illustrates the principle that at least some cardiovascular diseases and their complications are determined by cardiac anatomy and structure-function relationships.

Annulus

The fibrous ring that supports each of the 4 cardiac valves. The annulus for the tricuspid, mitral, and aortic valves is virtually a continuous structure arranged like a pretzel. The pulmonic valve annulus is somewhat separate from the other 3 (it arises from distinctly independent embryologic tissue, e.g. bulbus cordis). The valve base inserts into the annulus with inter-digitating connective tissue fibers. Infection of the valve tissue (endocarditis) can affect these connections thereby causing leaflet or cuspal dehiscence, or it can lead to an infection of the annulus itself (e.g. valve ring abscess). The proximity of the annulae of the 3 valves means that infection can spread readily from one to the other. The annulus also anchors the base of the heart through connective tissue attachment fibers that extend into the muscle of the ventricle. Sections of the base of the heart just below the annulus typically reveal fibrous tissue; however, this should not be interpreted as pathological scar since it represents normal anatomy. Dilatation of the ventricular or atrial chambers can stretch the annulae, most likely through side to side slippage of the connective tissue fibers. The dilatation may pull the valve base away from the center channel through which blood flows, and where there is closure with valve leaflet/cusp coaptation. The result is valvular insufficiency, as the valve tissue can no longer come together properly to close the orifice. By providing a surgical shortening of the annulus by placing crimping sutures, or by sewing in a prosthetic ring (annuloplasty), the annulus may be repaired with a decrease of insufficiency.

Aortic Valve

The 3 cusped valve separating the outflow tract of the left ventricle from the aorta. The cusps attach to the annulus, and insert as thin fibrous bands surfaced by endothelial cells (endocardium) into the aortic wall. These fibrous bands, immediately adjacent to each other but separated by less than 1 mm, form 3 commissures. Dilatation of the root of the aorta, the area immediately superior to the valve, may occur with connective tissue disease (e.g. Marfan's syndrome), atherosclerosis, or inflammation, and may lead to aortic valvular insufficiency. In particular, with syphilis, Takayasu's arteritis,

2

or rheumatoid arthritis, the inflammation and damage to these attachments leads to commissural separation, thus preventing cusp coaptation. The area behind the cusps, by the aortic surface, is a pocket known as the sinus of Valsalva (see below).

The sinuses are potential sites of stasis, and with aging, they may develop calcification followed by aortic valve degeneration with stenosis. The sinuses also contain the two coronary ostia (see below). The aortic valve is directly continuous with the ventricular surface of the mitral valve. Thus, infection, or degeneration of one valve can spread relatively easy to the other.

Apex, ventricle

A generally disregarded area of the heart, but one that may have important functional significance. It is composed of the most dependent portions of both left and right ventricles, with the myocardial fibers spiraling towards the tip of the chamber. The muscle and the associated connective tissue matrix (see below) come together as a button-like structure at this point. In fact, during normal contraction there is dimpling of the apex (dimples in the face are the result of connective tissue attachments between skeletal muscle and the dermis). It appears that the apex serves as a fulcrum for muscle shortening; thus, damage to the apex may have significant adverse consequences for ventricular contractile function, by 'untethering' the distal chamber attachments. Since the coronary supply to the apex is dependent on vessels derived from all 3 coronary arteries, obstruction of any one vessel may lead to either generalized infarction or no damage, depending on the collateral inter-connections between the vessels.

Atrio-ventricular node

A modified mass of myocardial cells that serves as the electrical pacemaker of the ventricles. Situated in the lower inter-atrial septum, it lies immediately superior to the tricuspid valve and its annulus and the mitral valve and its annulus. Blood supply is provided by a branch of the right coronary artery in most individuals, or a branch of the circumflex artery in the minority of cases. Thus disease of either vessel may lead to ischemic damage to the node, with the potential for conduction block. The node sends a bundle of fibers into the ventricles (the bundle of His, see below), by penetrating the annulus of the tricuspid and mitral valves. Thus, partial or complete heart block may occur with disease processes involving the annulus such as calcific degeneration of the annulus, infection, or surgical trauma following prosthetic valve replacement or repair of a congenital defect.

3

Bundle of His and conduction bundles

The bundle of His and conduction fibers are composed of modified cardiac muscle tissue. The bundle of His crosses through the annulus at the base of the cardiac septum. Upon reaching the ventricle, it divides into left and right divisions. The left division skirts around the membranous septum, where it then divides further into an anterior and posterior branch. The right bundle branch extends over the base of the septum into the right ventricle, where it runs superficially in a muscle known as the **moderator band** between the ventricular wall and the anterior papillary muscle. All of the conduction bundles are susceptible to damage or disruption, because they run superficially just below the endocardium. The bundle of His may be interrupted if the annulus develops degenerative calcification, or if it is affected by infection spreading from endocarditis of an adjacent heart valve. Left ventricular septal ischemia or infarction, high in the base around the membranous septum, may lead to left anterior or left posterior hemi-block. More proximal infarction may completely damage the bundle, leading to left, right, or complete heart block. Surgery for congenital heart disease, at or around the membranous septum may affect the bundle tissue in the surrounding myocardium. Aortic or mitral valve replacement surgery may lead to damage of conduction tissue if the prosthetic ring sewing sutures extend too deeply into the annulus.

Capillary loops

The myocardial microcirculation is an end-vascular system, which means that as the coronary arteries progressively branch into smaller ramifications, they reach a point where they no longer inter-connect. This lack of collaterals appears to occur when the vessels are approximately 25-50 microns in diameter, or at a level when they are pre-capillary arterioles. At that point, they give rise to an arcade of capillaries that do not inter-connect with adjacent arcades derived from other arterioles. The capillaries, usually 4-6 in number, provide oxygenated blood to individual myocytes looping around them, with the afferent arm draining into venules and then larger venous channels. This pattern of discrete capillary supply has several consequences. It provides an explanation for the very sharp histological and vascular border of ischemic myocardium, since there is minimal collateral blood flow at the cellular level. It also means that obstruction of arterioles (e.g. by spasm or microthrombosis), places a small number of myocytes at risk for necrosis defined by the arcade branching of the arteriole (generally about 10-20 myocytes, if examined in 3-dimensions).

Chordae tendineae

The fine fibrous bands that extend from the tips of the papillary muscles to the atrio-ventricular heart valves. The chordae branch at least 3 times and become smaller between the papillary muscle tip, known as the **myotendon** junction, and the valve. In total, there are approximately 120 chordae at the valve level. They insert on the undersurface of the valve, at the commissural junction, and at the free edge. With contraction of the ventricle, pressure within the cavity increases thereby forcing the leaflets of the mitral and tricuspid valves toward the midline. There is concurrent papillary muscle contraction, which pulls the chordae toward the mid portion of the ventricular chamber. This tethers the leaflets of the valves, prevents them from prolapsing into the atrium, and maintains their coaptation and orifice closure. The chordae from both papillary muscles in the left ventricle insert into both leaflets of the mitral valve. Therefore, partial disruption of the papillary muscle or dysfunction due to ischemia, may lead to a less severe degree of mitral valve insufficiency. Complete rupture of a papillary muscle, which may occur with infarction, generally causes massive mitral regurgitation, and usually rapid death due to pulmonary edema. Elongation or rupture of chordae can cause mitral regurgitation, and may occur as a result of connective tissue disease (e.g. Marfan's syndrome, and possibly the mitral valve prolapse syndrome). Rupture of one or multiple chordae can develop concomitantly with infection (endocarditis) or post-trauma. Chordae may also scar and shorten, or become adherent to adjacent chordae (so-called fusion) secondary to inflammation (typically seen in rheumatic heart disease). This may lead to valvular insufficiency by drawing the leaflets down into the ventricular cavity and preventing their coaptation.

Commissure

The commissures of the aortic valve have been described above; they are comparable for the pulmonic valve. The commissures of the atrio-ventricular valves are less well defined. The leaflets insert broadly into the annulae along a curved base; at the junction between one leaflet and the adjacent leaflet, they form a commissure. This is a potential site for damage. Inflammation, thrombus, and calcification may scar the commissure and prevent complete opening of the valve. This is typical of rheumatic heart disease with resulting mitral, or less commonly, tricuspid valve stenosis. Separation of these commissures may occur when the annulus is stretched or damaged; this results in valvular incompetence.

Conduction System

In addition to the atrio-ventricular node with the bundle of His and conduction bundles (see above), and the sino-atrial node (see below), the conduction system includes Purkinje fibers that course in the immediate subendocardium of the two ventricles. They serve as a fan-like projection of conductive fibers that rapidly transmit generated electrical impulses from the A-V node to the myocardium. Due to their subendocardial location, they are susceptible to damage from coronary artery ischemia that initially affects the inner wall of the ventricle. They also can be damaged with trauma (e.g. catheter-induced during invasive cardiology procedures; and open heart surgery), and endocardial injury secondary to inflammation or thrombosis. The conduction system is affected by external central neural influence through a network of nerves and ganglia in the outer atrial wall. Hormones and sympathetic and para-sympathetic transmitters also may affect it.

Connective Tissue Matrix

The myocardium is completely invested by a fine mesh-like network of connective tissue fibers that is virtually invisible with standard histologic sections, but can be visualized with special staining techniques or electron microscopy. This connective tissue wraps around single myocytes, attaches individual myocytes laterally, envelops groups of these cells, and maintains connections between myocyte layers in the ventricular wall. Although this skeletal framework is important for maintaining myocyte shape, it is critical for normal ventricular function. Damage or lysis of the matrix may result in ventricular dysfunction, even in the absence of significant myocyte injury. If the myocytes were not interconnected by matrix, they would be unable to generate a coordinated contraction to expel blood from the cavity. For the ventricular chamber to decrease its dimensions during systole, there must be both horizontal and vertical shortening. This is accomplished by a spiral movement of three obliquely oriented layers of myocardium that literally 'squeeze' the blood out of the chamber. To achieve this goal, there must be interconnection between the myocytes and the layers. There also must be tethering of the ventricle at both ends. In fact, there are parallel coiled fibers longitudinally oriented that run between myocardial cells that insert both as a 'button' at the apex (see above), and into the annulae at the base of the heart. Ischemia and inflammation, among other conditions, may lead to activation of local and systemic collagenolytic enzymes that may degrade the matrix. Degradation of matrix may cause localized or global remodeling of the ventricle with chamber dilatation. Increased synthesis of matrix, which occurs with aging and familial hypertrophic cardiomyopathy, among other conditions, decreases ventricular compliance and may lead to diastolic dysfunction.

Coronary Arteries

Muscular blood vessels lined by endothelium with a thin intima composed of 1-2 connective tissue cells at birth, and separated from the relatively thick media by an internal elastic lamella. The media usually has two obliquely oriented layers of smooth muscle. The outer coat of the artery is adventitia, or connective tissue that provides both innervation and blood supply to the coronary vessels (vasa nervorum and vasa vasorum, respectively). The diameter of the normal epicardial coronary artery, prior to its branching and entering the myocardium (where it is no longer susceptible to atherosclerosis) is usually 2-3 mm, but it can be variable. With progressive narrowing of the vessel secondary to atherosclerosis, there may be remodeling of the wall so that the overall diameter of the vessel may be increased, even when the functional lumen is decreased. Failure or inadequate remodeling has been suggested to be a contributing factor for coronary ischemia. The main condition that affects coronary arteries leading to disease is atherosclerosis; however, they are susceptible to inflammation (vasculitis), and non-atherosclerotic degeneration (calcification). The location of the major coronary arteries on the surface of the heart makes them vulnerable to blunt or penetrating chest trauma.

Coronary Ostia

The two openings for the left and right coronary arteries, usually located centrally at the upper portion of the sinus of Valsalva, approximately parallel to the free edge of the aortic valve. The location is variable. High insertion in the aortic wall has been associated with sudden cardiac death, presumably secondary to transient decrease of coronary flow (with high insertion, the ostium is affected by systolic pressure that can compress the opening, rather than diastolic pressure with which it is normally perfused). Lower insertion within the sinus of Valsalva may make the ostia more susceptible to stenosis by conditions that affect the aortic valve (e.g. degenerative calcification). Other acquired disease may lead to ostial stenosis. Atherosclerosis and/or inflammation of the ascending aorta, may cause narrowing of the ostium leading to myocardial ischemia, even in the absence of significant coronary artery disease. Syphilis is the classic cause of inflammatory ostial stenosis. Aortic dissection, when it leads to retrograde (e.g. towards the heart) splitting of the aortic wall, can disrupt the ostia.

Ductus Arteriosus

It represents one of the physiologic shunts of the fetal circulation (see also foramen ovale). It is the arterial connection between the left pulmonary artery and the aorta just distal to the origin of the left subclavian artery. The ductus allows for a bypass of the high-resistance pulmonary circulation, and the passage of oxygenated blood in the pulmonary artery into the aorta. It begins to close shortly after birth, and completes the closure within the first weeks of life. Persistence of a patent ductus arteriosus may lead to severe, irreversible pulmonary hypertension, if it is not closed.

In the newborn with certain congenital heart defects (e.g. ductal dependent lesions), the closure of the ductus arteriosus generally precipitates cardiovascular collapse. Therefore, it is usually kept open with medical therapy (prostaglandin E1), until surgical repair is possible.

Endocardium

The endothelial covering of the entire inner surface of the heart. This includes the cardiac chambers, both surfaces of the valves, and the chordae tendineae. The endocardium has functions similar to endothelium in vessels (the heart is really just a big muscular vessel). It can react to hormones (e.g. prostaglandins), and it has secretory capability with release of endothelin and nitric oxide. It most likely plays an active role in cardiac function, although it has not been studied extensively. The endocardium is susceptible to damage due to infection (e.g. endocarditis), thrombosis, and trauma from invasive procedures.

Foramen Ovale / Fossa Ovalis

Another one of the normal fetal circulation shunts (see ductus arteriosus). It refers to the opening in the mid-portion of the inter-atrial septum that allows oxygenated blood returning to the right heart from the placenta, to cross into the left atrium. The foramen is covered by a membrane, the septum secundum, which grows down on the left atrial side during embryogenesis, and overlies a separate membrane. During fetal development, when pressures are higher in the right atrium, there is flow from right to left, even when the membrane has completed its development. Following birth, when pressures become higher on the left side, the septum secundum is forced against the foramen, thereby maintaining it closed. Usually, the membrane fuses to the tissue, and there is an oval depression in the atrial wall (fossa ovalis). If the fusion is incomplete, one can put a probe through the foramen between the two membrane layers demonstrating the so-called 'probe-patent foramen'. This is usually of no clinical significance, and may only be an incidental finding at autopsy. However, if there is a marked increase of right-sided pressures as a result of pulmonary hypertension or other causes, the effects of the pressure and the dilatation of the right atrial cavity may lead to a progressive enlargement of the probe-patent foramen . This can then result in a clinically evident right to left shunt, or an acquired atrial septal defect (ASD).

Growth, Cardiac

The heart grows physiologically proportionally to body mass. The relationship is maintained from the fetus to the adult, and is equally true for all mammalian species. As a general rule, the heart weight can be estimated from the lean body mass. However, by multiplying the weight expressed in kilograms by 0.50% for a man, and 0.40% for a woman (because woman have a lower lean body mass), an approximation of the normalized heart weight can be determined. Physiological heart weight (e.g. without associated with fibrosis and myocyte damage) is maximized at 400-450 g for males, and 350-400 g for females, regardless of body size. Beyond these weight limits, there is virtually always pathology in the heart.

Heart Orientation

Although standard terminology suggests that the heart is oriented in a left-right direction, this is misleading. The heart is actually positioned so that the right ventricle is anterior, and lies just below the sternum. The major portion of the left ventricle lies posterior and lateral to the right ventricle, with the apex composed of the left and right ventricles obliquely pointing to the left. The right atrium is superior and posterior to the right ventricle. The left atrium is the most superior and posterior structure, lying as it does immediately anterior to the esophagus and vertebral column. This provides an explanation for why trans-esophageal echocardiography (TEE) is such a superior technique for visualizing the mitral valve; the TEE transducer introduced into the esophagus, is immediately adjacent to the valve. Another important consequence of the anatomical orientation is the effect of trauma. Blunt trauma to the chest wall (e.g. seat belt or steering wheel injury) may lead to contusion of the anterior surface of the heart below the sternum, or the right ventricle. If the trauma is more lateral and to the left, it may contuse the anterior surface of the left ventricle. Penetrating trauma (e.g. knife or gun shot) often leads to penetration of the anterior right ventricular wall, at a minimum. Marked compressive trauma to the chest wall may lead to rupture

9

of the thin-walled right ventricle, as the competent tricuspid valve allows for excessive pressure to develop in the ventricular cavity.

Interventricular Septum

The muscular separation between the left and right ventricles. The septum has a relatively smooth endocardial surface on the left ventricular outflow tract, whereas, the right ventricular surface of the septum is diffusely trabeculated. The septum is functionally considered to be a left ventricular structure. This is significant since endomyocardial biopsies of the septum are performed on the right side, for reasons of easy access through the jugular vein as well as increased safety; however, the biopsy findings usually reflect pathology present in the left ventricle (e.g. cardiomyopathy or myocarditis).

Jelly, Cardiac

The relatively acellular layer forming the wall of the embryologic cardiac tube, separating endothelial cells internally from an external layer of mantle cells. This tube forms the primitive ventricular tube and bulbus cordis.

Koch, Triangle

The triangle of Koch is the area defined inferiorly by the septal leaflet of the tricuspid valve inserting into the annulus, posteriorly by the coronary sinus, and superiorly by the ridge-like **tendon of Todaro.** The triangle is significant because it contains the atrio-ventricular node. For proper examination of the node, the triangle of Koch is sectioned, along with the annulus of the tricuspid and mitral valves, and the superior interventricular septum. This block of tissue permits examination of the node, and the bundle of His, as it penetrates the annulus.

Lambl's Excrescence

A small papillary frond-like vegetation that is found on the closing edge of valve cusps and leaflets. It is typically seen in the central closing edge of the aortic valve cusps. The excrescence resembles a fine thread-like structure. Microscopically, they have a fibrous core, and a surface of endothelial cells. They are thought to arise from localized trauma to the valve from repetitive closure, with organization of the resulting fibrin and platelet vegetation. They are related to the much less common, and larger, organized vegetation called **papillary fibroelastoma**. The latter lesions, for many years, were considered to be benign tumors or hamartomas. Structurally, however, they appear to be due to non-bacterial vegetation that undergoes replacement of the fibrin and platelets by fibrous and elastic connective tissue. Clinically, they are rarely significant. However, if a larger lesion, particularly on a stalk, prolapses into a coronary ostium, it may lead to sudden death or myocardial infarction. In contrast, the Lambl's excrescence is too small, and is only an incidental finding at autopsy.

Membranous Septum

The round or oval-shaped membranous area immediately below the aortic valve annulus. There are a number of congenital defects of this structure, particularly in association with endocardial cushion defects; however, isolated membranous septal defects also occur. Acquired defects may develop secondary to infective endocarditis of the aortic valve that extend to the aortic annulus and then to the septal base. Such defects typically present at or around the tricuspid valve. The membranous septum is the anatomic landmark where the atrio-ventricular conduction tissue progresses through the annulus at the base of the septum, and then branches into left anterior and posterior divisions. Infection of the membranous septum, or surgical repair of a defect, may lead to interruption of the bundle tissue and the development of acquired left heart block.

Mitral Valve

The only valve with 2 leaflets. The mitral valve has an unusual configuration, with marked asymmetry of the leaflets. The **anterior leaflet** is a broad, shield-shaped structure that fills approximately two-thirds of the valve orifice, but only one-third of the annular circumference. It extends much deeper into the ventricular chamber than the **posterior leaflet**. The latter is a shallow, usually scalloped leaflet that has a broad annular attachment, but comprises only one-third of the orifice area. Together, the 2 leaflets have approximately equal surface areas. Both are tethered on their undersurfaces by chordae tendineae and two papillary muscles, which maintain them in a flat orientation relative to the annulus during ventricular systole. When seen from the atrial surface, the 2 leaflets have a curvilinear convex-concave apposition, with the convex surface from the anterior leaflet; resembling a 'fish-mouth'. The mitral valve orifice is large, thereby allowing a high volume of blood to be passed into the ventricle at low pressure. The commissural attachments of the 2 leaflets are poorly defined areas of junction, but important sites for inflammation (e.g. rheumatic heart disease) and infection.

Nuclei, Myocyte

Myocytic nuclei are relatively large, round to oval-shaped structures at birth. During embryogenesis, mitotic division of nuclei and cells can be easily appreciated. Shortly after birth, mitoses become exceedingly rare. For years it has been assumed that myocytes are terminally differentiated cells, with no new cell proliferation after birth. Recent evidence suggests that limited numbers of cells may proliferate in adulthood around areas of injury (e.g. healing myocardial infarction). It is known that myocyte nuclei may divide without cytokinesis, thereby giving rise to myocardial cells with 2 nuclei. This is common with increasing age, particularly in association with myocardial hypertrophy. Also with age and hypertrophy, myocyte nuclei may increase their chromosome number by meiosis without nuclear division. This gives rise to heteroploid nuclei, typically with a doubling of chromosomes. On routine section, stained with hematoxylin, the nuclei have a larger configuration with increased blue staining intensity.

Organization, Myocardium

As discussed in **connective tissue matrix,** the myocardium is composed of obliquely oriented layers that 'wrap' around the ventricular cavity. This is particular obvious in the left ventricle, with 3 layers; whereas, the thinner, low-pressure right ventricle generally has 2 less well-defined layers. Since the layers in the left ventricle are oriented obliquely to each other, sectioning through the ventricular wall reveals groups of myocardial cells parallel to each other, but oriented at approximately 45 degrees to adjacent parallel bundles of cells. Thus, a section across the left ventricle wall has myocytes oriented longitudinally, obliquely, and in cross-section. These layers are attached to each other by connective tissue matrix fibers as previously discussed. Contraction of the ventricle takes place in a screw-like manner, as the obliquely oriented layers shorten in a curvilinear pattern from apex to base. Upon diastolic relaxation, since the layers and the individual myocytes are interconnected, and because there are spring-like connective tissue fibers running along the axis of the ventricle, negative pressure develops enhancing diastolic filling by 'sucking' blood from the atrial cavities.

Papillary Muscle

There are 2 papillary muscles in the left ventricle, an anterolateral and a posteromedial. They are broad, finger-like projections into the cavity that enlarge with ventricular hypertrophy, and therefore may contribute to a decreased cavity volume in association with conditions such as hypertension. The papillary muscles also have a terminal coronary circulation with little or no collaterals. Ischemia associated with the left anterior descending or circumflex coronary arteries makes them particularly susceptible to necrosis or focal scarring. This may lead to papillary muscle dysfunction, and without the tethering effect of the muscle, mitral valve regurgitation. Typically, each papillary muscle has multiple smaller heads giving rise to chordae tendineae. The main papillary muscle body is known as the belly. The chordae from both papillary muscles fan out to support both leaflets of the mitral valve. The chordae from the 2 right ventricular papillary muscles support the anterior and middle leaflet. The septal leaflet chordae insert directly into the ventricular septum without a papillary muscle. In the right ventricle, the papillary muscles are less prominent, appearing more like hypertrophied trabeculae.

Pericardium

A thin fibrous sac that envelops the heart and extends along the ascending aorta to the brachiocephalic artery. Thus, rupture of the ascending aorta (often as a result of aortic dissection) can lead to pericardial tamponade. The pericardium is structurally considered as 2 surfaces: a visceral layer made up of mesothelial cells overlying the epicardial fibroadipose tissue, and a parietal layer with an inner lining of mesothelial cells, a fibrous body, and an outer layer that blends with the connective tissue of the mediastinum. The mesothelial cells secrete a small volume (usually 10-20 cc) of thin serous fluid that serves to lubricate pericardial and cardiac movement. The pericardial sac is drained by lymphatic channels. Increased secretion (e.g. associated with inflammation), or reversal of lymphatic flow (e.g. associated with elevated pressure in the venous and lymphatic system that occurs in right-sided congestive heart failure) leads to increased fluid volume in the pericardial sac. A slow accumulation of volume allows the fibrous pericardium to accommodate; whereas if it occurs acutely, the volume and pressure can cause tamponade. The fibrous pericardium stretches by a slippage of 2-3 obliquely oriented collagen fiber layers attached by connective tissue matrix fibers, and also elastic fibers within the tissue. An increase of pericardial sac volume is possible between 1-2 liters, as long as it occurs slowly. This volume includes the actual fluid within the sac, as well as the mass of the hypertrophied heart.

Pulmonary Valve

Structurally it is similar to the aortic valve, with 3 cusps. The sinuses behind the cusps are shallower than the sinuses of Valsalva. Compared to the aortic valve, the pulmonary valve is rarely susceptible to degeneration, inflammation, or infection; presumably because it is not chronically damaged by a high pressure system. The valve is the site of congenital anomalies particularly that associated with **tetralogy of Fallot**.

Right Ventricle

As described in the organization of the myocardium, the right ventricle is a thin-walled structure with several poorly defined layers of myocardium. The free-wall and septum are heavily trabeculated. The free-wall is often infiltrated by fibroadipose tissue that extends between the muscle fibers from the epicardial fat towards the endocardium. This tends to increase with obesity, and is often associated with diabetes mellitus. There is generally no functional consequence of this increase of adipose tissue, but it may lead to confusion on endomyocardial biopsy interpretation with a relatively rare condition known as right ventricular cardiomyopathy. The latter condition, is associated with a marked increase of fat and connective tissue in the ventricle, and is associated with sudden cardiac death.

The right ventricle undergoes significant remodeling after birth since it is relatively hypertrophied compared to the left ventricle, and is usually equal in thickness. Within months of delivery it becomes proportionally one-third to one-half the thickness of the left ventricular wall. It can hypertrophy, however, in association with pressure overload usually due to persistent or acquired pulmonary hypertension.

Sinoatrial Node

An elongated, fusiform collection of modified cardiac muscle cells and connective tissue lying immediately below the epicardium at the junction of the superior vena cava and the right atrial wall. The node is supplied by a branch of the right coronary artery or a branch of the left circumflex coronary artery in about equal numbers of people. Degeneration of the node may occur with ischemia, inflammation, or in association with increased atrial pressure.

Tricuspid Valve

Although structurally considered to have 3 leaflets, the tricuspid valve frequently has a diffusely scalloped appearance with numerous small leaflets. This appearance is enhanced if associated with fibromyxomatous valve disease (e.g. 'floppy' mitral valve, or mitral valve prolapse). In general the most common cause of tricuspid valve regurgitation is secondary to dilatation of the tricuspid annulus in association with right ventricular chamber dilatation and failure. The tricuspid valve commissures are also poorly defined. Typically there are 3 leaflets: anteriosuperior (or anterior leaflet), posteroinferior (mid or mural leaflet), and septal. As noted previously, the septal leaflet has chordal attachments that insert directly into the septal wall. The orifice of the tricuspid valve is the largest of the 4 valves, ranging from 11.0-13.0 mm, compared to the mitral valve 8.0-10.0 mm, the aortic valve 7.0-8.5 mm, and the pulmonic valve 7.5-9.0 mm.

Ultrastructure

The ultrastructural appearance of the myocardium is complex and would take an entire atlas to describe. Several unique features will be outlined here. Myocardial cells are generally elongated, with lateral branches that attach at each end and at the end of the branches to adjacent cells by electron-dense **intercalated disks**. The **sarcolemma** or myocardial cell membrane is lined by a basal lamina. Invaginations of the sarcolemma at the level of the **Z-band** extend deeply into the myocyte along with a thinner basal lamina. This is called the **T-tubule** which permits access of electrolytes into the myocyte where there is interaction at the **sarcoplasmic reticulum** (a series of fine tubules that extend along the contractile fibrils) to release or uptake calcium necessary for myocyte contraction and relaxation. The contractile unit is known as the **sarcomere**. It includes myosin, actin, and a number of associated fibrils. The margins of the sarcomere are the lateral **Z-Band** into which the thick myosin filaments attach. The central portion of the sarcomere is the **A-Band**, composed of actin filaments. Although far too complex to describe here, the actin and myosin filaments slide over each other during each contractile cycle, powered by adenosine triphosphate (ATP). The mitochondria supply the ATP, and lie between the myofibrils (groups of myofilaments. Not surprisingly, comparable to the microscopic anatomy of ventricular muscle contraction, the myofilaments and myofibrils are interconnected through a cytoskeletal framework. These cytoskeletal fibers are attached to the sarcolemma and, through it, to the extracellular space. Other structures of note, that have a potential role in storage diseases affecting heart muscle, are lysosomes. These are typically found adjacent to both ends

15

of the nucleus in the cell center. In adults, the lysosomes usually contain lipid droplets and cell debris.

Valves

The four valves have a similar microscopic appearance, despite their different gross anatomy. Each is surfaced entirely by endocardium. Beneath the endocardial layer, there is a fibrous layer (fibrosa) of variable thickness, which increases with age. The fibrous layer is also thicker in the left-sided valves, than those on the right side. The central region of the valve is composed of a myxoid layer with scattered spindled and stellate connective tissue cells, and loose mucopolysaccharide (spongiosa). There is expansion of both the fibrous and the myxoid layer in fibromyxomatous valve degeneration with a proportionally greater increase in the myxoid zone. Moreover, there are relatively severe changes seen in association with hereditary connective tissue conditions such as Marfan's syndrome, or Ehlers-Danlos syndrome. In clinically less severe forms of valve degeneration, associated with most cases of floppy mitral valve disease, both the fibrosa and the spongiosa increase to a variable degree. As a general rule, in association with fibromyxomatous valve degeneration, the surface area of the valve leaflets or cusps increases, with the development of tissue redundancy. This is not the sole explanation for valvular insufficiency, since the chordae tendineae also increase in length, in the more severe forms. Comparable to the development of vascular thrombosis, degeneration or injury to the endocardial layer is the initiating event in all forms of valvular vegetation (infective or non-infective). However, some virulent bacterial organisms may directly adhere to the valvular endocardium, thereby initiating infective endocarditis.

Wall-Thickness

Cardiac organization and structure has been discussed in detail; however, the wall thickness of the left and right ventricles can provide useful clues to underlying disease, and correlation with clinical symptomatology. The ventricle should be measured from endocardium to inner epicardium, with the measurement not including trabeculae, papillary muscles, or epicardial adipose tissue. The measures are usually carried out in a standard location: the outflow tract of both ventricles. However, if there is asymmetrical hypertrophy (e.g. septal hypertrophy associated with hypertrophic cardiomyopathy, or a subaortic hypertrophy associated with hypertensive heart disease), it is worthwhile to measure in multiple sites. Some prefer measuring the mid-portion of the left ventricle, since it can provide useful correlation with echocardiographic measurements. For a 'normal-sized' heart of 350-400 g in an adult, the left ventricle should measure between 1.3-1.5 cm in thickness, and the right ventricle 0.3-0.4 cm. Obviously, this is variable, since as discussed previously, heart weight is proportional to body weight, in general. Increases of wall thickness above these limits are associated with hypertrophy. Then, it is necessary to determine the etiology of the hypertrophy, and whether it is diffuse (concentric) or focal (eccentric). Furthermore, the absence of hypertrophy, or subnormal thickness is also meaningful. A markedly enlarged heart (e.g. increased cardiac mass) with a 'normal' wall thickness of 1.5 cm is not necessarily a positive finding. It generally implies that there has been ventricular remodeling and cavity dilatation, associated with ventricular dysfunction and, possibly, congestive heart failure. Subnormal measurements almost always indicate dysfunction or mural damage. Cardiac wall thinning also may occur with loss of cardiac mass (atrophy associated with malnutrition or cachexia), but usually the wall maintains proportionality with the cardiac mass.

Z-Band

This has been discussed previously under ultrastructure. It represents the borders of the sarcomere, visible under the light microscope as cross-striations. It is composed of a structural protein known as α-actinin. Normally the Z-band is a relatively straight electron dense line that runs perpendicular to the sarcolemma. In myocellular damage, or in hypertrophy, the Z-band may increase in volume, and may take on an irregular streaming appearance, losing its straight borders. The distance between two Z-bands defines the sarcomere, and it is a relatively fixed measurement ranging between 1.6 and 2.2 microns. This is a physiologically critical distance in which there is maximal overlap of the cross-bridges between actin and myosin filaments. Longer distance virtually always indicates cell damage. Thickening of cross-striations is typically seen in **contraction band necrosis**, which is an irreversible form of cell necrosis associated with reperfusion injury. It represents a hypercontraction of the cell secondary to an influx of calcium ions across the sarcolemma, leading to a herniation of the actin and myosin filaments in the central portion of the cell. It does not usually include the Z-band.

Chapter 2

ATHEROSCLEROTIC HEART DISEASE AND ISCHEMIA

Case # 1

Clinical Summary

This is the case of an 84 year old man who was admitted with complaints of chest pain and shortness of breath for 2 hours. The pain started at 2:30 AM and he was brought to the hospital at 4:00 AM. His past medical history was remarkable for insulin-dependent diabetes mellitus. There was no history of cerebro-vascular accident (CVA), myocardial infarction (MI) or peripheral vascular disease (PVD). He was an alcohol user, but not a smoker. On admission, the vital signs were: BP 140/70 mmHg, T 37°C, P 87, R 32. The physical exam was significant for jugular vein distention and on cardiac auscultation an S4.

Laboratory data and other tests

Laboratory: WBC 11, Hg/Hct 11/34; BUN/Creat 23/1.8, SGOT/SGPT 51/41, LDH 172, CPK 22; PT/PTT 10/17. The ECG showed 1st degree AV block, and ST elevation in V2-V5.

Hospital course: a diagnosis of anterior myocardial infarction was made. The patient was given the thrombolytic agent TPA (tissue plasminogen activator), aspirin (ASA) and nitroglycerin, with which he had an initial improvement. No cardiac arrhythmias were recorded. At 7:30 am, he suddenly went into cardiopulmonary arrest. Resuscitation efforts were unsuccessful.

Gross Description

The autopsy exam was limited to the chest. The body weighed 70 kg and measured 173 cm. The heart weighed 430 g. The pericardium was smooth and there was no pericardial effusion. The walls of the left and right ventricle measured 1.4 and 0.4 cm in thickness, respectively. The size of the chambers was normal. The leaflets and cusps of the valves as well as the chordae tendineae appeared normal. The myocardium revealed a hemorrhagic infarct involving approximately 60% of the left ventricular wall

(Figure 1). The coronary arteries showed severe atherosclerotic changes with up to 95% occlusion of the left main coronary artery, 85% occlusion of the left anterior descending and circumflex arteries, and 60% occlusion of the right coronary artery. There was no evidence of acute thrombosis of these vessels. The aorta showed moderate atherosclerosis, but no aneurysms were identified. The lungs weighed 1200 g combined and were congested.

Microscopic Description

Sections from the left ventricle showed myocyte swelling, contraction bands, interstitial hemorrhage and neutrophilic infiltration involving 80% of the left ventricular wall. This finding was consistent with recent hemorrhagic (reperfusion) infarct (6-12 hours old) (Figure 2). In addition, there was evidence for severe myocardial hypertrophy, interstitial and perivascular fibrosis, and multiple areas of replacement fibrosis and hyaline eosinophilic material distinct from scar tissue. The latter finding was consistent with remote infarct and multifocal deposition of amyloid. Sections from the left main and left anterior descending coronary arteries showed severe calcific atherosclerosis with lumen occlusion and ruptured plaque.

The lung revealed severe pulmonary hypertension, interstitial fibrosis with chronic inflammation, parenchymal congestion, emphysema and diffuse anthracosis.

Case Analysis

This is an instructive case for understanding the pathophysiology and the pathogenesis of acute myocardial infarction. A number of critical events took place over a brief period of time, in someone who was seemingly healthy despite being an insulin-dependent diabetic (presumably type II diabetes mellitus). He developed a fulminant course that led to his death within hours of symptom onset. The analysis of these events can teach us much about ischemic heart disease.

We know little about this man prior to his presentation to the emergency room early in the morning. He had complaints of chest pain that were not characterized in the record as to their nature or radiation, but clearly sufficient to bring him to the hospital. It is noteworthy that the pain developed in the early morning hours, obviously when he was at rest, since this is the most common time for acute myocardial ischemia to develop. Although this is counterintuitive in that it is often assumed that myocardial infarction is most often associated with exercise; development of acute ischemia and/or sudden arrhythmia leading to death occurs more frequently in the hours between midnight and 6 A.M. Why this is so, is not entirely understood, but some postulate that there may be acute hormonal or neural effects on the coronary circulation, possibly related to rapid eye movement (REM) sleep. We do know about his diabetes mellitus, but there is no report as to whether he was chronically hypertensive. This is an important piece of information lacking in the record, since it may affect the decision to use thrombolytic therapy, which carries somewhat more risk in hypertensive patients because of the potential for hemorrhagic cerebral infarctions. Regardless, we are told that his blood pressure was normal in the emergency room (140/70 mmHg), but this may represent a fall in pressure in someone with evidence of left ventricular failure.

He did have findings that were strongly suggestive of heart failure despite maintaining normal blood pressure and pulse rate. His complaints of chest pain were associated with shortness of breath, consistent with pulmonary congestion secondary to left heart failure. The chest X-ray demonstrated an enlarged heart, which may be secondary to pre-existing cardiomegaly, or to an increase of the cardiac silhouette due to dilatation. However, it also showed increased vascular congestion and interstitial edema, which is one of the earliest signs of elevated left atrial pressure, presumably due to increased end-diastolic pressure in a failing left ventricle. Moreover, he had an S4 gallop rhythm, which is a pre-systolic extra sound due to atrial contraction with blood forced into a less compliant left ventricle. Myocardial infarction decreases the compliance of the left ventricle due to the stiffness of non-contracting myocytes, and the presence of interstitial edema. Although not specific for myocardial infarction because other conditions may lead to stiffness of the ventricular wall (e.g. sarcoidosis and scarring), an S3 and/or S4 gallop is a frequent finding in patients with myocardial infarction. In addition, the patient presented with jugular venous distention, which is a sign of elevated pressure in the right atrium, most likely due to right ventricular failure.

On clinical grounds, was there sufficient information to support the diagnosis of an acute myocardial infarction? The acute onset of heart failure with chest pain is presumptive evidence; however, unstable angina pectoris may be associated with ventricular failure due to stunned myocardium (e.g. ischemia-induced contractile dysfunction without myocardial necrosis), and cannot be used as an absolute indicator of infarction. The electrocardiographic findings of ST elevation in the anterior leads V2-V5 are supportive of acute ischemia, but whether the ischemia was transient or associated with actual tissue damage cannot be determined from this information. The creatine kinase (CK) was within normal limits (22 U/L). Does this mean there was no myocardial necrosis, or was the enzyme drawn too early in the course of events to be abnormal? Creatine kinase is an intracellular enzyme that is only released into the interstitium from necrotic cells. It is then mobilized in the cardiac lymph, where it is eventually drained

21

from cardiac lymphatics into the venous system through the thoracic duct. The measured enzyme activity of CK is thus dependent on the volume of myocardium undergoing damage, the time it takes for the enzyme to reach the circulation, and the velocity of the lymphatic drainage. The latter is at least, partially dependent on blood flow and interstitial pressure in the affected tissue. This generally correlates with whether there is blood flow (e.g. in an infarction due to coronary occlusion with profound ischemia, versus a transient occlusion of the coronary artery with subsequent re-perfusion). In the situation where profound ischemia develops, the CK may peak at 12-24 hours after the onset of infarction. In contrast, with a reperfusion infarction, the CK may be "washed out" of the tissues more rapidly, thereby leading to an earlier peak elevation, which by 12-24 hours post- injury may already return to baseline values. The fact that the CK was normal within several hours after the onset of pain may be due to the early time course of events. Within the last several years, another more sensitive, early marker for myocardial necrosis has been identified: Troponin I enters the serum earlier than CK, and it persists there longer. The other clinical laboratory finding in this man that may support a presumptive diagnosis of myocardial infarction is the elevated white blood count (WBC) of 10,900 cells/nL. Non-specific mild elevations of the WBC are often present in early myocardial infarction but generally not with anginal chest pain without myocardial necrosis.

Therefore, based on the initial presentation, it is not absolutely certain that a completed myocardial infarction had developed by the time the patient reached the emergency room. This may explain why the physicians elected to treat him with TPA, despite the potential risks in an older patient with diabetes mellitus and possible hypertension. The efficacy of treatment with TPA or streptokinase is directly related to the time in which re-perfusion is achieved, and this is dependent on the pathophysiology of myocardial infarction. Myocardial infarction is the end result of tissue damage, which is blood flow and time dependent. What this means is that when coronary flow to the tissue is suddenly interrupted, the tissue supplied by that vessel becomes acutely ischemic. Assuming that the tissue is not protected by sufficient collateral blood flow to prevent ischemic injury (a situation that is not common in the human heart), or that the myocardium has not been pre-conditioned with previous transient episodes of ischemia in the hours or days prior to the acute coronary occlusion (this may have the effect of providing partial myocardium protection, and eventually slow the progression of the injury), then the myocardium will begin to undergo necrosis.

Myocardial necrosis occurs sequentially from the inner subendocardial layer of the ventricular wall, through the mid and subepicardial layers of the ventricle until the infarction is transmural (more than 50% of the ventricular thickness). This process of inner wall to outer wall progression is known as the 'wave-front' phenomenon. Originally described by Reimer and Jennings, it relates the necrosis of the myocardium to the blood flow and the time in which the blood flow is decreased below a critical level. The progression of the 'wave-front' phenomenon is accelerated by severe ischemic conditions, mainly low collateral blood flow, hypotension, or increased myocardial oxygen demand (i.e. tachycardia, fever). In contrast to experimental infarctions where a coronary artery can be occluded suddenly in a completely normal heart, humans will have variable amounts of time required for actual necrosis. In addition, this time can be affected by other coexistent medical conditions (i.e. coronary atherosclerosis, hypertension, myocardial hypertrophy, and ventricular scarring). Nonetheless, in most cases, the infarction of the inner myocardial layers ensues within hours. The clinical implications of the wave-front phenomenon are profound, for it explains why some individuals develop a subendocardial and others a transmural myocardial infarction. Spontaneous interruption of coronary occlusion (e.g. intrinsic thrombolysis, or relaxation of a coronary artery spasm) leads to a cessation of the myocardial ischemia, and reperfusion of the necrotic tissue by blood. Hence, subendocardial myocardial infarctions are generally hemorrhagic. Complete coronary occlusion by thrombus, may be treated by thrombolysis or emergency angioplasty, leading to patency of the vessel, and the transformation of what would have been a transmural infarction into a subendocardial infarction. However, this is only effective if the reperfusion occurs within a time frame in which all of the myocardium destined to die has not done so. If the tissue is already necrotic, reperfusion only leads to the development of a hemorrhagic transmural infarction, which also has some increased risk because such infarctions are somewhat more susceptible to the fatal complication of ventricular rupture. It is particularly difficult in clinical situations to be cognizant of the time course of myocardial ischemia and infarction, because, as in this case, it is not clear that the symptoms were secondary to unstable angina pectoris, or actual myocardial infarction.

The treatment of this patient with TPA appeared to lead to initial improvement, suggesting that thrombolysis had been achieved. It is only a suggestion because his improvement may have been the result of treatment with nitroglycerin and subsequent anginal pain relief. It is noteworthy that he did not develop acute arrhythmias when TPA was infused, as sudden reperfusion following thrombolysis may decrease the sensitivity of the ischemic but not infarcted myocardium to electrical instability, leading to ventricular tachycardia or fibrillation, among other rhythms. It is also possible that the absence of initial arrhythmia was related to delayed thrombolysis, and that the sudden cardiac arrest he developed three hours after TPA administration was due to sudden reperfusion of the tissue at that point. Had CK enzymes been drawn sequentially every hour after TPA administration, it is possible that the time course of thrombolysis might have

23

been marked by a sudden elevation of the enzyme as it was washed out of the necrotic myocardium. It is also conceivable that the TPA played no role in his death, and that the sudden arrhythmia was a spontaneous event associated with extensive myocardial infarction.

The autopsy clarified some of the pathophysiological and pathogenetic events. He had mild cardiomegaly; a 70 kg male should have a heart that weighs no more than 350-400 g (approximately 0.5% of the body weight expressed in kilograms). The heart weight of 430 g is most likely a reflection of pre-existent hypertension and prior myocardial damage. He had critical atherosclerotic narrowing (generally defined as more than 75%) of his entire left coronary artery system (left main, left anterior descending, and left circumflex), with moderate stenosis of his right coronary artery. With such severe disease of his left coronary artery, he was at extremely high risk for myocardial infarction and/or sudden cardiac death. The fact that he may not have experienced prior symptoms could be related to his diabetes mellitus, which is frequently associated with silent ischemia. The microscopic observation of multifocal replacement fibrosis was consistent with remote, presumably silent myocardial infarction, as well as myocardial damage associated with intramyocardial small vessel disease (a frequent finding in diabetic patients). He had a transmural myocardial infarction that grossly involved 60 % of the ventricular wall thickness, and microscopically was up to 80 %; however, its appearance clearly indicated it was a reperfusion infarction, since it was hemorrhagic. Thus, it would appear that the TPA had been effective, but it most likely was given too late to prevent a transmural infarction. On the other hand, since the infarction had been aborted at only 60-80% of the ventricular wall, and had he not developed a sudden arrhythmic death, the treatment might have had a positive effect on his subsequent ventricular function.

The marked coronary atherosclerosis and the observation of a ruptured atherosclerotic plaque, provide insight into a pathophysiologic conundrum regarding coronary artery disease. How can patients, such as this one, progress for years with significant occlusive coronary artery disease, and then suddenly have an acute event that takes place over minutes to hours leading to myocardial infarction and sudden arrhythmic death? The simple answer, but one that has only become evident over the last approximately 25 years, is that the chronic atherosclerotic plaque must be affected by a sudden acute event, such as plaque rupture with or without luminal thrombosis, or plaque rupture with spasm of the vessel. It is now recognized that the atherosclerotic plaque is not stable, particularly when it is composed of cholesterol, fibrous tissue, calcium, and inflammatory cells (the so-called complex plaque). The plaque contents are often overlain by a fibrous cap, that may be thick and relatively immune to rupture, or thin and susceptible to rupture. The thin fibrous cap may be affected by the plaque materials, and

24

specifically collagenases (tissue metalloproteinases, or TMPs), elaborated by inflammatory cells, and capable of degrading the cap collagen. This may lead to plaque rupture, and the release of thrombosis promoting material into the coronary lumen. Alternatively, the plaque may be affected by mechanical disruption secondary to spasm of intact smooth muscle in the coronary artery wall (particularly if the plaque is eccentrically localized in the vessel circumference). Thus, stimulation of vessel contraction that may occur secondary to the release of stress related hormones, or secondary to vasogenic substances such as nicotine or cocaine, can lead to plaque rupture, also. The ruptured plaque in this case was not associated with luminal thrombosis, which may be explained by the efficacy of the TPA that led to thrombolysis. However, as noted by the presence of a transmural myocardial infarction, there must have been complete left coronary artery occlusion for at least two to four hours before TPA treatment was instituted. It would appear that the treatment was appropriate but the extent and severity of the infarction, particularly in a patient with underlying, and probably silent, myocardial disease, led to his death.

A final comment pertains to the microscopic incidental finding of multifocal amyloid deposition in the myocardium. In the absence of systemic amyloidosis associated with a plasma cell dyscrasia, or chronic inflammation, it is most likely that this amyloid represents the so-called senile amyloidosis. This condition, which tends to increase in frequency with age, is of unknown etiology. It is generally due to the abnormal accumulation of transthyreitin, which develops the beta pleated sheet conformation of all of the amyloid proteins, and therefore stains with Congo red dye, producing apple-green birefringence when viewed by polarized microscopy. Why this particular type of amyloid has a predilection for the myocardium is unknown. It usually is asymptomatic, but it may occasionally be associated with a restrictive cardiomyopathy characterized by diastolic dysfunction. It is unlikely that amyloidosis played a direct role in this patient's course, although it may have made him more susceptible to develop acute congestive heart failure when his myocardial infarction developed.

Suggested Readings

1. Jennings RB, Steenbergen C Jr, Reimer KA. Myocardial ischemia and reperfusion. Monogr Pathol. 1995; 37:47-80.
2. Reimer KA, Vander Heide RS, Jennings RB. Ischemic preconditioning slows ischemic metabolism and limits myocardial infarct size. Ann N Y Acad Sci. 1994; 723:99-115.
3. Jennings RB, Reimer KA. The cell biology of acute myocardial ischemia. Annu Rev Med. 1991; 42:225-46.
4. Reimer KA, Jennings RB. The "wavefront phenomenon" of myocardial ischemic cell death. II. Transmural progression of necrosis within the framework of ischemic bed size (myocardium at risk) and collateral flow. Lab Invest. 1979; 40:633-44.
5. Brockington CD, Lyden PD. Criteria for selection of older patients for thrombolytic therapy. Clin Geriatr Med. 1999; 15:721-39.
6. Hamm CW. New serum markers for acute myocardial infarction. N Engl J Med. 1994; 331:607-8.
7. Straznicky IT, White HD. Thrombolytic therapy for acute myocardial infarction in the elderly. Coron Artery Dis. 2000; 11:299-304.
8. Zhao M, Zhang H, Robinson TF, Factor SM, Sonneblick H, Eng C. Profound structural alterations of the extracellular collagen matrix in post-ischemic dysfunctional ("stunned") but viable myocardium. J Am Coll Cardiol 1987; 10:1322-34.
9. Factor SM, Bache R. " Pathophysiology of Myocardial Ischemia". In Hurt's The Heart. Ninth Edition. Alexander WR, Schlant RC, and Fuster V eds. McGraw-Hill Co, Inc., 1998.

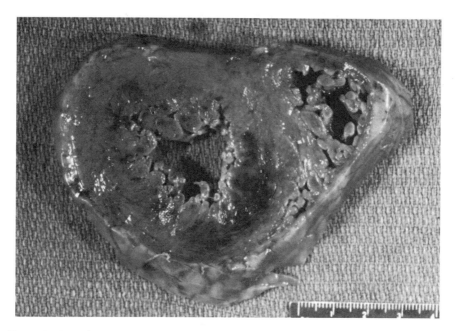

Figure 1. Reperfusion injury. A hemorrhagic infarct is evident in the anterior wall of the left ventricle extending to the septum.

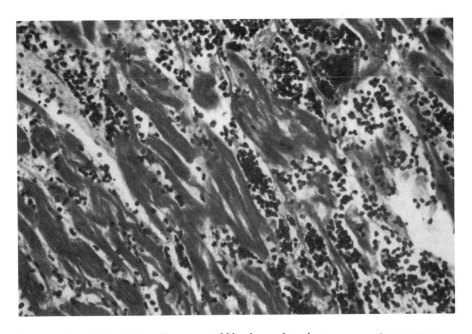

Figure 2. Reperfusion injury. Extravasated blood percolates between necrotic myocytes (Hematoxylin and Eosin, 40X)

Case # 2

Clinical Summary

The patient was a 60 year old woman who was found unresponsive at home. Paramedics were called. Her initial electrocardiogram (ECG) rhythm was asystole followed by a brief period of ventricular fibrillation. Cardiopulmonary resuscitation (CPR) measures were unsuccessful and the patient was pronounced dead at the time of her arrival to the hospital.

The patient's medical history was significant for hypertension, hypercholesterolemia and severe coronary artery disease (80-90% stenosis of left anterior descending coronary artery and 50-60% occlusion of right coronary artery). Eight months prior to her death, the patient underwent percutaneous transluminal coronary angioplasty (PTCA) of the left anterior descending coronary artery (LAD). Four months later, because of post-angioplasty re-stenosis, she underwent coronary artery bypass graft (CABG) using the left internal mammary artery to the LAD (Figure 3).

Gross and Microscopic Description

The patient measured 154 cm and weighed 64 kg. The heart weighed 450 g. The pericardium was thickened. The left ventricle revealed concentric hypertrophy consistent with long-standing hypertension (wall thickness 1.9 cm). The lateral wall of the left ventricle had an area of discoloration, which on histologic examination consisted of multiple foci of fibrosis and granulation tissue consistent with subacute and remote myocardial infarcts. The right ventricle was of normal thickness (0.5 cm). Both atria were dilated. The aortic and mitral valves were thickened and calcified, but were relatively pliable. All coronary arteries showed severe stenosis with up to 90% occlusion. Sectioning of the right coronary artery revealed 100 % occlusion by an organized thrombus. The left circumflex also had fresh thrombi within the lumen, and the distal left anterior descending showed evidence of re-stenosis, proximal to the bypass graft. Severe atherosclerosis involved the aorta and main branches, and a 3 cm fusiform aneurysm was found in the abdominal portion. The lungs, liver and spleen were congested. The right kidney was small and weighed 35 g. The left kidney was enlarged and weighed 100 g. The surface of both was granular. Moderate to severe atherosclerosis was also noted in the circle of Willis with up to 60% occlusion in the right middle cerebral artery. Multiple old infarcts were found in the lower thoracic/upper lumbar spinal cord (watershed area).

Case Analysis

This woman, with a known history of significant coronary artery disease, died suddenly at home. In general, because of the possibility of illegal circumstances, the determination of the cause of death for someone who dies outside of a medical facility would be the responsibility of the Medical Examiner's Office. However, in this case, the history of cardiovascular disease was sufficiently strong to suggest that death was due to natural causes.

Sudden cardiac death (SCD) is virtually always arrhythmic, and is usually caused by a so-called malignant ventricular rhythm such as ventricular fibrillation (VF, often following episodes of ventricular tachycardia or runs of premature supraventricular or ventricular contractions). Asystole also may occur, either as the initial event of cardiac arrest, or following VF. Electro-mechanical dissociation (EMD) is another pattern, in which a normal or non-fatal electrical pattern is maintained, but there is an uncoupling of electrical activity and muscular contraction. Although this may occur following VF with resuscitation attempts including defibrillation, it can often be seen in the setting of hemopericardium due to ventricular rupture (as a result of myocardial infarction) or aortic rupture (due to aortic dissection). In this case, the patient was initially asystolic, followed by VF shortly thereafter, with unsuccessful resuscitation attempts.

She had a number of risk factors for SCD, all of which are positively and independently associated with this outcome. It is noteworthy that SCD is by far the most common cause of death due to heart disease, and it accounts for 500,000 to one million deaths per year, with the majority occurring outside the hospital. Only a small percentage of individuals experiencing an arrhythmic cardiac arrest will have resuscitation attempted on them, and of those, less than 5-10% are resuscitated successfully to reach a medical facility. Many of the survivors have significant anoxic brain injury that subsequently leads to death or disability. Of the risk factors predisposing to SCD, the following are the most important:

1. left ventricular hypertrophy
2. occlusive coronary artery disease
3. acute coronary artery thrombosis
4. myocardial scarring
5. acute or organizing myocardial infarction
6. cardiomyopathy
7. myocarditis

Of these risk factors, this patient had all except #6 and #7: She had significant cardiac hypertrophy with a gross heart weight of 450 g, and a left ventricular wall measuring 1.9 cm in greatest thickness (normal up to 1.5 cm). The estimated cardiac mass for a woman who weighed 63 kg is between 250-300 g. The calculation is estimated by taking the weight of the individual in kilograms and multiplying by 0.4%. For males, with somewhat greater lean muscle mass, the multiplier is 0.5%. More precise estimates can be obtained by using the body surface mass-index, but for practical purposes, a 0.4-0.5% multiplier gives a reasonable approximation. The upper limits are equally significant, and are considered pathological, regardless of body size, if more than 350-400 gm in a woman, or more than 400-450 gm in a man. The proviso that the hypertrophy is non-physiologic is also an important consideration. In a well-trained athlete, particularly one performing isometric exercise (e.g. weight lifting), cardiac hypertrophy may ensue; however, it is a physiologic response not associated with myocardial scarring. In general, the difference between pathologic hypertrophy and physiologic hypertrophy is dependent on the presence or absence of fibrosis.

The etiology of this patient's hypertrophy is most likely secondary to longstanding hypertension, although compensatory hypertrophy of the non-infarcted heart may have played a role. Even without the medical history of hypertension, it would be possible to deduce that she was hypertensive based on her kidney pathology. The kidneys were discrepant in size (35 gm and 100 gm), and they had granular cortices. The discordant renal mass was most likely the result of a "Goldblatt kidney" phenomenon. The latter occurs when one kidney is chronically ischemic (usually as a result of renal artery stenosis), and produces excess renin with increases of circulating angiotensin. The angiotensin causes an elevation of the systemic blood pressure that leads to arterionephrosclerosis of the contralateral kidney (e.g. damage and sclerosis of intrarenal arteries and arterioles with secondary localized ischemia and fibrosis of the glomeruli and tubules). The ischemic kidney is "protected" from the effects of hypertension by the renal artery stenosis. Thus, in a classic Goldblatt kidney, the diffusely ischemic kidney is small and generally has a smooth cortex, with the other kidney showing features of a granular cortex consistent with nephrosclerosis. In this case, although one kidney was smaller than the other, even the larger of the two was moderately shrunken (normal kidney weight is approximately 150-200 gm), and both were granular. This suggests that the patient was chronically hypertensive thereby causing nephrosclerosis of both kidneys, and then subsequently she developed renal artery stenosis leading to superimposed ischemia. Thus, she did not have a classic Goldblatt kidney phenomenon, though she did have hypertensive renal disease.

This patient had severe chronic coronary artery disease secondary to atherosclerosis, with predominant involvement of the LAD (e.g. single vessel

31

disease), although her right coronary artery was also affected. The 50-60% narrowing of the RCA is below the critical level of stenosis (defined as greater than 65%), because that level of narrowing at rest will have an associated pressure drop across the stenotic segment. Sub-critical narrowing can certainly be significant during exercise, or if there is an acutely unstable vessel. Furthermore, such sub-critical vessels can progress to critical stenosis over time, or they can be associated with thrombosis.

The autopsy revealed obvious disease progression in the RCA (e.g. 90% occlusion), and it showed changes of LAD re-stenosis proximal to the CABG. Re-stenosis is a commonly recognized complication of balloon angioplasty that occurs in up to 40% of patients within 3-4 months following the procedure. The precise explanation of why it occurs preferentially in some patients, while sparing others, is not understood; nor are there predictors of who will re-stenose. The process of re-stenosis is an exuberant proliferation of smooth muscle cells and myxomatous stroma in the intimal layer of the ballooned vessel, leading to a neo-intima that impinges on the lumen. The pathogenesis of this tissue proliferation is complex. It is partially dependent on the injury to endothelial cells following the balloon damage to the vessel wall that generally causes a local compression and dissection of the occluding plaque. The balloon injury leads to an "uncovering" of subendothelial connective tissue with adherence of platelets that release the prostaglandin thromboxane (TXa, a smooth muscle vasoconstricting agent), and platelet-derived growth factor (PDGF, which is a mitogen for smooth muscle cell proliferation), thereby stimulating smooth muscle cell migration into the intima. Additionally, there is release of endothelin-1, a potent vasoconstrictor, and other hormones and cytokines, which can also stimulate smooth muscle and connective tissue proliferation.

In this case, the patient did re-stenose following the balloon angioplasty, and then she underwent an internal mammary artery to LAD graft. The internal mammary artery is a useful arterial graft that is relatively devoid of atherosclerosis, and does not develop atherosclerosis when interposed in the coronary circulation. Its major limitation is that it can only be grafted to the anterior heart surface, because of its location and length; therefore it is primarily used for LAD grafts. At autopsy, the native LAD was severely narrowed proximal to the patent graft, and it showed evidence of re-stenosis.

Prior to her death, this woman had several other significant conditions that made her susceptible to a sudden fatal arrhythmia. She had evidence of a healed scar in lateral left ventricle, which was at least 3 months old (it takes a minimum of 3 months for scar tissue to mature). In the same geographic area of the ventricle as the scar tissue, she had granulation tissue, which represents a healing response to myocardial necrosis composed of endothelial cell and fibroblastic proliferation. Granulation tissue generally begins to form at 7-10 days after tissue injury, and then it progressively matures for several weeks until immature scar tissue develops. Thus, this region represents a subacute infarction that presumably developed silently (e.g. without clinical signs and symptoms) at least several weeks prior to her death. The temporal changes link this area of necrosis to the organizing right coronary artery thrombus, which was also approximately 1-2 weeks in age. Individuals with myocardial scarring are at risk to develop cardiac arrhythmias; however, those with healing infarction are at markedly higher risk. The myocardial tissue immediately adjacent to a healing infarction has increased irritability as a result of inflammation, interstitial edema, and slight hypoxemia, and is therefore more likely to cause a generalized arrhythmic event.

It is most probable that the sudden arrhythmia that led to this woman's death was a direct result of the acute event that was temporarily related to her cardiac arrest. We are referring to the acute thrombosis of the left circumflex coronary artery. Sudden occlusion of this vessel, together with prior complete occlusion in the right coronary artery, made her ventricle ischemic, and susceptible to generate fatal electrical rhythms. It is noteworthy that she developed an acute thrombosis of her circumflex artery within a few weeks of an RCA thrombus. It is not that rare for patients to develop thrombi in multiple vessels, sometimes concurrently. This suggests an increased tendency for thrombus formation in already diseased atherosclerotic arteries, possibly as the result of enhanced plaque instability and/or systemic or local hormonal factors. In this case, no specific etiology could be determined.

Suggested Readings

1. Levine GN, Ali MN. The role of percutaneous revascularization in the treatment of ischemic heart disease: insights from published reports and randomized clinical trials. Chest. 1997; 112:805-21.
2. Kawasuji M, Sakakibara N, Takemura H, Tedoriya T, Ushijima T, Watanabe Y. Is internal thoracic artery grafting suitable for a moderately stenotic coronary artery? J Thorac Cardiovasc Surg. 1996; 112:253-9.
3. Jensen J, Eriksson SV, Lindvall B, Lundin P, Sylven C. Women react with more myocardial ischemia and angina pectoris during elective percutaneous transluminal coronary angioplasty. Coron Artery Dis. 2000; 11:527-35.
4. Friesinger GC, Ryan TJ. Coronary heart disease. Stable and unstable syndromes. Cardiol Clin. 1999; 17:93-122.
5. Cishek MB, Gershony G. Roles of percutaneous transluminal coronary angioplasty and bypass graft surgery for the treatment of coronary artery disease. Am Heart J. 1996; 131:1012-7.
6. Tennant M, McGeachie JK. A biological basis for re-stenosis after percutaneous transluminal angioplasty: possible underlying mechanisms. Aust N Z J Surg. 1992; 62:135-4.
7. Weiner DA. Significance of silent myocardial ischemia after coronary artery bypass surgery. Am J Cardiol. 1992; 70:35F-38F.
8. Factor SM, Minase T, Cho S, Fein F, Capasso JM, Sonneblick EH. Coronary microvascular abnormalities in the hypertensive-diabetic rat. A cause of cardiomyopathy? Am J Pathol 1984; 116:9-20.

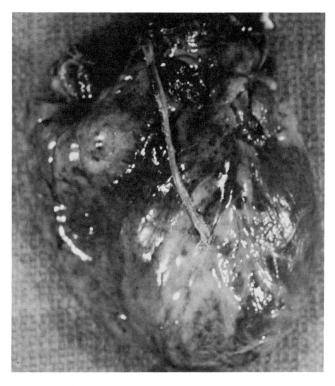

Figure 3. Coronary artery bypass graft (CABG). A segment of internal mammary artery is connected to the left anterior descending coronary artery (LAD)

35

Case # 3

Clinical Summary

The patient was a 77 year old obese, Hispanic man who presented to the emergency room with a 2 hour history of shortness of breath. The patient had a past medical history significant for hypertension and a myocardial infarction 10 years previously. The day prior to his current admission, he was seen by a physician, who diagnosed bronchitis and prescribed antibiotics as well as a non-steroidal anti-inflammatory medication for his back pain.

On admission to the ER, his vital signs were BP 100/64 mmHg, HR 116/min, and RR 24/min. Shortly after his arrival to the hospital, he developed severe chest pain radiating to his upper right back. A chest-x-ray showed widened mediastinum with interstitial markings. A CT of the thorax with contrast revealed a thoracic aortic dissection with questionable leak.

The patient developed respiratory distress and hypotension, which progressed to a cardiorespiratory arrest. He was successfully resuscitated and transferred to the CCU where vasopressors and fluids were administered. In addition, the patient required a transfusion with a unit of packed red blood cells (PRBC). The attending cardiologist suggested immediate surgical intervention; however, the patient deteriorated rapidly, had a second cardiorespiratory arrest and died.

Gross Description

Permission was granted for a complete autopsy. The heart weighed 600 g. The pericardial sac had minimal amount of serous fluid. The pericardium and epicardium were smooth and glistening. The atria were of normal size and free of thrombi. The foramen ovale was closed. The left ventricle was hypertrophic (wall thickness 2cm) and the right ventricle showed severe dilatation and hypertrophy. The valves were partially calcified. The tricuspid valve was hemorrhagic. The postero-lateral papillary muscle of the left ventricle was ruptured with consequent prolapse of the mitral valve (diameter of the ring 11.5 cm). (Figure 4) The chordae tendineae were focally thickened. The myocardium was red-brown with average consistency, and the endocardium was thin and shiny.

Examination of the coronary arteries showed complete occlusion of the right coronary artery as well as acute thrombosis of the left circumflex artery. The aorta showed severe atherosclerosis with thrombi and ulceration, especially in the thoracic and abdominal portions. The major branches were unremarkable except for aneurysmal dilatation of the right iliac artery.

The lungs were heavy (2250 g combined), but no discrete lesions were identified. The liver was congested (1530 g). Other significant findings included severe nephrosclerosis with cyst formation, and hemorrhagic adrenals, pancreas and intestine. The brain weighed 1255 g and was grossly unremarkable except for severe atherosclerosis of the circle of Willis.

Microscopic Description

Sections from the heart revealed a recent apical-lateral myocardial infarction involving the papillary muscle. Remote infarcts in both anterior and posterior walls were also noted. Sections from the left circumflex showed plaque hemorrhage with associated inflammation. Significant findings in the lungs included moderate emphysematous change, early focal bronchopneumonia and intimal vascular proliferation consistent with pulmonary hypertension. The kidneys, adrenals, pancreas, intestines and bladder revealed diffuse hemorrhage in keeping with shock. The brain was remarkable for acute anoxic changes and multiple, old areas of encephalomalacia involving cerebellum, cortex and white matter.

Case Analysis

Although this patient does not fit the classical definition of sudden cardiac death (sudden collapse without symptoms, or death within one hour of symptom onset), essentially this is a sudden death case. He had acute respiratory distress of only a few hours duration. In retrospect, his complaints the day prior to admission were almost certainly related to the events that led to his death. When he presented to the hospital he had a low blood pressure (even if he was adequately treated for his longstanding hypertension, 100/64 mmHg is hypotensive), tachycardia, and tachypnea. This suggests significant acute compromise of his cardiopulmonary system. He then developed severe, acute chest pain radiating to his upper back. Together with a widened mediastinum on chest X-ray, the physicians evaluating him in the emergency department suspected an aortic dissection. A CT scan of the thorax with contrast was ordered which confirmed the diagnosis. Although this was the appropriate diagnostic modality to evaluate a suspected aortic dissection, the interpretation of the scan was inaccurate, thereby providing a false positive result. Soon thereafter, he deteriorated and developed shock and cardiac arrest. He died in a short period of time despite resuscitative measures. In retrospect, the inaccurate diagnosis of aortic dissection, and the treatment that may or may not have been instituted as a result of the diagnosis, did not play a role in his death. Before addressing the actual disease process that led to this patient's demise, it is worthwhile to address whether the suspicion of aortic dissection was reasonable.

Dissection of the aorta has multiple etiologies. One group of entities is the congenital or inherited abnormalities of the aortic connective tissue, most commonly represented by Marfan's syndrome. The latter is an autosomal dominant disease, with high penetrance, that results from a mutation in the fibrillin-1 gene on chromosome 15. Although the penetrance is high, the phenotypic features of Marfan's syndrome are variable, related to the greater than 50 different mutations of the fibrillin gene. Fibrillin is a 10-15 nm microfibrillar protein component of elastic tissue. Abnormal fibrillin affects connective tissue throughout the body, thereby leading to elongated skeleton, subluxation of the lens, annuloectasia of the aortic valve ring, and fibromyxomatous cardiac valve degeneration, among other conditions. Classically, Marfan associated aortic dissection occurs in the 2nd to the 4th decades of life. In contrast, non-Marfan's dissection is a disease of unknown etiology, often associated with hypertension, and occurring most often in individuals in the 5th through the 7th decades. There is no known hereditary predisposition, and no mutations of connective tissue have been identified. However, it is noteworthy that aortic tissue from Marfan's syndrome and non-Marfan's dissections has an increased friability and increased ease in separating the tissue layers (e.g. split the media). This suggests that even non-Marfan's syndrome dissections are secondary to some type of connective tissue defect.

Although the patient had hypertension by history, the likelihood of a spontaneous dissection leading to his cardiovascular collapse is significantly less likely due to his age. More specifically, someone 77 years old, with recognized atherosclerotic cardiovascular disease (a myocardial infarction 10 years before admission), is virtually precluded from developing dissection. This broad statement is predicated on the fact that such a patient is almost certain to have aortic atherosclerosis; and, this condition, even if moderately severe, leads to intimal and medial plaque formation. The atherosclerotic plaque destroys the normal lamellar structure of the media, and replaces it with scar and plaque material. Intact elastic lamellae are a necessary requirement for dissection, as the dissecting channel of blood splits apart the layers comprising the media. Although localized plaque hemorrhage and focal dissection may occur in an atherosclerotic aorta, spread of the dissection is stopped when the channel of blood reaches an adjacent scarred region. In a similar way, aortitis with scarring (e.g. syphilitic aortitis) precludes dissection. Rupture of an atherosclerotic aneurysm is far more likely in a patient in his 8th decade, than a ruptured aortic dissection. Thus, on clinical and pathological grounds, the consideration of aortic dissection as a possible diagnosis in this patient should not have been high on the differential diagnosis list.

The rapid downhill course of this patient with cardiogenic shock and pulmonary edema is explained by the postmortem findings of acute coronary occlusion, acute posterolateral wall myocardial infarction, and a ruptured papillary muscle. Statistically, the two most likely causes of cardiogenic shock in this age group would be a massive myocardial infarction with extensive damage of the myocardium, and a myocardial infarction with tissue disruption (e.g. acquired ventricular septal defect or papillary muscle rupture). With tissue disruption, the infarction may be relatively small, yet have disproportionate effects on ventricular function. In the current case, that is precisely what occurred, with a rupture of the posterolateral papillary muscle. This event accounted for the acute mitral regurgitation (new holosystolic 3/6 murmur) followed by rapid development of cardiogenic shock, and respiratory distress due to pulmonary edema. It is not clear why the clinical staff considered the diagnosis of acute aortic dissection with this constellation of findings. An aortic dissection, even if it led to aortic valve insufficiency due to annular disruption, would be associated with a diastolic murmur. Furthermore, aortic dissection is only rarely associated with cardiogenic shock, and pulmonary edema. It is most often associated with sudden death due to rupture and pericardial tamponade. If it extends retrograde towards the aortic annulus, it can dissect or occlude a main coronary artery at the ostium, and under those circumstances it could cause massive myocardial injury and cardiogenic shock.

Rupture of the myocardium can affect 3 main sites: free left ventricular wall, interventricular septum, and papillary muscle. Ruptures tend to occur more frequently in patients in their 6th to 7th decades, in a background of hypertension, and often with no prior history of myocardial infarction. Ruptures of the free wall lead to rapid death with pericardial tamponade. Either the interventricular septum or papillary muscle rupture can lead to cardiogenic shock. The latter, can affect the entire papillary muscle body (the so-called 'belly'), any of the separate muscular heads (there are often as many as six separate heads), or at the myotendon junction where it can lead to disruption of a primary chorda tendineae. With complete disruption of the entire papillary muscle, massive mitral valve regurgitation and overwhelming pulmonary edema ensues rapidly, often leading to death before surgical intervention. Rupture of a single head or of a chord may permit surgical repair. In such conditions, either replacement of the entire mitral valve with prosthesis, or more recently, chordal plication or repair in order to salvage the native valve, may be attempted.

In this case, the rupture of the papillary muscle was not diagnosed, but even if it had been, it is unlikely that there would have been sufficient time to permit surgical intervention. An echocardiogram, if it had been performed rather than a CT scan, would have revealed segmental left ventricular wall motion abnormalities, and either papillary muscle dysfunction

39

or rupture with a freely moving papillary muscle fragment in the ventricular chamber. In addition, severe mitral valve regurgitation would have been detected. Papillary muscle rupture, as is true with other forms of ventricular rupture associated with myocardial infarction, frequently occurs between the first to 4th day after infarct inception. True to form, the infarction in this case was approximately 2 days old, based on the presence of well-defined coagulative necrosis and a heavy infiltration of neutrophils.

Suggested Readings

1. Nienaber CA, Von Kodolitsch Y. Therapeutic management of patients with Marfan syndrome: focus on cardiovascular involvement. Cardiol Rev. 1999; 7:332-41.
2. Libby P, Sukhova G, Lee RT, Liao JK Molecular biology of atherosclerosis. Int J Cardiol. 1997; 62 (Suppl 2):S23-9.
3. Leopold JA, Loscalzo J. Clinical importance of understanding vascular biology Cardiol Rev. 2000; 8:115-23.
4. Samman B, Korr KS, Katz AS, Parisi AF. Pitfalls in the diagnosis and management of papillary muscle rupture: a study of four cases and review of the literature. Clin Cardiol. 1995; 18:591-6.
5. Reeder GS. Identification and treatment of complications of myocardial infarction. Mayo Clin Proc. 1995; 70:880-4.
6. Buda AJ. The role of echocardiography in the evaluation of mechanical complications of acute myocardial infarction. Circulation. 1991; 84 (3 Suppl):I109-21.
7. Prieto A, Eisenberg J, Thakur RK. Nonarrhythmic complications of acute myocardial infarction. Emerg Med Clin North Am. 2001; 19: 397-415.
8. Robinson TF, Geraci MA, Sonneblick EH, Factor SM. Coiled perimysial fibers of papillary muscle in rat heart; morphology, distribution, and changes in configuration. Circ Res 1988; 63:577-92.

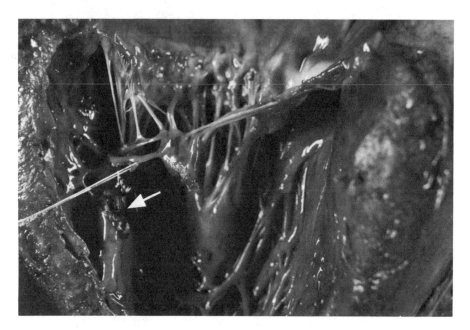

Figure 4. Infarcted papillary muscle with rupture (arrow)

Case # 4

Clinical Summary

Mr. S was 45 years old at the time of his death. He had smoked cigarettes for 25 years, had hypertension, and was a known non-insulin dependent diabetic (type II) controlled with oral hypoglycemic drugs. He was moderately obese, weighing 105 kg and 175 cm length (BMI 34 kg/m^2). He also had a history of illicit intravenous drug use with scarred veins in the antecubital fossa. He had clinical evidence of diabetic neuropathy, and peripheral vascular disease (intermittent claudication and sexual dysfunction). He was admitted to the hospital because of complaints of indigestion and progressive discomfort radiating to both arms. The presumptive diagnosis was acute inferior wall myocardial infarction, and he was treated with tissue plasminogen activator (TPA). The patient slowly became clinically stable after his creatine kinase (CK) peaked at 1555 U/L. On medication, and 3 days later, he had a low level stress exercise ECG, which was negative for ischemia. He was discharged home with a plan for a stress thallium test in one month. A week later, he was admitted again with a provisional diagnosis of unstable angina pectoris. During this hospitalization, he was clinically stable, the cardiac enzymes were normal and the ECG had no significant change. He was discharged with a plan to return to his doctor's office within 2 days for follow up. However, the next morning, he was found unresponsive. Resuscitation efforts were unsuccessful.

Gross Description

The post mortem examination revealed cardiomegaly (heart weight. 510 g, normal between 400 and 450 g). The heart had 4 chamber dilatation, with hypertrophy of the left ventricular wall (2.0 cm, normal 1.5 cm). There was discoloration of the posterior wall and the interventricular septum, with an area of softening extending to the base of the heart measuring 6 x 2.5 cm. There was marked subendocardial hemorrhage and wall thinning. The right coronary artery was severely narrowed and contained a 1.0 cm long intraluminal thrombus. The left coronary artery and branches were occluded up to 50% with no acute lesions. The lungs were heavy and edematous.

Microscopic Description

The heart revealed extensive subendocardial myocardial infarction (SEMI) with granulation tissue, organizing myocytolysis, and focal immature connective tissue. All findings consistent with a 10-14 day old healing

43

infarction. In addition, in the same region of subendocardial myocardial infarct, there was an acute myocardial infarction with extension toward the epicardial surface. This acute transmural infarction extension had predominantly occurred within the past 12-24 hours. Moreover, there were few foci with active neutrophilic inflammation, and thus consistent with 24-48 hours duration. This pattern of SEMI with acute transmural extension was apparent in multiple sections of the left ventricle. The pathologic findings consistently dated the subendocardial infarction between 10-14 days, and the acute transmural extension to 1-2 days.

In addition to the acute and organizing necrosis, there was evidence of myocellular hypertrophy and multiple foci of interstitial and replacement fibrosis; all consistent with chronic diabetic and hypertensive heart disease. Larger zones of scarring were noted, particularly in the subendocardial myocardium. The sections of the right coronary artery showed focal high grade atherosclerotic complex plaques with intraplaque hemorrhage and focal plaque rupture (Figures 5 and 6). The acute plaque rupture led to fresh thrombus and plaque material in the lumen of the vessel. The acute occlusion of the vessel was consistent with the acute transmural extension of the previous subendocardial infarction.

Case Analysis

Mr. S. had a large subendocardial myocardial infarction (SEMI) that showed organizational changes that dated the infarct to approximately 10-14 days before death. Subsequently, he had transmural extension of the original SEMI that occurred 1-2 days before death. The extension resulted from acute thrombotic occlusion of a severely atherosclerotic coronary artery affected by plaque hemorrhage and rupture. Since the thrombus was 1-2 days old, it was temporally related to the infarct extension. We will focus on several aspects of this case in this discussion:

1. Subendocardial versus transmural myocardial infarction;
2. Transmural extension of an infarction, and why this is different from lateral extension;
3. Coronary artery lesion(s) accounting for the myocardial pathology;
4. Histological dating of infarction and thrombus

This case illustrates basic cardiac pathophysiology and pathology. It reflects what occurs *in vivo* in humans, as a counterpart of what has been demonstrated convincingly in the animal laboratory. It also provides a rationale for some of the interventional approaches currently being employed to prevent the unfortunate outcome that resulted in the death of Mr. S. As we have discussed earlier, myocardial infarction is not a sudden, 'all-or-none' phenomenon. There is a progression of necrosis across the ventricular wall from the endocardium towards the epicardium. It develops in stages or waves, giving rise to the term 'wavefront', described by Reimer and Jennings in several classic papers. Although based on experimental studies, the concept has been amply verified in humans. It represents the conceptual underpinning for the use of thrombolytic agents, acute catheterization with balloon angioplasty and stenting, and acute coronary artery bypass grafting, during myocardial infarction. In the present case, Mr. S. received the thrombolytic agent TPA, and this led to the development of a SEMI. The reasons for this will become obvious.

Acute myocardial infarction occurs with temporal and spatial determinants. This means that the progression across the ventricular wall is time-dependent, and the volume of myocardium affected by ischemia and its evolution to necrosis, is spatially limited by the coronary artery anatomy and flow. The myocardium affected by ischemia is also referred to as **myocardium at risk**, or **vulnerable myocardium**. Not all of the myocardium at risk will infarct; the actual volume will depend on the collateral circulation to support it, and whether intervention(s) allow reperfusion of the obstructed coronary vessel. As long as reperfusion occurs sufficiently early in the course of the MI, the wavefront will be aborted and a potential transmural infarction will be limited to the subendocardium. Consequently, a SEMI by definition represents a reperfusion injury, whereas transmural infarctions are ischemic lesions resulting from the total absence or marked diminution of blood flow to the tissue.

There are other implications that result from this pathophysiology. SEMIs are hemorrhagic, and are associated with ischemic injury to capillaries, which results in interstitial leakage of blood. Since there is reperfusion that follows a period of ischemia, the re-introduced oxygenated blood interacts with damaged sarcolemmal proteins and lipids. This generates oxygen and hydroxyl free radicals that irreversibly perforate the sarcolemma, leading to a massive influx of extracellular fluid and calcium. The perforations prevent the myocardial cell maintenance of fluid and electrolyte balance, and the calcium causes hypercontraction of the actin-myosin filaments. The end result is contraction band necrosis, which is a characteristic feature of SEMI (Figure 7). Moreover, since the infarction process has been aborted by the reperfusion, a pathological definition of a SEMI is an infarct that extends less than 50% through the ventricular wall (starting from the subendocardium).

The clinical definition of a SEMI depends on its electrocardiographic findings. It generally does not produce Q-waves in the leads identifying the area of ischemia. Accordingly, it is clinically termed a **non-Q-wave MI**. In practical terms, some non-Q-wave infarctions may progress beyond 50% of the ventricular wall. Consequently, there may not be an absolute correlation between the clinical and pathological terminology. The explanation for the absence of Q-waves is of significant interest: the Q-wave represents the negative deflection below the iso-electric line on the ECG. Necrotic muscle does not generate any electrical impulses, positive or negative (the dead muscle is electrically invisible). It allows the ECG leads to 'see through' the necrotic tissue to the viable myocardium on the opposite side of the ventricular wall, which is able to generate upward positive deflections, or R-waves, in the ECG leads directly facing this zone. In the opposite leads, and facing the electrically negative infarct zone, the deflections are downward negative, or Q-waves. Since a SEMI has a viable zone of myocardium overlying the infarct, it is not electrically neutral. Therefore, no Q-waves are seen.

The SEMI is hemorrhagic and initially is composed of myocardium with contraction band necrosis. Time-dependent necrosis of the ventricular layers extending towards the epicardium is associated with time-dependent survival of the immediate subendocardial layers. Normally, if one examines the myocardium just under the endocardium from a heart with a transmural infarction, there will be 3-5 myocardial cell layers that survive. They are maintained viable by direct diffusion of oxygen across the endocardium into the tissue (oxygen can diffuse approximately 30-50 microns, or about the distance of 3-5 myocardial cell diameters). If the myocytes are hypertrophied, the endocardium is fibrosed, or the zone underlying the infarction is blocked by a mural thrombus, there is no myocardial cell survival. Although these cells probably have no functional role, the immediate subendocardial zone is also where the Purkinje cells are found; thus, the survival of this tissue through oxygen diffusion may permit normal ventricular conduction. The same zone, in a SEMI, is initially much larger, representing as many as 10-20 myocardial cells, which are potentially ischemic and represent vulnerable myocardium. Furthermore, this subendocardial myocardium is most likely 'stunned', is non-contractile, and with time, may even undergo necrosis. However, it can generate electrical activity, and as such may be a source of malignant and possibly fatal arrhythmias. Hence, the association of SEMI and lethal rhythm disturbances.

The other consequence of the different pathophysiology between a SEMI and a transmural myocardial infarction (TMMI), is that the TMMI occurs following complete occlusion of a coronary artery. In contrast to contraction bands characteristic of SEMI, the myocardium undergoes coagulative necrosis, which is a denaturing process of the cellular proteins secondary to oxygen deprivation. This leads to a smudgy 'cooked' appearance of the myocardium, with intense red staining with the dye eosin, or hypereosinophilia. Since this may take as long as 4-6 hours to become evident, it may be very difficult to ascertain whether any patient dying suddenly actually had a myocardial infarction as the precipitating event.

Clearly, then, there are pathophysiological, pathological, and functional differences between a SEMI and a TMMI. We will next turn to the issue of infarct extension:

Ordinarily, coronary vessels in humans have limited collateral branches. This is particularly true when the obstruction is more distal in the coronary artery, thereby providing fewer branches to bridge the zone of ischemia. However, the prediction as to whether any patient will or will not have adequate collaterals to support the myocardium is not possible prior to obstruction. Generally, collaterals are more likely to be present in the immediate subepicardial myocardium, decreasing from epicardium to endocardium. Accordingly, the myocardium at risk following coronary occlusion is spatially determined in an inside-outside dimension, and is sharply delimited along the lateral margins. The infarction is broader along the endocardium, and angles inward toward the epicardium. There are minimal collaterals that maintain the lateral margins. This means that there is no significant lateral border zone. The latter observation was a source of major controversy 20 years ago, but now is a widely accepted concept.

The myocardium at risk for infarction remains vulnerable even if the initiating coronary artery occlusion is transformed into a patent vessel. Even after reperfusion, the surviving subepicardial myocardium remains vulnerable to necrosis. If the vessel re-occludes at the same level, the surviving myocardium will then infarct as if the coronary artery was initially blocked in its entirety, and remained so for many hours. This is what is known as **transmural extension**; and it is precisely what occurred in the present case. Mr. S. had re-establishment of flow with TPA, and then he re-occluded many days later leading to a TMMI found at autopsy. The vulnerable infarct zone does not extend laterally, since distinct and separate vessels or branches supply that myocardium. If the myocardium lateral to an infarct undergoes necrosis, it would represent an extension to a new vascular territory. It is not unusual for additional vessels to become thrombosed or occluded by spasm in the setting of a TMMI. This would lead to new lateral or distant lesions from the initial focus.

As a final point, there is one concept that relates to post-occlusion modification of an MI and that is the term **infarct expansion**. It refers to the modification of the ventricular wall affected by a TMMI that undergoes remodeling. This leads to mural thinning and aneurysmal bulging of the wall. This process has significant effects on ventricular function, susceptibility to endocardial thrombus, and the potential for ventricular rupture. Expansion is usually associated with a large TMMI, but not a SEMI. When it occurs, it has a relatively poor prognosis.

47

The coronary lesion that accounted for the events affecting this patient is fairly common. He had a high-grade atherosclerotic plaque, which presumably led to an acute luminal thrombosis. The thrombus was then lysed with TPA, re-establishing adequate coronary flow and aborting the infarct progression across the ventricular wall. Subsequently, the same plaque ruptured leading to re-thrombosis of the vessel at the same level, extending his SEMI into a TMMI. This was a clinically silent event, most likely because of his diabetes mellitus. If these events had occurred today, he would have undergone coronary catheterization following the development of the SEMI. An angiogram would have demonstrated persistent high-grade coronary occlusion, and he would have had balloon angioplasty and stent placement, if clinically feasible. If not, he might have had coronary artery bypass grafting. With either approach, the vulnerable myocardium would have been well-perfused, and he would not have extended his SEMI.

The pathology of the initial infarction and the subsequent extension could be dated histologically. This is possible because of the use of well-established criteria that define the time course for the inflammatory response, the development of granulation tissue, and the deposition of connective tissue until the entire infarct is replaced by mature scar tissue. Similar dating of the thrombi can be done, as documented in this case with the coronary artery thrombus that correlated with the TMMI. Although the dating is not precise to the minute and hour (in contrast to the frequent impression one gets from television or fictional depictions of pathological investigation, where the fatal event is identified to the minute and hour), it can provide a rough 6-12 hour time frame for most of the cellular events affecting the infarcting myocardium. It is beyond the scope of this book to provide the details of the dating procedure, although they are adequately described in numerous pathology and cardiology texts. In most cases, such an evaluation is of academic interest, with some clinical implications. It is often of great importance in the medico-legal sphere where the determination of the precise time of an infarct and correlation with clinical signs and symptoms may be significant. For instance, this approach may help establish whether a fatal motor vehicle accident occurred due to a MI and fatal arrhythmia, or trauma directly caused the death of the driver.

In summary, the extension of a SEMI into a TMMI in this patient, serves as clinical verification for many of the major insights into myocardial ischemia and coronary thrombosis, which have been developed over the past 2 decades with animal studies. These insights have provided a firm scientific grounding for the interventional cardiology and cardiac surgery treatments of coronary ischemia and myocardial infarction. Over the last years, these treatment options have had a tremendous impact on disease prognosis, quality of life and survival of patients with ischemic coronary artery disease.

Suggested Readings

1. Villablanca AC, McDonald JM; Rutledge JC. Smoking and cardiovascular disease. Clin Chest Med. 2000; 21:159-72.

2. Reimer KA, Jennings RB. Biologic basis for limitation of infarct size. Adv Exp Med Biol. 1986; 194:315-30.

3. Ravn HB, Falk E. Histopathology of plaque rupture. Cardiol Clin. 1999; 17:263-70.

4. Schroeder AP, Falk E. Pathophysiology and inflammatory aspects of plaque rupture. Cardiol Clin. 1996; 14:211-20.

5. Becker RC, Bovill EG, Seghatchian MJ, Samama MM. Pathobiology of thrombin in acute coronary syndromes. Am Heart J. 1998; 136:S19-31

6. Stern S, Cohn PF, Pepine CJ. Silent myocardial ischemia. Curr Probl Cardiol. 1993; 18:301-59.

7. Okun EM, Factor SM, Kirk ES. End-capillary loops in the heart: An explanation for discrete myocardial infarctions without border zones. Science 1979; 206:565-67.

8. Factor SM, Okun EM, Kirk ES. The histological lateral border of acute canine myocardial infarction: a function of the microcirculation. Circ Res 1981; 48:640-49.

9. Factor SM, Okun EM, Minase T, Kirk ES. The microcirculation of the human heart: end capillary loops with discrete perfusion fields. Circulation 1982; 66:1241-48.

10. Forman R, Cho S, Factor SM, Kirk ES. Acute myocardial infarct extension into a previously preserved subendocardial region at risk in dogs and patients. Circulation 1982; 67:117-24.

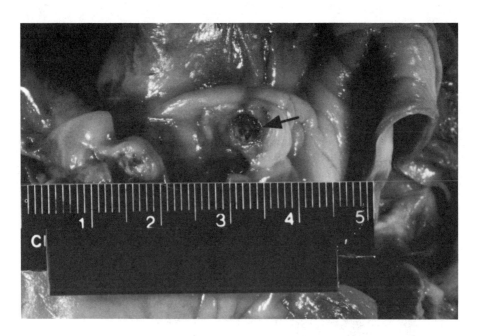

Figure 5. Transverse section of the right coronary artery showing intraplaque hemorrhage and luminal thrombotic occlusion.

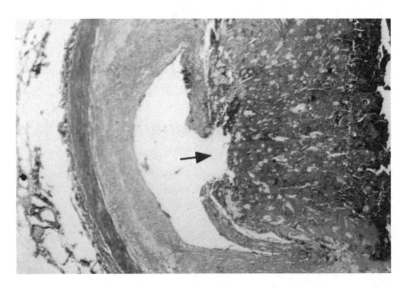

Figure 6. Section of right coronary artery partially occluded by a ruptured atheromatous plaque with hemorrhage (arrow) (Hematoxylin and Eosin, 40X). Distal sections of the artery revealed lumen thrombosis secondary to plaque rupture.

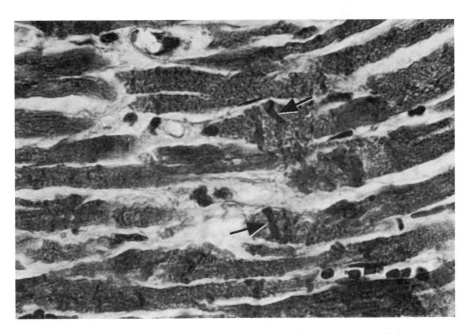

Figure 7. Contraction bands (arrows) are present in reperfusion injury, catecholamine-induced damage and as a result of resuscitation efforts. (Hematoxylin and Eosin, 60X)

Case #5

Clinical Summary

The patient was a 69 year old man with a history of hypertension and chronic obstructive pulmonary disease, who three days prior to admission to the hospital experienced exertional chest pain relieved by rest. The patient presented to the emergency room with complaints of substernal chest pain of a few hours duration that radiated to the shoulder, and was not relieved by nitroglycerin.

Laboratory data and other tests

Laboratory: WBC 10.3 (S 53%, L 39%, M 7%, E 1%), Hb/Hct 16/51, Plt 293; SGOT 384 U/L, LDH 751 U/L, CK 1875 U/L (CK-MB 11%). ECG: sinus tachycardia at 107 and ST elevation V1-V5.

The diagnosis of acute myocardial infarction was made. The patient was given thrombolytic therapy (tissue plasminogen activator, TPA) in the ER with resolution of the chest pain and clearance of the cardiac enzymes over the following 3 days. On the 5th hospital day, the WBC was noted to be increasing to 14 (S 77% and Bands 9%). He was afebrile and the blood and urine cultures were negative. A chest X-ray was done which showed a right upper lobe infiltrate, which resolved in few days. The patient was feeling better and he was scheduled for a cardiac catheterization. The procedure was postponed due to worsening abdominal and left hip pain. Within the next two days the hematocrit dropped to 29% and subsequently to 17%. On the 14th day of hospitalization, the patient suddenly developed shortness of breath and hypotension. Resuscitation efforts were unsuccessful and the patient was pronounced dead.

Gross Description

The patient measured 157 cm and weighed 59 kg. External examination revealed no clubbing, cyanosis or edema. The heart weighed 450 g and the shape was normal. The pericardium was smooth. The atria were unremarkable. Both ventricular chambers were dilated and hypertrophic. The myocardium showed a hemorrhagic subendocardial and focally transmural infarct of the antero-septal wall, approximately 2 weeks old. Other foci of scarring were also noted. The coronaries showed severe atherosclerosis with 100% occlusion of the left anterior descending artery and right coronary artery, and up to 70% stenosis of the left main and left circumflex arteries.

No acute thrombosis was identified. The lungs weighed 1050 g combined. Pleural plaques were noted in the left upper lobe. Emphysematous changes as well as anthracosis were moderate to severe. The liver, weighing 1200 g, was congested. The kidneys were unremarkable; however, a large left retroperitoneal hematoma was noted, enveloping the left kidney and extending to the psoas muscle and left diaphragmatic region.

Microscopic Description

The heart showed transmural myocardial necrosis of the anteroseptal wall with hemorrhage, fibrosis and granulation tissue consistent with a 12-14 days old infarct. There was severe calcific atherosclerosis of the coronaries with 100% occlusion of the left anterior descending and right coronary arteries. Another significant finding was the large retroperitoneal hematoma involving the psoas muscle (Figure 8). The lungs showed mild congestion, severe emphysematous change, chronic bronchitis, focal scarring and granulomatous reaction with calcification consistent with old pulmonary tuberculosis. The pulmonary vessels were thickened consistent with pulmonary hypertension. The liver showed fatty infiltration, congestion and portal inflammation with bridging fibrosis.

Case Analysis

This case illustrates the major complication of thrombolytic therapy, which is bleeding. The patient was admitted with the diagnosis of a myocardial infarction based on the clinical symptoms, ECG changes, and elevated cardiac enzymes. ST elevations are often seen as the earliest expression of a transmural myocardial infarction, and are followed by the development of abnormal Q waves. Since most transmural myocardial infarctions (~ 90%) are the result of coronary thrombosis, administration of TPA was indicated to avoid further myocardial damage. TPA converts plasminogen to plasmin, which in turn is responsible for the lysis of fibrin and fibrinogen, the main components of an acute thrombus. The use of TPA followed by intravenous heparin has been successful in restoring blood flow after an acute coronary occlusion. To maximize results, TPA must be administered within a period of less than 6 hours after the onset of symptoms, as was done in this case. Reperfusion was successful since the chest pain disappeared and the enzymes normalized. Adjuvant therapy with heparin was started to prevent re-occlusion.

Sudden onset of abdominal pain in a patient that is receiving anticoagulant therapy should alert the clinician of the possibility of bleeding. Potential sources include a gastric or duodenal peptic ulcer, hemorrhagic pancreatitis, and a dissecting or ruptured abdominal aortic aneurysm. Upper GI bleeding was unlikely in the absence of hematemesis or melena. Acute pancreatitis is associated with leukocytosis, but there was no evidence of increased levels of serum amylase and lipase. Abdominal aortic aneurysms are common in patients with atherosclerosis and hypertension. These patients often develop saccular dilatations below the renal and above the iliac arteries. Aortic dissection can occur in patients with a history of hypertension, but are rare in the context of severe atherosclerosis due to the protective effect of substantial medial scarring and fibrosis. Rupture of an aortic aneurysm can cause excruciating pain, but this is a catastrophic event with massive blood loss and rapid death. There is no time for development of progressive pain with subsequent radiation to the hip and dropping hematocrit within a 48 hours period, unless the aneurysm was leaking slowly. Bleeding within a third space (pleura, pericardium and retroperitoneum) has been reported following anticoagulant therapy, although fatal bleeding is rare. Pleural and pericardial hemorrhages usually cause chest pain. Patients with a large pericardial effusion present with symptoms of cardiac tamponade. Dysphagia and dyspnea may result from esophageal or lung compression due to mediastinal or pleural hemorrhage.

Retroperitoneal hematomas are more likely to cause abdominal pain that radiates to the extremities. Pain in the hip and leg are the result of entrapment of the lumbar plexus and femoral nerve, and the dissection of the planes of the psoas muscle. The retroperitoneum is a relatively large and expansible space that allows a gradual accumulation of blood and changes in the hematocrit values. Retroperitoneal hematomas may occur even with controlled prothrombin time (PT) and partial thromboplastin time (PTT) values; therefore a CT scan is indicated if the patient develops abdominal pain associated with progressive normochromic, normocytic anemia. In this case, the bleeding was most likely caused by heparin rather than by TPA. The adverse effects of TPA are evident early after administration and include stroke, intracerebral hemorrhages and less often, bleeding from vascular access sites. Therapeutic heparin dose has been associated with an estimated bleeding risk of 5%. The risk increases if the dose is given intermittently rather than continuously, and in patients with chronic illnesses such as pulmonary or liver diseases. Interestingly, our patient was a heavy smoker with both severe COPD and evolving cirrhosis. Nonetheless, he had enough spared and functional liver parenchyma to maintain normal coagulation and unremarkable levels of bilirrubin and alkaline phosphatase. The sudden onset of shortness of breath was due to the extension of the hemorrhage into the left diaphragmatic region. The cause of death in this case was most likely hypoxemia followed by a cardiac arrhythmia.

Suggested Readings

1. Hirsh J. Coronary thrombolysis: hemorrhagic complications. Can J Cardiol 1993; 9:505-11.
2. Sleight P. Thrombolysis: state of the art. Eur Heart J 1993; Suppl G:41-7.
3. Simoons ML. Risk-benefit of thrombolysis. Cardiol Clin 1995; 13:339-45.
4. Jafri SM, Walters BL, Borzak S. Medical therapy of acute myocardial infarction: Part I. Role of thrombolytic and antithrombotic therapy. J Intensive Care Med 1995; 10:54-63.
5. Indications for fibrinolytic therapy in suspected acute myocardial infarction: collaborative overview of early mortality and major morbidity results from all randomised trials of more than 1000 patients. Fibrinolytic Therapy Trialists' (FTT) Collaborative Group. Lancet 1994; 343:311-22.

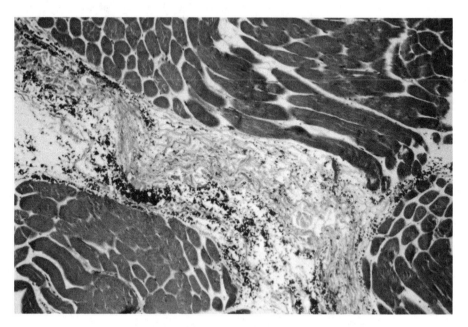

Figure 8. Dissecting hematoma of the psoas muscle. Blood is present in the interstitium between skeletal muscle fibers (Hematoxylin and Eosin, 10X)

NON-ATHEROSCLEROTIC ISCHEMIA

Case # 6

Clinical Summary

This is the case of a 45 year old Hispanic woman with a 30 pack/year smoking history, and a six year history of Hepatitis B seropositivity. She had suffered from migraines for the past 11 years, and had had several syncopal episodes. She presented to the hospital after acute onset of left-sided chest pain of 15 minutes duration. It was described as sharp with radiation to the left arm, which felt numb and weak with associated paresthesias ('tingling'). She had no shortness of breath, diaphoresis, dizziness, nausea, vomiting or diarrhea. She did not have a history of hypertension, diabetes mellitus, angina or myocardial infarction. Prior to her arrival to the hospital she had a brief period of arm weakness and unconsciousness.

Her past medical history was also remarkable for sinus problems, and hay fever. Both parents were alive and healthy. She had two sisters, one of whom had a history of coronary artery disease and myocardial infarction. Her brother, age 50 y, had colon cancer.

On admission her vital signs were BP 112/52, P 85, T 37°C, and RR 20. The patient was hydrated, alert, with normal mental exam, and in no significant distress. The neurological exam was grossly normal. Her skin had no lesions. There was no mouth erythema or exudate. The neck was supple, with a diffusely enlarged thyroid, and no bruits or jugular venous distension (JVD). The heart had regular rhythm, and the lungs were clear to auscultation. The abdomen had normal bowel sounds, was soft, non-tender, non-distended, with no hepatosplenomegaly or masses. The extremities had no clubbing, cyanosis or edema, and the peripheral pulses were 2+ bilaterally.

Laboratory data and other tests

Laboratory: WBC 5.9 (S 35%, L 49%, M 10%, E 5%), Hb/Hct 12/35, Plt 348; SGOT/SGPT 25/18 U/L, Cholesterol 108, PT/PTT 13/26. CXR normal. ECG: sinus rhythm at 82, normal axis and ST elevation in II, III and avF.

The patient was admitted to rule out myocardial infarction and to work up her syncopal episodes. The day after admission she complained of chest pain, which subsided with sublingual nitroglycerin. Her ECG at the time showed ST elevations in many leads. Soon thereafter, she began gasping and became pulseless. Resuscitation efforts were unsuccessful

Pre-Autopsy Evaluation and Analysis

Crucial clinical information can be derived from the first sentence of the history: 1) a 45 year old woman, 2) a smoker, 3) seropositive for hepatitis B, 4) affected by migraine headaches, and 5) someone who had experienced multiple episodes of syncope (although the time frame is not indicated). Her presentation was suggestive for acute ischemic heart disease. The quality and characteristics described are very specific for coronary pain (~95 % specificity, and a high positive predictive value). Electrocardiograms at first revealed ST segment elevations in II, III, and avF; and then diffuse ST elevations across the precordium. Her death was rapid, and it was not associated with cardiac enzyme increases. Thus, we are trying to establish the cause of apparent ischemic heart disease in a relatively young woman. Several questions about this case can easily be raised:

1. Is this really ischemic heart disease?
2. If so, is it more likely to be typical or atypical?
3. If it is typical, what is the differential diagnosis?
4. If it is atypical, what is the differential diagnosis?

Ischemia vs. Non-ischemia

It would certainly appear that the presentation is most consistent with ischemic heart disease. The acute onset of chest pain with radiation to the left arm is strongly suggestive of this conclusion. She did not have diaphoresis, nausea, or vomiting, all signs and symptoms of ischemic heart disease, but very variable in their presence. Furthermore, as described below, the ischemia may not have been persistent. Although one must consider other causes of chest pain, it is difficult to explain the nature of these complaints with chest wall disease (e.g. costochondritis, or myositis), muscle strain, pericarditis, pleuritis, or parenchymal pulmonary disease (including pulmonary embolism). When one adds the electrocardiographic findings to the clinical complaints, it strengthens the association even further with ischemia. The fact that the cardiac enzymes were within normal limits, simply indicates that the ischemia was transient and did not persist for sufficient time to irreversibly injure the myocardium. It is possible that today, with the use of the more sensitive early marker of myocardial damage, troponin I, that there would have been evidence of myocardial injury, but this marker was not in general use in 1994 when this case occurred. Additionally, the clinical history of multiple episodes of syncope, and the brief period of unconsciousness associated with the acute chest pain events leading to her hospitalization, suggests that ischemia may have been intermittent and causing transient cardiac arrhythmia. Thus, it appears entirely reasonable to assume that this patient had ischemic disease based on her presentation to the hospital; in fact, she was admitted with the working diagnosis of rule out myocardial infarction (ROMI).

Typical vs. Atypical Ischemia

Once we consider it more likely than not that this patient had ischemic disease, the question of whether it was typical or atypical is somewhat more difficult to ascertain. First, it is necessary to define these two terms. Typical ischemic heart disease is generally considered secondary to coronary atherosclerosis, with atherosclerotic plaque (s) narrowing the lumen and causing damage to the coronary artery wall. The presence of atherosclerosis may increase the possibility of superimposed coronary artery lesions including acute plaque hemorrhage or rupture, luminal thrombosis, and/or coronary artery spasm. The presence of atherosclerosis does not provide information concerning the pathogenesis of the plaque, whether it is idiopathic but associated with cigarette smoking, hypercholesterolemia, hypertension, or diabetes mellitus (or combinations of all of these), or whether it may be secondary to less common risk factors such as hyperhomocysteinemia, cocaine use, or radiotherapy (chest irradiation for neoplastic disease).

Atypical ischemia is discriminated from typical angina pectoris, because it is considered to be non-atherosclerotic coronary artery disease. This implies different pathophysiological mechanisms, primarily secondary to coronary artery spasm, which may be spontaneous or caused by pharmacological agents including drugs such as cocaine. Other causes include hypercoagulable states, leading to coronary artery thrombosis; direct or indirect coronary artery infection (e.g. herpes virus or cytomegalovirus infection in immunosuppressed patients; salmonella infection of endothelial cells; or direct extension of bacterial infection from active endocarditis or pericarditis, leading to mycotic coronary artery aneurysm); mechanical disruption of the coronary artery, such as spontaneous or post-traumatic dissection (e.g. the trauma may be related to blunt force chest wall injury, or iatrogenic injury during interventions such as coronary angiogram or angioplasty); and finally, inflammatory diseases such as vasculitis. It is of particular importance to recognize that combinations of these various etiologies may occur simultaneously, making the assessment of the situation even more difficult.

Based on the previous definitions, did this patient have typical or atypical coronary artery ischemia? She was a relatively young woman. Atherosclerosis begins to increase in women in their fifth decade, but it is relatively uncommon unless they are postmenopausal, or affected by atypically high cholesterol levels or diabetes mellitus. Accelerated atherosclerosis, even in women with adequate ovarian hormonal function, can occur with hypercholesterolemia, diabetes mellitus, and rarely hypothyroidism with myxedema. We are not informed of this patient's menstrual history, a critical piece of information that is often not investigated during acute presentations with serious complaints in emergency rooms. However, it is reasonable to assume that at age 45 she was not postmenopausal. Moreover, she did not have a history of diabetes mellitus or hypertension. However, her physical examination did reveal a diffusely enlarged thyroid gland, but she had no complaints or physical signs of significant hypo or hyperthyroidism. Her serum cholesterol was low, which may even be secondary to hyperthyroidism, but it certainly rules out hypercholesterolemia. Despite this, she had a positive family history, with one sister (unknown whether she was older or younger) with coronary artery disease and myocardial infarction. Furthermore, the fact that her parents were alive and well, and a 50 year old brother was not reported to have coronary disease, strongly mitigate against the diagnosis of any familial condition that might have predisposed her to coronary artery disease. The significant smoking history put her at higher risk for coronary artery atherosclerosis, but it is rarely associated with this diagnosis in pre-menopausal women in the absence of hypercholesterolemia and hypertension.

Could there be any association with hepatitis B seropositivity? First of all, we are not informed whether she actually was infected previously, and if so, whether she was core or surface antigen positive. Regardless, there is no direct relationship with hepatitis B infection and coronary artery disease. There have been some loose associations with hepatitis B infection and the subsequent development of polyarteritis nodosa, but generally, most investigators do not consider this to be a convincing etiologic relationship. Polyarteritis nodosa is a vasculitis that can affect coronary arteries and could lead to ischemia with or without coronary thrombosis, but as an isolated event causing an acute presentation such as in this case, is very unlikely.

Could there be an association with her eleven year history of migraine headaches? This issue is somewhat more promising as an area of investigation. There have been cases of acute ischemic heart disease associated with several classes of agents used to treat migraine or vascular headaches. These include ergotamine derivatives, methysergide, and the newest class of serotonin receptor agonists. However, with all of these drugs that can potentially stimulate smooth muscle contraction and lead to coronary artery spasm, it is generally accepted that the rare coronary events are secondary to superimposed drug use in the presence of pre-existing coronary atherosclerosis. There are also anecdotal reports of patients with migraine headaches who have spontaneous coronary artery spasm, presumably due to hyper-reactivity of their coronary circulation. In the current case, there was no history of pre-existing migraine headache for which she had taken medication. Since patients with migraines are so exquisitely sensitive to their symptoms and affected by their condition, it is unlikely she would have not reported her symptoms or drug use, if she had had a migraine episode. Thus, it appears unlikely that migraine headaches, or their treatment, could explain her coronary ischemia. It is possible, however, that migraines could have been the etiology of the multiple episodes of syncope she reported previously.

Does the limited clinical information give us any additional clues, either positive or negative? There doesn't seem to be a condition associated with an increased tendency to thrombosis. There was no history of recurrent thromboemboli or thrombophlebitis. We are not informed as to whether she was using oral contraceptives, which might increase the risk of a thrombosis (along with smoking cigarettes). Her prothrombin time and partial thromboplastin time were completely normal, along with her platelet count. She was mildly anemic, but this is not associated with an increased tendency to thrombosis. Although we are not informed about her serum homocysteine levels, significant elevations of homocysteine are often associated with an increased thrombogenic tendency, and a higher risk for generalized development of atherosclerosis.

What about illicit drugs? One must always consider the possibility of prior or current drug use (specifically cocaine) in the context of a relatively young patient who should not be affected by typical coronary artery ischemia. Since cocaine is used by all strata of society as a recreational drug, it cannot be discounted regardless of socioeconomic class. Cocaine can affect the coronary circulation acutely or chronically, at any dose, and by any means of intake. Chronically, it can lead to damage of the vessel wall through hyper-stimulation of vascular smooth muscle, endothelial damage, and subsequent atherosclerotic plaque development. Acutely, it can cause coronary artery spasm, either superimposed on a previously damaged vessel or in a normal vessel. In all circumstances, the mechanism is through binding to α-2 adrenergic receptors, leading to inhibition of catecholamine re-uptake at the neuromuscular junction, and subsequent increased contractile stimulation of smooth muscle. In this case, the patient was not asked specifically whether she had used cocaine previously, or shortly before her presentation; therefore, this possible cause for her symptoms cannot be assessed.

Two other etiologies have to be evaluated. Could this presentation be secondary to an inflammatory cause? There was no history or clinical findings consistent with a collagen vascular disease such as systemic lupus erythematosus, which may be associated with coronary artery vasculitis. She was not in the age-range of patients affected by Kawasaki disease (mucocutaneous lymph node syndrome, which is exclusively a pediatric condition), or temporal arteritis (a disease of the elderly, which as a giant cell

61

arteritis can affect coronary arteries). She is in the appropriate age range for Takayasu's arteritis, but without other clinical complaints and with normal peripheral pulses, this is an extremely unlikely diagnosis. Could this be a mechanical event? Coronary artery dissection can occur in patients with connective tissue disorders such as Marfan's syndrome and Ehlers-Danlos syndrome, but both are generally associated with skin, joint, and skeletal abnormalities, in addition to a family history. Other connective tissue disorders, such as pseudoxanthoma elasticum, can lead to calcification and atheromatous plaque formation in the coronary artery; however this condition is usually associated with skin lesions. Spontaneous dissections also occur in pregnancy, or shortly after delivery. The current case had no such history. Rarely, coronary artery dissections occur spontaneously, without a history of iatrogenic intervention, trauma, pregnancy, or underlying connective tissue disorder.

Thus, we are left with a rapid onset of acute coronary ischemia in a relatively young woman, with no definite cause for her symptoms and sudden death. In this case, we can say that without an autopsy, the cause of her terminal events would remain a mystery, but would most likely be ascribed to coronary artery atherosclerosis. However, for a number of the reasons addressed above, it is more likely that the coronary artery ischemia was secondary to an atypical, non-atherosclerotic cause. The rapid course of her disease, and the failure of the admitting physicians to question her about her menstrual history and illicit drug use, makes the diagnosis not attainable on clinical grounds alone. Even if she had survived for a period of time after admission, it is not likely that a stress test or coronary angiography would have been able to pinpoint the etiology of her condition.

Gross Description

The autopsy was limited to the heart. The heart weighed 275 g and was of the expected shape. The pericardium was smooth and glistening. The epicardium had moderate amount of epicardial fat. The atria were normal in size and free of thrombi. The foramen ovale was closed. The right and left ventricular walls measure 0.3 and 1.2 cm in thickness, respectively. The valve leaflets were delicate and pliable. The chordae tendineae were slender. The endocardium was thin and glistening. The coronaries had normal distribution. The myocardium appeared grossly unremarkable with average consistency, except for an area of hemorrhage surrounding the left anterior descending artery at 3.5 cm from the ostium and extending along the artery for a distance of 0.5 cm. (Figure 9). There were no occlusions. The coronaries and the aorta showed no evidence of atherosclerosis.

Microscopic Description

The endocardium was unremarkable. Multiple representative sections from the myocardium failed to reveal histologic evidence of remote or acute ischemic injury. Sections from the abnormal area of the left anterior descending coronary artery showed accumulation of blood within the outer media compressing the lumen. The blood was contained within the external elastic lamina. The intima was intact. The changes were consistent with left anterior descending coronary artery dissection (Figure 10). There was no evidence of cystic medial necrosis. Surrounding the vessel and extending into the epicardial fat was an inflammatory infiltrate composed predominantly of eosinophils. There was no inflammation in areas of the LAD unaffected by the dissection or in sections of other coronary arteries.

Post-autopsy Evaluation and Analysis

The post mortem examination revealed a limited dissection of the left anterior descending coronary artery, with no intimal disruption, but compression of the true lumen by a medial hematoma. The dissection was associated with eosinophilic inflammation in the vessel wall and in the surrounding tissues. There was no atherosclerosis.

The spontaneous dissection of a coronary artery, in the absence of iatrogenic instrumentation or external trauma, is a rare but well-recognized cause of coronary ischemia and sudden death. It most often occurs in women of child bearing age, during pregnancy or following delivery. The association with eosinophilic vasculitis is not incidental, as is the also case with peripartum cardiomyopathy and myocarditis, in which eosinophilic inflammation is common. Although the etiology of the eosinophilic infiltration of the vessel wall is unknown, it is likely that collagenolytic eosinophilic enzyme release leads to a disruption of the media. In the current case, there was no history of recent pregnancy, nor was there any systemic increase of eosinophils. The inflammation of the coronary artery wall, with the subsequent disruption of the media and medial hematoma, probably stimulated coronary artery spasm thereby accounting for the intermittent nature of her complaints, and the lack of myocardial necrosis. Although spontaneous coronary artery dissection with or without eosinophils is a rare cause of coronary ischemia, the lesson derived from this case is that unusual etiologies for ischemia have to be considered when patients do not have the usual and expected causes for the common conditions.

Suggested Readings

1. Elming H, Kober L. Spontaneous coronary artery dissection. Case report and literature review. Scand Cardiovasc J. 1999; 33:175-9.
2. Atay Y, Yagdi T, Turkoglu C, Altintig A, Buket S. Spontaneous dissection of the left main coronary artery: a case report and review of the literature. J Card Surg. 1996; 11:371-5.
3. Waller BF, Fry ET, Hermiller JB, Peters T, Slack JD. Nonatherosclerotic causes of coronary artery narrowing--Part II. Clin Cardiol. 1996; 19:587-91.
4. Jouriles NJ. Atypical chest pain. Emerg Med Clin North Am. 1998 Nov; 16:717-40.
5. Borczuk AC; van Hoeven KH; Factor SM. Review and hypothesis: the eosinophil and peripartum heart disease (myocarditis and coronary artery dissection)--coincidence or pathogenetic significance? Cardiovasc Res. 1997; 33:527-32.
6. Hahn IH, Hoffman RS. Cocaine use and acute myocardial infarction. Emerg Med Clin North Am. 2001; 19:493-510.
7. Rump AF, Theisohn M, Klaus W. The pathophysiology of cocaine cardiotoxicity. Forensic Sci Int. 1995; 71:103-15.

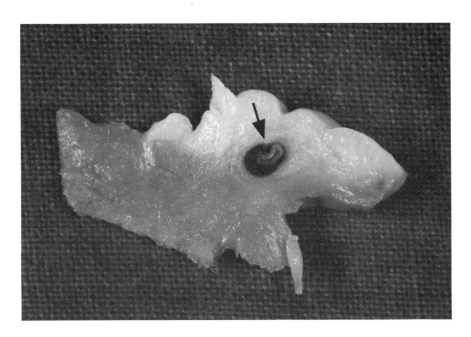

Figure 9. Coronary artery dissection. Notice the blood in the adventitia compressing the lumen of the vessel (arrow).

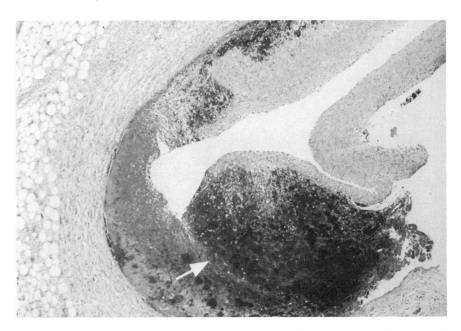

Figure 10. Coronary artery dissection, histologic section. Blood is dissecting the layers of the artery (arrow) (Hematoxylin and Eosin, 10X)

Chapter 3

DIABETES AND THE HEART

Case # 7

Clinical Summary

This is the case of a 43 year old Hispanic woman with more than a 20 years history of diabetes mellitus, hypertension, congestive heart failure, and gastritis associated with Helicobacter pylori infection. She developed nephropathy, neuropathy and retinopathy secondary to her diabetes, and was legally blind and wheelchair bound. She was brought to the hospital after 24 hours of localized colic-type epigastric pain, nausea and vomiting of "coffee-ground" material. Her medications before admission included NPH insulin, furosemide and atenolol.

Significant findings on her physical exam were: Vital signs BP 168/94, HR 86, RR 12, T 37°C. Heart: normal S1S2 and an S3 with no murmurs. Clear lungs. Abdomen: bowel sounds present; distended and soft with mild tenderness, no guarding and no rebound. Positive stool test for blood. Extremities: bilateral pretibial edema, left foot with healing ulcer on plantar surface, and the right first toe tip had evidence of dry gangrene. Neurologic: blind; decreased sensation on both lower extremities knee to foot distribution (stocking).

Laboratory data and other tests

Laboratory: WBC 19 (S 90%, L 5%), Hct 37, Plt 270; PT/PTT 10/29; amylase 6.1; glucose 320; BUN/creat 37/1.3; UA pH 7, protein 300, glucose 1000, WBC/RBC 3/heavy, bacteria 5-10 and epithelial cells 10-20/HPF.

The patient continued to vomit, the bloody diarrhea persisted and the bowel sounds diminished. Infection or ischemic bowel disease were the clinical diagnoses considered. An abdominal CT-scan showed occlusion consistent with thrombus in the superior mesenteric artery (SMA), which was confirmed by angiography. Thrombectomy of the SMA and Goretex patch angioplasty were performed. In addition, the patient was transfused. Soon after surgery, acute renal failure developed. Hemodialysis and anticoagulation therapy were started. However, 10 days later she had an episode of gastrointestinal bleeding and the heparin was discontinued. The following day the blood pressure suddenly dropped and the patient expired.

Gross Description

The heart weighed 500 g and showed dilatation of the right and left atria, and hypertrophy of the left ventricle (1.6 cm in thickness). The tricuspid valve measured 12.6 cm in length. The coronary arteries were partially occluded (60–90%) by atherosclerosis with calcification. The aorta had moderate atherosclerosis. The lungs were congested (850 g combined). Two ulcers were noted in the body of the stomach, each measuring 1 cm in diameter. The distal portion of the jejunum and the proximal portion of the ileum had serosal purple discoloration consistent with ischemic bowel disease. The luminal content was bloody. The vascular graft of the superior mesenteric artery was partially occluded by a thromboembolus. The kidneys weighed 450 g combined and had a finely granular surface. The cut surface was unremarkable.

Microscopic Description

The cardiovascular examination confirmed right and left ventricular hypertrophy with mild perivascular fibrosis and multifocal interstitial and replacement fibrosis. Sections from the superior mesenteric artery and its branches revealed medial calcific sclerosis (Monckeberg's) with recent hemorrhage in the portion where fragments of synthetic graft were identified. The lumen was 60% occluded by a hyaline plaque showing signs of remote and recent hemorrhage.

Sections from the lung revealed congestion as well as numerous hemosiderin-laden macrophages, the so called 'heart failure cells', and signs of mild pulmonary hypertension. The small bowel had segments of transmural ischemic and hemorrhagic infarction with focal areas of mucosal regeneration. The kidneys exhibited areas of nodular and diffuse glomerulosclerosis (Kimmelstiel-Wilson). The central nervous system revealed acute hippocampal hypoxic and degenerative changes. The remaining organs were unremarkable; except for the liver which showed mild steatosis and centrilobular congestion.

Case Analysis

This case classically depicts a number of features of diabetic cardiovascular disease. The patient had Type I, insulin-dependent diabetes mellitus (IDDM, juvenile onset) for more than 20 years, with hypertension, and complications affecting multiple organ systems. Primarily, she had diffuse vascular disease affecting a wide range of different caliber blood vessels, from the smallest to the largest. This is a crucial feature of longstanding diabetes for 10 or more years, whether it is insulin dependent or not (types I and II, respectively), and particularly when it is associated with systemic hypertension. Even the autonomic and peripheral diabetic neuropathy, which has been associated with metabolic derangements that affect neural transmission, may have an ischemic component mediated by microvascular damage to nerve fibers.

The classification of blood vessel calibers by size as macrovascular, small, and microvascular is an arbitrary one, and varies between investigators. Nevertheless, it is useful because pathological injury is generally limited to one class of vessel (e.g. atherosclerosis affects the macrovasculature), and tissue damage may depend on the size of the vessel affected in the process. In general, macrovascular blood vessels are the major elastic capacitance vessels including the aorta and the iliac arteries (these have a media composed of multiple lamellae or layers of elastic tissue and smooth muscle cells), and the muscular arteries including the aortic branch vessels (e.g. coronary, carotid, femoral, popliteal, renal, celiac, superior mesenteric, etc.). The muscular arteries have an intima separated from the media by an internal elastic lamella, and the media is composed of smooth muscle tissue. The macrovasculature is primarily affected by atherosclerosis. Microvascular vessels are the small arteries below 100-200 µm (micrometers or microns), although some investigators would consider vessels beginning at 50-100 µm and smaller. The microvasculature includes vessels identified as arterioles, capillaries, and venules. These vessels are affected by smooth muscle hypertrophy, and increased connective tissue deposition (fibrillar and non-fibrillar collagen).

In diabetes mellitus, it is common to find increased basement membrane material surrounding capillaries, and intercalated around smooth muscle cells in the media of small vessels. In addition, the microvasculature may have endothelial cell dysfunction, and hyper-reactivity (e.g. spasm) of the endothelial and smooth muscle cells, which may lead to tissue damage. The small vessels are arteries with calibers ranging between 50-100 µm and 1000 µm. These are muscular vessels, easily identified by microscopic tissue examination, that are generally affected by "sclerosis" not atherosclerosis. This means that they are 'stiffer' or hardened (literal definition of sclerosis) due to the deposition of connective tissue and smooth muscle hyperplasia. The end-result is an increase in resistance to blood flow, and with severe proliferative changes, there is decreased luminal caliber, thereby causing chronic obstruction and tissue ischemia. Essentially, diabetic vascular injury is ubiquitous and diffuse, eventually affecting all blood vessels, leading to extensive tissue and multiorgan damage.

The patient in this case had macrovascular disease with significant atherosclerosis of coronary arteries, the aorta and its branches. It was the disease of the superior mesenteric artery that precipitated the ischemic bowel disease, requiring surgical intervention. Histologically, there was an atherosclerotic plaque with remote and recent hemorrhage, which can trigger vascular instability or dynamic changes in the vessel, leading to acute luminal occlusion (thrombosis) and subsequent ischemia. There were also changes of sclerosis, with features of Monckeberg's medial sclerosis and calcification. This is a degenerative change that involves the internal elastic lamella with spread of calcium and scar tissue into the media. Monckeberg's medial sclerosis is a common finding in diabetic patients, particularly in the lower extremities where it may lead to vascular insufficiency and gangrene.

She had evidence of small vessel disease, with thickened small arteries in the heart, and in the kidneys. The latter are associated with arterionephrosclerosis secondary to hypertension, which leads to chronic cortical ischemia, scarring, and renal dysfunction. Although her renal dysfunction was also related to microvascular disease, it is not uncommon in diabetic patients to develop ischemia due to vascular pathology affecting all sizes of vessels (e.g. renal artery, small arteries, arterioles, and capillaries). In the heart, small artery disease may lead to focal areas of ischemia with subsequent scarring, which may contribute to the hypertensive and diabetic cardiomyopathy (see below). The ulceration and dry gangrene on her extremities may also have been secondary to disease of small arteries in the muscle and skin.

There was also evidence of microvascular disease in different organs. She had retinopathy leading to blindness. This is often secondary to rupture of capillary microaneurysms with retinal and vitreous hemorrhage and proliferation of new vessels and scar tissue obliterating the retina (e.g. proliferative retinopathy). Ischemic damage may also result from hypertensive sclerosis and narrowing of arterioles. In the kidney, in addition to hypertensive arterionephrosclerosis, she had nodular diabetic glomerulosclerosis or Kimmelstiel-Wilson disease. The latter causes marked nodular thickening and ultimate obliteration of glomerular capillary loops. Only recently has it been shown to be secondary to damage to the glomerular capillaries leading to microaneurysms with ultimate thrombosis and reorganization. These microaneurysms, which occur due to localized injury to the capillary endothelial cells with outpouching of the lumen, are similar to those found in the eye and in the heart.

The patient had a clinical history of congestive heart failure, and her heart was hypertrophied (500 g, normal up to 350 g), with microscopic changes of interstitial and replacement fibrosis. The left and right ventricles were hypertrophied. These findings were characteristic of hypertensive and diabetic cardiomyopathy, with thick-walled chambers and microscopic scarring. Pathophysiologically, the chamber dimensions are small (e.g. decreased end-diastolic volume), and generally the contractility of the ventricle is normal or super-normal. The congestive heart failure symptoms

70

result from diastolic dysfunction. The ventricles are stiff with poor compliance; they pump adequately but fill poorly. As seen in the present case, the description of the ventricular chamber sizes, and the dilation of both atria are typical of a heart with diastolic dysfunction (the atria dilate because of the poor compliance of the ventricles).

The pathogenesis of hypertensive and diabetic cardiomyopathy is complex and multiple factors contribute to its development. Though the diabetic heart is often affected by significant coronary artery atherosclerosis, large vessel ischemia may not be sufficient to account for the disease. In this patient, there was no evidence of large areas of scarring secondary to coronary artery disease. However, small vessel sclerosis certainly contributes to microscopic areas of scarring. These hearts have significant microvascular disease, with microaneurysms present in arterioles and capillaries (Figure 11). In addition, the microvasculature is hyper-reactive (e.g. spasm) and leads to multiple areas of reperfusion damage in the myocardium, with eventual replacement by scar tissue (Figures 12 and 13). Finally, the effects of hypertension also lead to hypertrophy of myocardial cells. The combination of scar tissue and hypertrophy contributes the major component of the diastolic dysfunction, although metabolic cellular considerations (e.g. poor relaxation of cells due to abnormal calcium flux) also play a role.

Despite the fact that the immediate cause of death in this patient could be directly attributed to the mesenteric artery thrombosis, and bowel ischemia, there was significant evidence for systemic disease affecting multiple organs. This is a very typical scenario in diabetic patients, because the disease affects vessels of all calibers, leading to tissue damage throughout the body.

Suggested Readings

1. Drouet L. Atherothrombosis in diabetes--its evolution and management. Diabetes Obes Metab. 1999; 1 (Suppl 2):S37-47.
2. Calles-Escandon J, Cipolla M. Diabetes and endothelial dysfunction: a clinical perspective. Endocr Rev. 2001; 22:36-52.
3. Mazzone T. Current concepts and controversies in the pathogenesis, prevention, and treatment of the macrovascular complications of diabetes. J Lab Clin Med. 2000; 135:437-43.
4. Donnelly R, Emslie-Smith AM, Gardner ID, Morris AD. ABC of arterial and venous disease: vascular complications of diabetes. BMJ. 2000; 320:1062-6.
5. Goldberg RB. Cardiovascular disease in diabetic patients. Med Clin North Am. 2000; 84:81-93.
6. Modena MG, Barbieri A. Diabetes mellitus and cardiovascular complications: pathophysiological peculiarities and therapeutic implications. Cardiologia. 1999; 44:865-77.
7. Factor SM, Okun EM, Minase T. Capillary microaneurysms in the human diabetic heart. .N Eng J Med 1980; 302:384-8.
8. Factor SM, Bhan R, Minase T, Wolinsky H, Sonneblick EH. Hypertensive-diabetic cardiomyopathy in the rat: an experimental model of human disease. .Am J Pathol 1981; 102:219-28.
9. Factor SM, Sonneblick EH. Microvascular spasm as a cause of cardiomyopathies. Cardiovasc Rev Rep 1983; 4:1177-82.
10. Eng C, Cho S, Factor SM, Sonneblick EH, Kirk ES. Myocardial micronecrosis produced by microsphere embolization. Role of an alpha adrenergic tonic influence of the coronary microcirculation. Circ Res 1984; 54:74-82.

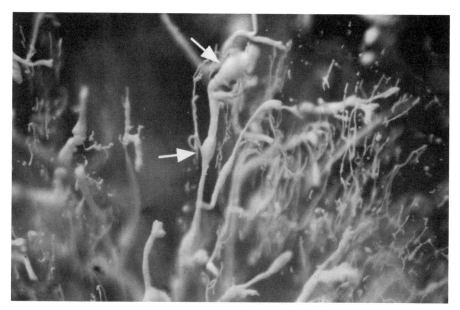

Figure 11. Silicone rubber (Microfil) perfused diabetic heart after "clearing" the tissue so that it is semi-translucent. The microcirculation vessels are examined with epi-illumination, thereby providing a 3-dimensional appearance. There are several fusiform microaneurysms (arrows) in arterioles and capillaries characteristic of diabetic human hearts, and similar to microaneurysms in the diabetic retina and renal glomerulus (30X).

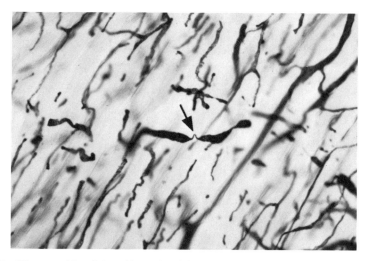

Figure 12. Silicone rubber (Microfil) perfused diabetic heart photographed with trans-illumination. This field shows aneurysmically dilated capillaries with focal narrowing (arrow) consistent with microvascular spasm that persisted after death (30X)

73

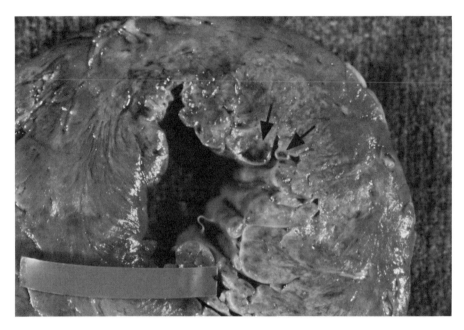

Figure 13. Left ventricular cross section demonstrating typical features of hypertensive and diabetic cardiomyopathy. There is left ventricular hypertrophy, extensive multifocal myocytolytic necrosis (the darker areas in the subendocardium and mid-wall), and multifocal fibrosis (the paler areas involving the papillary muscle, trabeculae, and ventricular wall). The recent and organizing necrosis, together with remote scarring, leads to replacement of large areas of functional myocardium, equivalent to myocardial infarction.

Chapter 4

CARDIOMYOPATHIES

Case # 8

Clinical Summary

A 52 year old woman with past medical history significant for dilated cardiomyopathy and hypertension was found at home by paramedics pulseless and with no respirations. Despite resuscitation efforts, she was pronounced dead.

Gross Description

The patient weighed 64 kg, and measured 163 cm. The heart weighed 760 g and showed concentric left ventricular hypertrophy (wall thickness 2.7 cm). Focal fibrosis of the epicardium was noted and was consistent with remote pericarditis. The atria and right ventricle were mildly dilated. The myocardium was scarred with multiple foci of interstitial and replacement fibrosis. Examination of the valves revealed fibrous thickening of the aortic valve cusps with a remote, organized vegetation of the non-coronary cusp. There was evidence of subaortic thickening of the left endocardial surface, consistent with the contact lesion of systolic anterior motion of the mitral valve (SAM). The mitral valve also showed fibrous thickening of the anterior leaflet with thickening and fusion of the chordae tendineae in keeping with SAM. The coronaries were up to 50% occluded by atheromatous plaques. The lungs weighed 980 g and were congested. The liver was smooth and soft (weight 1300 g). The kidneys weighed 160 g combined and had a finely granular surface. There were several scars bilaterally consistent with remote infarcts.

Case Analysis

Cardiac pathology tends to be a descriptive specialty, but it also allows for an analysis of cardiac function (e.g. pathophysiology) based on the interpretation of changes in the heart and blood vessels. In some instances, one can even identify specific genetic abnormalities based on the pathology alone. This case is an example where even without meaningful clinical history, the diagnosis is reachable, and the genetic defect can be predicted.

Therefore, and most importantly, guidance can be provided for family members to possibly prevent future adverse outcomes.

The patient was a relatively young woman who died suddenly at home. The only significant medical history was hypertension (unknown whether it had been treated), and a diagnosis of dilated cardiomyopathy (DCM). It is unclear how the diagnosis of DCM was made, and what it was based on. Regardless, after the autopsy, it seemed certain that she did not have DCM, though it is possible that she had symptoms of congestive heart failure (CHF). Perhaps, because of CHF symptoms, she was classified clinically as having DCM, although this diagnosis usually requires sophisticated cardiological tests including echocardiography, and studies to rule out ischemic coronary disease. Endomyocardial biopsy is the confirmatory test. We do not know whether any cardiac work-up was carried out. However, with the autopsy findings, we can deduce the condition that presumably led to this woman's sudden death; and we can infer what her pre-mortem cardiac function was.

This woman had severe concentric left ventricular hypertrophy, with a total cardiac mass of 760 g, and a left ventricular wall of 2.7 cm (Figure 14). She weighed 64 kg, and therefore an expected heart weight for her should have been 250-300 g, and the wall thickness should have been less than 1.5 cm. Could the hypertrophy have been due to hypertension? It is certainly possible, though with the other findings discussed below, it would be very unlikely. Hypertension, in some predisposed individuals, can lead to severe concentric hypertrophy, associated with myocardial fibrosis and potentially CHF. In this case, she had several other alterations that are not typically seen in hypertensive cardiac disease. In particular, there was fibrous thickening of the sub-aortic endocardium, also known as the outflow tract of the left ventricle. There was fibrous thickening of the ventricular surface of the anterior leaflet of the mitral valve, with fibrosis and focal fusion of chordae tendineae attached to that leaflet. The posterior leaflet and its chordae were unaffected. The sparing of the posterior leaflet rules out a diffuse valvulopathy of the mitral valve, such as rheumatic heart disease. There was also mild fibrous thickening of the aortic valve cusps, with sparing of the commissures. These findings were not characteristic of a specific valvulopathy, but most likely were secondary to outflow tract turbulence. Finally, microscopic examination of the myocardium revealed severe myocyte hypertrophy; multiple foci of interstitial and replacement fibrosis; markedly thickened small muscular arteries; and numerous foci of myocyte disorganization, known as whorls (Figures 15 and 16). The totality of the pathological changes allows us to make a specific diagnosis. This woman had hypertrophic cardiomyopathy (HCM), which is also known as familial hypertrophic cardiomyopathy (FHC). The features are absolutely diagnostic, as described below. In addition, the strong association of HCM with fatal arrhythmia, provides an explanation for this woman's sudden death.

The findings of massive left ventricular hypertrophy in association with a subaortic endocardial plaque and anterior mitral valve leaflet thickening, indicate that this woman had obstructive HCM. This means that during systolic contraction, there was a rapid expulsion of blood across the prominent subaortic bulging muscle, which led to two related phenomena. The anterior leaflet of the mitral valve was literally swept or sucked into the outflow tract where it came in contact with the outflow tract endocardium. This is called systolic anterior motion of the mitral valve, or SAM. The markers of this process are the fibrous thickening of the outflow tract (endocardial plaque), and the fibrosis of the anterior leaflet. The pathological degeneration results from the trauma of the leaflet striking the endocardium during each systolic contraction, but particularly during periods of increased heart rate and more forceful contraction (e.g. during stress or exercise). Why does the anterior leaflet, which normally moves in a posterior direction to coapt with the posterior leaflet occluding the atrial-ventricular orifice, move in the opposite direction to strike the septum? Although there is still controversy over the explanation, most investigators believe that the rapid expulsion of blood over the convex bulging septum leads to a pressure drop over the curved surface (Venturi effect, similar to the decreased pressure over the curved upper surface of an airplane wing). The movement of the leaflet in the anterior direction, together with the hypertrophied muscle that narrows the outflow tract, leads to late systolic obstruction. The obstruction, together with turbulence causes a late systolic ejection murmur (the obstruction occurs late in systole because sufficient acceleration of the blood has to occur before the leaflet is sucked anteriorly).

The obstruction and the murmur can be accentuated by tachycardia, increased contractility, and decreased end-diastolic volume. Increasing the velocity of the flow leads to a greater pressure fall across the septum, and decreasing the chamber dimensions shortens the distance the valve leaflet must traverse to strike the septum. End-diastolic volume can fall if there is a decrease in circulating blood volume, which may result from the inappropriate use of diuretics in a patient with congestive symptoms who is not identified as having HCM. End-diastolic volume will also decrease transiently during the Valsalva maneuver (increasing intra-thoracic pressure against a closed glottis), which is a good way to accentuate the murmur when auscultating the heart in a patient suspected of having HCM. In contrast, a patient with structural aortic stenosis may have a diminution of murmur intensity with a fall in end-diastolic volume. Any process that increases end-diastolic volume, thereby increasing the left ventricular dimensions and enhancing the separation of the anterior mitral valve leaflet and the septal endocardium, will lead to a decrease of the subaortic obstruction and the late systolic murmur. Similarly, decreasing contractility or slowing the heart rate (as with calcium channel blocking agents or beta adrenergic blockers) will decrease the obstruction and the murmur. The concomitant effect of the anterior mitral valve leaflet being swept into the outflow tract, is that it does not coapt with the posterior leaflet. Thus, individuals with SAM, also have mitral regurgitation, which may further compromise cardiac function and may enhance pulmonary congestion.

Usually, individuals with HCM who have CHF, do not have significant symptomatology due to the subaortic obstruction or the mitral valve regurgitation. Rather, they generally have severe diastolic dysfunction as a result of the marked ventricular hypertrophy, in association with extensive scarring in the myocardium. These hearts are also affected by an increased interstitial connective tissue matrix, although the pathogenesis of this process is not understood. The result is a markedly stiffened ventricle, with small ventricular volumes. The ventricle fills poorly, and there is an elevation of left atrial pressure, which is increased even further if there is significant mitral valve regurgitation. Thus, congestive symptoms are secondary to diastolic dysfunction. In fact, systolic function is relatively well maintained and even super-normal, in most patients with HCM. The pathophysiologic problem is one of inadequate ventricular filling. It is likely that the diagnosis of DCM in this case was based on congestive symptoms that she had secondary to diastolic dysfunction. Had an echocardiogram been performed, it would have been obvious immediately that she did not have DCM, but she had HCM.

Microscopically, patients with HCM have extensive areas of disorganized muscle fibers called whorls. This pattern of disorganization is not pathognomonic of HCM, as it can be seen in normal hearts and in areas around myocardial scars; but its extent in HCM is greater than in any other condition. Ordinarily, myocardial fibers are aligned in parallel within the 3 layers of the ventricular wall (each of the layers is oriented obliquely to the adjacent layer, but within the layers, the myocytes line-up in parallel). However, in myocyte whorls, the fibers are arranged at random, and are therefore unlikely to be capable of generating meaningful forceful contraction. The etiology for this fiber disposition is unknown, but one possible explanation is that it develops as a result of localized abnormal contraction patterns in the myocardium, secondary to the basic defect in this disease (see below).

The other microscopic finding typical of HCM, is that these patients generally have extensive myocardial scarring with areas of interstitial fibrosis, and infarct-like replacement fibrosis. Some of the scarring may in fact be related to myocardial ischemia, as the increased stiffness and thickness of the ventricular wall, and the enhanced contractility, lead to increased wall stress, which in turn may diminish myocardial perfusion. In addition, the intramyocardial muscular arteries are abnormally thickened and sclerotic, thereby causing a structural limitation to tissue perfusion. Patients with HCM may have complaints of atypical chest pain, and may have electrocardiographic abnormalities consistent with ischemia. However, although ischemic injury may be significant, and may even provoke arrhythmias, the most significant complication of this condition is sudden fatal arrhythmia. As in this patient, sudden death can be entirely unexpected, and may be the very first manifestation of the disease. Despite the relative rarity of HCM in the general population, it attains great notoriety because of it strong association with sudden death, often in otherwise healthy young people. Sudden death is also very predictable in individuals from families with known genetic mutations that have been shown to be particularly lethal.

Hypertrophic cardiomyopathy is an autosomal dominant hereditary disease. It can occur sporadically, presumably due to a unique mutation, but it occurs in families, often with variable penetrance. Prior to the last decade, HCM was thought to be due to a single mutation of the gene that codes for myosin heavy chain (MHC, a structural component of myosin, which is part of the contractile apparatus of the heart cell) in cardiac myocytes. A number of single amino acid mutations of MHC have now been identified in numerous families. Of interest, a particular mutation leads to similar phenotypic expression, including enhanced tendency to sudden death (thereby allowing for prediction and potential treatment in affected family members). The disease, however, has become far more complex than originally thought. Affected patients or families that did not have mutation of the MHC gene on chromosome 14 were identified. However, linkages to mutations on other chromosomes were found. This suggested that HCM is not a disease, but it is a syndrome.

In fact, 7 different forms of the condition have been found, often with phenotypic variability, and not all associated with marked ventricular hypertrophy, outflow tract obstruction, or other related findings. All 7 defects involve the sarcomere, thereby leading to the concept that HCM is a sarcomeric cardiomyopathy. The two most significant, and apparently most frequent in the population, are those that affect MHC, and troponin T. The latter is interesting because it does not lead to significant ventricular hypertrophy and obstruction, but it is associated with a very high prevalence of sudden death. Six of the 7 different abnormal proteins that cause HCM have been identified, with their specific mutant gene. The seventh that leads to HCM in association with a conduction defect known as the Wolf-Parkinson-White (WPW) syndrome is most likely the one that affected the patient in this case. This form of HCM has been linked to a gene on chromosome 7. Recently, an abnormal protein kinase encoded by this gene was identified.

At the completion of this autopsy, the family was contacted due to the fact that HCM was the final diagnosis, and because of the concern that other family members unknowingly might be affected. The patient had no siblings, and no other close relatives who had either been diagnosed with HCM, or had died unexpectedly and suddenly as a result of heart disease. However, she did have a single 29 year old daughter. Discussion with the daughter led to the information that she had been diagnosed with WPW as a child. Although WPW can occur sporadically, the association of HCM and WPW in first degree relatives did not appear to be a coincidence. Based on the likelihood of both mother and daughter having HCM, it was strongly suggested to the daughter that she have a cardiac work-up, including echocardiography. If the diagnosis was confirmed, then appropriate monitoring and treatment would be instituted. Pharmacologic treatment has been shown to be beneficial in symptomatic patients, although it may not prevent sudden arrhythmic death. To prevent the latter complication, an automated implantable defibrillator has been used with some success.

As a final note, WPW is an arrhythmic condition that can occur independently of HCM. It represents accelerated transmission of electrical activation from the atrium to the ventricle through an abnormal bypass (accessory) pathway. Thus, the ventricle is activated faster than normal, which may lead to disruption of the atrio-ventricular coordination. Electrophysiologically, the result is a shortened PR interval, and a slurring of the upstroke of the QRS complex leading to the formation of a delta wave. This delta wave is thought to represent the combined rapid transmission through the accessory bundle, and the normal transmission from the sino-atrial node through the atrial wall into the atrio-ventricular node. Drug treatment of WPW is available, along with surgical or interventional cardiologic ablation of the accessory bundle, if it can be identified. Sudden death may be a rare but recognized complication of WPW. It is not known whether sudden death in patients with HCM and WPW results from the WPW alone.

Suggested Readings

1. Wigle ED. Novel insights into the clinical manifestations and treatment of hypertrophic cardiomyopathy. Curr Opin Cardiol 1995; 10:299-305.
2. Wigle ED, Rakowski H, Kimball BP, Williams WG. Hypertrophic cardiomyopathy: clinical spectrum and treatment. Circulation 1995; 92:1680-92.
3. Posma JL, van der Wall EE, Blanksma PK, van der Wall E; Lie KI. New diagnostic options in hypertrophic cardiomyopathy. Am Heart J. 1996; 132:1031-41.
4. Lakkis N. New treatment methods for patients with hypertrophic obstructive cardiomyopathy. Curr Opin Cardiol. 2000; 15:172-7.
5. Basso C, Corrado D, Thiene G. Cardiovascular causes of sudden death in young individuals including athletes. Cardiol Rev. 1999; 7:127-35.
6. Maron BJ. Hypertrophic cardiomyopathy. Lancet. 1997; 350:127-33.
7. Davies MJ, McKenna WJ. Hypertrophic cardiomyopathy--pathology and pathogenesis. Histopathology. 1995; 26:493-500.
8. Tardiff JC, Factor SM, Tompkins BD, Hewett TE, Palmer BM, Moore RL, Schwartz S, Robbins J, Leinwand LA. A truncated cardiac troponin T molecule in transgenic mice suggests multiple cellular mechanisms for familial hypertrophic cardiomyopathy. J Clin Invest 1998; 101:2800-11.
9. Gollob MH, Green MS, Tang ASL, Gollob T, Karibe A, Hassan A, Ahmad F, Lozado R, Shah G, Fananapazir L, Bachinski LL, Roberts R. Identification of a gene responsible for familial Wolff-Parkinson-White syndrome. N Engl J Med 2001; 344:1823-31.

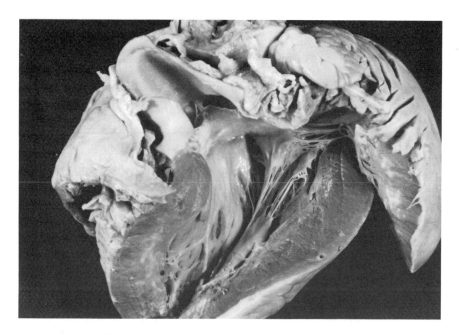

Figure 14. Hypertrophic cardiomyopathy. The heart shows severe generalized left ventricular hypertrophy and asymmetric septal hypertrophy with a reduced ventricular cavity and marked endocardial thickening.

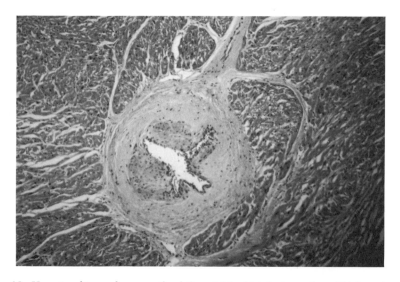

Figure 15. Hypertrophic cardiomyopathy, left ventricle, histologic section. Thickened and sclerotic muscular artery. There is significant perivascular fibrosis (Hematoxylin and Eosin, 40X).

82

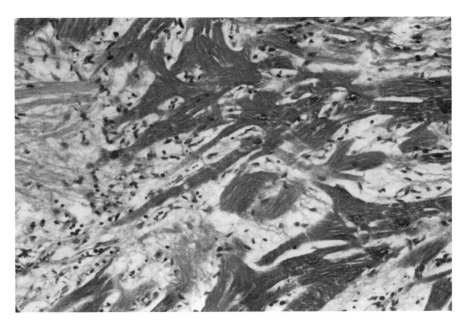

*Figure 16. Hypertrophic cardiomyopathy. Haphazardly-arranged myocardial fibers
(whorls) and interstitial scarring (Hematoxylin and Eosin, 40X)*

Case # 9

Clinical Summary

This is the case of a 55 year old woman with no significant past medical history who was found at home unresponsive by her daughter. She was transferred to a nearby emergency room where she was pronounced dead on arrival. In the last few days she had complained of fatigue, weight gain and shortness of breath that awakened her suddenly at night.

Gross Description

The body measured 160 cm and weighed 68 kg. On external examination there was peripheral edema, but no evidence of clubbing or cyanosis. The heart weighed 400 g. The pericardium was smooth. Both atria and ventricles were dilated and hypertrophied (RV 0.7 cm, LV 1.9 cm). No mural thrombi were present (Figure 17). The valve rings had the following measurements: tricuspid 12.5 cm, pulmonic 10 cm, mitral 11 cm and aortic 7.5 cm. The leaflets were pliable. The myocardium was flabby and mildly scarred. There was no significant atherosclerosis of the coronaries and aorta.

The lungs weighed 1450 g. Bilateral pleural effusions were noted with adhesions more prominent on the right side. The parenchyma had a red, congested appearance, but no discrete lesions were noted. The liver weighed 1920 g and had a dark red cut surface. The kidneys weighed 280 g combined and exhibited multiple cortical scars in keeping with remote renal infarctions. The spleen weighed 280 g. The thyroid weighed 25 g and had a multinodular appearance.

Microscopic Description

Sections from the heart showed adipose tissue infiltration of the atria, myocyte hypertrophy more prominent in the left ventricle and replacement and perivascular fibrosis. In addition, there were myxomatous changes of the mitral valve with subvalvular thickening of the mural endocardium. The lungs showed mild emphysematous changes and hemosiderin-laden macrophages within alveolar spaces. Sections from the liver revealed moderate centrilobular fatty change, congestion and mild periportal lymphocytic infiltrates. The thyroid was multinodular with a lymphocytic infiltrate.

Case Analysis

As previously discussed, sudden cardiac death is virtually always arrhythmic and has several predisposing factors. The post-mortem exam excluded all of them (occlusive coronary disease, myocardial infarction, myocardial fibrosis) except for one, cardiomyopathy. This is defined as a disease of the myocardium associated with cardiac dysfunction. Specifc cardiomyopathies refer to heart muscle diseases related to particular cardiac (e.g. ischemic, valvular, or hypertensive) or systemic disorders.

The finding of cardiomegaly (400 g vs. normal 270 g), and four chamber dilatation associated with mild ventricular hypertrophy, is characteristic of one type of cardiomyopathy known as dilated cardiomyopathy (Table 1, 1995 WHO/IFSC classification of cardiomyopathies). Dilated cardiomyopathy (DCM) has numerous and different etiologies that include: ischemia, myocarditis, sarcoidosis, connective tissue disorders, alcohol, drugs, metabolic and neuromuscular diseases. In a significant number of patients there is no obvious cause, hence the term "idiopathic dilated cardiomyopathy". DCM is characterized by the gradual development of cardiac failure associated with heart enlargement. Patients with this condition may be asymptomatic for years due to the compensatory mechanisms of the heart. This patient, for example, had no significant past medical history until she presented with fatigue, weight gain due to accumulation of fluid in third space and paroxysmal nocturnal dyspnea, which are all symptoms of heart failure. The autopsy findings of peripheral edema, pleural effusions and chronic passive congestion of lungs, liver and spleen were also in keeping with cardiac decompensation.

The progressive myocardial thinning and dilatation in DCM decreases the contractile function of the ventricles and therefore the cardiac output (CO). Compensation is achieved in several ways. One of the most important mechanisms is the Frank-Starling law of the heart, in which CO is maintained by increasing the stroke force. In addition, reduced CO activates the adrenergic and renin-angiotensin system. In low CO situations, the stimulated adrenergic system leads to increased heart rate and contractility; and the increased production of renin and angiotensin results in systemic vasoconstriction. Unfortunately, the outcome is enhanced wall stress and oxygen consumption in an already impaired myocardium. Thus, further myocyte damage ensues leading to failure. It is unknown what causes the myocardial dysfunction in the first place. Possible explanations include abnormal expression of genes responsible for the contractile function of the myocyte, loss of myocytes due to apoptosis (individual pre-programmed cell death), and abnormal cellular and chamber remodeling. In the latter, there is degradation of the connective tissue matrix and slippage of the cell layers

85

with the myocytes aligning in series rather than in their normal oblique and overlapping fashion. The heart assumes a less elliptical shape and becomes more round, which augments the wall tension and makes the myocyte less effective in managing increases in oxygen demands. Enlargement of the chambers also results in dilatation of the valve rings leading to insufficiency. Both mitral and tricuspid valves may become incompetent. This patient had an increased mitral valve diameter of 11 cm and a tricuspid valve diameter of 12.5 cm. In addition, she had thickening of the mural endocardium and a mitral valve jet lesion that resulted from the turbulence of the regurgitant blood. Although we do not know if she was ever diagnosed with a murmur, we can be certain, based on the autopsy findings that she had a holosystolic murmur. In addition, she must have had a third heart sound (S3) of left ventricular failure. The ECG would have shown cardiomegaly, conduction abnormalities, repolarization defects, and perhaps Q waves due to the interstitial and replacement fibrosis noted in her myocardium.

Despite the dilatation, she had significant hypertrophy of both sides, likely the result of the sustained increase in systemic pressure from the renin-angiotensin compensatory mechanism. We are unaware of a prior history of hypertension.

A common complication of patients with DCM is intracavitary thrombosis due to blood stasis. These thrombi may reach the systemic and pulmonary circulations depending on the cavity where they form, and reach the brain, kidneys and lungs. Although we did not find mural thrombi in this case, there is evidence that she was embolizing since the renal cortices showed scarring of prior infarctions.

The main question in this case is: What is the etiology of her DCM? Is it idiopathic or does it have a specific cause? As mentioned before, there are numerous causes of dilated cardiomyopathy. We can definitely exclude ischemia and myocarditis because she did not have significant coronary artery disease, inflammatory infiltration or myocardial necrosis. Other causes such as drugs, AIDS and alcohol are unlikely. Familial predisposition has been documented in some cases (the genetic abnormality is generally unknown), but she lacked a positive family history for heart disease. An interesting hypothesis, however, may be obtained from the autopsy findings. She had a nodular thyroid with a lymphocytic infiltrate. Lymphocytic thyroiditis is considered an autoimmune disease that can cause hypothyroidism, one of the endocrinologic disorders that is known to cause DCM. She had some of the features of Hashimoto's disease with gross lobulation of the gland, scant colloid, Hurthle cell changes and lymphoplasmocytic infiltrate. The differential diagnosis is "nonspecific" thyroiditis, an entity frequently diagnosed on post-mortem examination that occurs in older patients without symptoms and low levels of antithyroid antibodies. This condition is more prevalent in females and has increased in the United States population after the addition of iodine in the water. Thyroid tests were never performed in this patient, but it has been described that clinical manifestations of hypothyroidism may be subtle and insidious in elderly patients. Microscopically, changes associated with hypothyroidism are basophilic degeneration of the myofibers, and accumulation of interstitial mucopolysaccharide-rich fluid (myxedema). These changes occur in advanced hypothyroidism, and were not seen in this case. It is unlikely that she had hypothyroidism, and if she did it was not severe enough to cause a cardiomyopathy. Patients with hypothyroidism also have hypercholesterolemia and hypertriglyceridemia. It would be unusual to have DCM secondary to hypothyroidism in the absence of coronary atherosclerosis. At the other end of the spectrum, apathic hyperthyroidism occurs in elderly patients, is usually silent and is frequently associated with atrial arrhythmias. Furthermore, these patients are at a high risk for thromboembolic events associated with atrial fibrillation.

In summary, this patient died of an arrhythmic event secondary to a dilated cardiomyopathy of unknown etiology. Treatment of her condition would have included diuretics for her CHF, angiotensin-converting enzyme inhibitors and arteriolar as well as venous vasodilators. Cardiac transplant is a consideration in patients with severe DCM.

Table 1. Classification of cardiomyopathies. Modified from the Report of the 1995 WHO/ISFC Task Force (Circulation. 1996; 93:841-42).

FUNCTIONAL CLASSIFICATION	UNCLASIFIED CARDIOMYOPATHY	SPECIFIC CARDIOMYOPATHY
Dilated	Fibroelastosis	Ischemic Cardiomyopathy
Hypertrophic	Noncompacted Myocardium	Valvular Cardiomyopathy
Restrictive	Mildly Dilated Cardiomyopathy	Hypertensive Cardiomyopathy
Arrhythmogenic Right Ventricle	Mitochondrial Cardiomyopathy	Inflammatory Cardiomyopathy
		Metabolic Cardiomyopathy
		Others

Suggested Readings

1. Pathak SK, Kukreja RC, Hess M. Molecular Pathology of Dilated Cardiomyopathies. Curr Probl Cardiol. 1996; 21:99-144.
2. Thiene G, Angelini A, Basso C, Calabrese F, Valente M. The new definition and classification of cardiomyopathies. Adv Clin Path. 2000; 4:53-7.
3. Richardson P, McKenna W, Bristow M; Maisch B, Mautner B; O'Connell J, et al. Report of the 1995 WHO/ISFC Task Force on the definition and classification of cardiomyopathies. Circulation. 1996; 93:841-42.
4. Bristow MR, Bohlmeyer TJ, Gilbert EM. "Dilated Cardiomyopathy". In Hurt's The Heart. Ninth Edition. Alexander WR, Schlant RC, and Fuster V eds. McGraw-Hill Co, Inc., 1998.

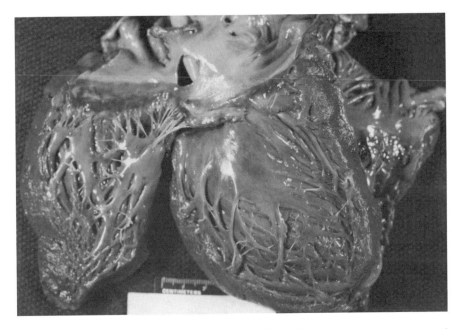

Figure 17. Dilated cardiomyopathy. The heart has a "flabby" appearance and the ventricular walls are thin. The ventricular cavity is very large corresponding to a high end-diastolic volume.

Case # 10

Clinical Summary

This is the case of a 30 year old woman who was 7 months post-partum with no significant past medical history. The present illness began 6 weeks after delivery, when tachycardia, palpitations and exophtalmos led to the diagnosis of Grave's disease. Treatment with propylthiouracil (PTU) and propranolol was prescribed. Her palpitations decreased initially, but after a few months her symptoms worsened. She suffered 3 syncopal episodes within the 3 months prior to admission, each lasting a few seconds. Her liver enzymes increased mildly, and the PTU was discontinued. She developed orthopnea, fever of 39°C, weight loss, diarrhea and decreased urine output.

The physical exam on admission revealed a young woman in moderate respiratory distress. Vital signs: P 210, RR 32, BP 90/palpation, and T 37.5°C. HEENT: exophtalmos, hyperemic throat without exudate. Neck: jugular venous distension up to mandible and diffuse thyromegaly without stridor, carotid bruit or lymphadenopathy. Chest: right lower third dull to percussion with decreased breath sounds, but no egophony; left base with rales. Heart: S1S2, no murmurs. Abdomen: distended with normal bowel sounds, ascites present, and liver span approximately 16 cm. Extremities: 3+ pitting edema up to distal thigh, bilaterally. Sacral edema. Neuro: normal mental status; grossly non-focal; hand tremor bilaterally.

Laboratory data and other tests

Laboratory: WBC 11.5 (S 67%, L 22%); Hb/Hct 10/31, Plt 236; bilirubin T/D 4.9/3.7, SGOT/SGPT 41/27 U/L, glucose 110, cholesterol 63, PT/PTT 19/27; free thyroxine 4.7 (normal 0.7-2), T3 RIA 476 (normal 90-180), TSH 0.03 (normal 4-4.6). CXR: enlarged cardiac silhouette, large right pleural effusion and/or infiltrate. ECG: SVT at 264/min, regular (atrial flutter).

In the ER, her heart rate was slowed to 140/min by test doses of adenosine followed by diltiazem in 3 divided doses. She was admitted to the CCU with a heart rate of 136 and a BP 102/65, fully oriented and receiving oxygen by nasal cannula. She was given furosemide IV and propranolol P.O. One and a half-hours after admission, the patient complained of severe shortness of breath and became restless and agitated, and shortly thereafter, hypotensive and unresponsive. CPR and fluids were given and she was intubated. Cardioversion and administration of glucagon elevated her blood pressure to 100 mmHg, but still she remained unresponsive. Vasopressor therapy with norepinephrine and dopamine was started. Her serum potassium was 7.1 mEq/L, which was treated with CaCl2, NAHCO3, insulin and glucose IV. An echocardiogram showed global hypokinesis with all chambers markedly enlarged and dilated, moderate to severe mitral and tricuspid regurgitation, large pleural effusion, but no pericardial effusion. The Swan-Ganz catheter showed the following pressures RA 10 mmHg, PCWP 20 mmHg and PA 38/20. Supraventricular tachycardia (SVT) and hypotension recurred several times and resolved every time after cardioversion and adjustment of pressor therapy. Follow-up neurologic examination revealed absence of brainstem reflexes. A CT scan of the head was consistent with anoxic encephalopathy. The WBC rose to 19,700 with 89% granulocytes. Cultures of blood, sputum, CSF, pleural fluid and urine were all negative. Urine output was scant. Apnea test showed absence of spontaneous respiration. Nine days after admission, bradycardia developed, her blood pressure fell and her heart stopped. Resuscitation efforts were unsuccessful.

Gross Description

The body was that of a well-nourished, well-developed black woman appearing the stated age of 30 years. The heart weighed 420 g and was of expected shape. The pericardium was smooth and glistening. The epicardium was shiny with moderate amount of subepicardial fat. The atria and ventricles were dilated, more significantly in the right side. The right and left ventricular walls measured 0.3 and 1.2 cm in thickness, respectively. The right atrium contained 2 organizing mural thrombi measuring 0.5 to 1.0 cm in diameter. The foramen ovale was probe-patent. The valve rings measurements were as follows: tricuspid valve 12 cm, pulmonic valve 9 cm, mitral valve 10 cm, and aortic valve 7 cm. The valve leaflets were delicate and pliable. The chordae tendineae were slender. The endocardium was thin and glistening. The myocardium was brown-red and mildly softened. The coronary arteries were of normal caliber and distribution, with no sclerosis or occlusion. The superior and inferior caval veins and major tributaries were grossly unremarkable. The aorta showed no atherosclerosis. The lungs weighed 1400 g and were essentially similar in appearance with patchy as well as confluent areas of increased firmness. The tracheobronchial tree, as well as the pulmonary vessels, were unremarkable. The liver weighed 1400 g with a smooth surface. The cut surface revealed centrilobular congestion without necrosis. The thyroid weighed 70 g and was of average shape. On section, the parenchyma was uniformly tan-brown with no apparent colloid cysts. The right ovary contained a 4 cm tumor, which on section showed many cysts containing gelatinous yellow-brown material.

Microscopic Description

Sections from the heart revealed myocyte hypertrophy, mild interstitial and replacement fibrosis, and organizing thrombi in the right atrium (Figures 18 and 19). The lungs showed bilateral acute bronchopneumonia with areas of intra-alveolar hemorrhage.

Sections from the thyroid showed diffuse thyroid hyperplasia with colloid depletion consistent with Grave's disease. The tumor found in the right ovary consisted of thyroid tissue consistent with the diagnosis of struma ovarii. No colloid depletion was noted in the tumor.

Case Analysis

This 30 year old woman had a sudden arrhythmic cardiopulmonary arrest occurring within 7 months post-partum, and in a setting strongly suggestive of hyperthyroid disease. The question to be addressed is whether her presentation and death were the result of peri-partum cardiomyopathy, or whether she had an additional element of hyperthyroid cardiomyopathy.

Peri-partum cardiomyopathy (PPC) is a syndrome that, by definition, occurs between the last trimester of pregnancy and the first 6 months following delivery. However, the timing of the disease is somewhat variable, since the acute symptomatic presentation may extend beyond the 6 months post-partum. In other words, there may be damage to the myocardium in the immediate peri-partum period, but ventricular dysfunction may not ensue for many months later. The reason that PPC represents a syndrome rather than a specific disease, is because there may be several different pathogenic mechanisms that lead to cardiac damage. In approximately one half of cases, endomyocardial biopsies taken during the peri-partum period reveal the presence of active myocarditis, often characterized by an abundant myocardial eosinophilic infiltrate (Figure 20). This suggests that the myocarditis is allergic in etiology. It remains unknown if the antigenic stimulation derives from the fetus, or represents cross-reactivity against myocardial tissue from the gestational uterine tissue. There are no animal models of the disease, and our knowledge is based on limited human tissue from biopsy material or autopsy. In the rest of the cases without myocarditis, there are features of cardiomyopathy with myocellular hypertrophy and fibrosis. Further studies are needed to determine whether these degenerative changes develop during pregnancy, or are pre-existing and only become manifest because of the hemodynamic and hormonal stresses of pregnancy. Logically, one would assume that if there was cardiomyopathic damage prior to the pregnancy, then the disease would become manifest during pregnancy at the maximal hemodynamic stress period, when the intravascular volume and cardiac output are the greatest (second trimester). Yet, as noted above, the disease is defined by its presentation during the third trimester, suggesting that myocardial damage before the onset of pregnancy is an insufficient explanation for most cases.

In our patient, although she presented to the hospital 7 months after delivery, her symptoms began 6 weeks post-partum. Accordingly, her disease could be secondary to PPC. The question is whether PPC can present with tachycardia and palpitations? The answer is that these are usually not common manifestations; however, tachyarrhythmias and paroxysmal atrial fibrillation may be secondary to cardiomyopathy. Therefore, PPC cannot be ruled out on clinical grounds alone as a cause of this young woman's complaints and death.

There is an association of thyroid disease in the peri-partum period (although generally with hypothyroidism). In this case, it would difficult to overlook the likelihood of hyperthyroidism. Her complaints were typical with tachycardia, palpitations, and exophthalmos. Weight loss might not be a helpful sign post-partum, as she would be expected to lose weight; however, she continued to lose weight 4 months after delivery. She also had fever and diarrhea, which may be secondary to hyperthyroidism. The episodes of syncope are suggestive of sudden ventricular arrhythmias. Her shortness of breath and complaints of orthopnea were symptoms of CHF. It is noteworthy that when she presented to the hospital she had a pulse of 260 and hypotension (BP 90/palpation). On physical examination, she had jugular venous distension, fluid overload, and signs of pulmonary congestion with rales. She had features of both left heart failure (hypotension and pulmonary congestion), and right heart failure (jugular venous distension, pleural effusion, ascites, liver congestion, and peripheral edema). Her laboratory studies were confirmatory of severe hyperthyroidism, with elevated free thyroxine and T3, and markedly reduced thyroid stimulating hormone. Her electrocardiogram revealed significant SVT at 220/min, and atrial flutter. Despite slowing of her heart rate to 140 with adenosine and calcium channel blocker (diltiazem), she had a sudden cardiac arrest. Subsequently, she developed several more episodes of SVT and hypotension, and despite resuscitation and slower heart rate, she died secondary to anoxic encephalopathy due to her initial cardiorespiratory arrest.

The post-mortem findings were consistent with hyperthyroid heart disease with bi-ventricular failure. The heart was enlarged (420 g, normal 300-350 g), both ventricular walls were thinned, and all 4 chambers were dilated. She had mural thrombi in the right atrium, most likely secondary to atrial flutter and stasis in the chamber, but also consistent with cardiomyopathy. Microscopically, the myocytes were hypertrophied, and there was evidence of interstitial and replacement fibrosis. These are non-specific features of cardiomyopathy; but in the absence of inflammation and

94

with evidence of a hypertrophied and dilated heart, the findings are much more consistent with hyperthyroidism than peri-partum cardiomyopathy.

Hyperthyroidism causes a cardiomyopathy through several related mechanisms. It leads to the so-called high output heart failure, similar to the effects of an arteriovenous malformation or severe anemia, where the cardiac output is markedly increased. However, in hyperthyroidism there is hypermetabolism with increased circulating blood volume, low peripheral vascular resistance, and tachycardia. Another characteristic feature is the development of a hypermetabolic state, which has direct and indirect thyroid hormone effects on the myocardium. Furthermore, thyroid hormone stimulates myocyte hypertrophy through its actions as a growth hormone on myosin synthesis; and hyperthyroidism can also lead to hypertension, which can cause secondary hypertrophy of the heart. Moreover, catecholamine levels are high in hyperthyroidism, which can further stimulate hypertrophy and tachycardia.

The pathogenesis of the hypertrophied and dilated heart (signs of cardiac remodeling) has only become clear recently with experimental studies on prolonged tachycardia. Thyroid hormone stimulates rapid ventricular and atrial rhythm, leading to supraventricular tachycardia (e.g. atrial flutter or fibrillation). Animals with electrical pacing-induced tachycardia develop a high-output dilated cardiomyopathy over several weeks, even with normal thyroid hormone levels. The tachycardia causes global hypertrophy, chamber dilatation, mural thinning, and microscopic features of myocyte hypertrophy and focal fibrosis. There is evidence of remodeling of the ventricular chamber mediated through damage to the interstitial connective tissue matrix, (via activated metalloproteinases or collagenolytic enzymes) that allows for "slippage" of myocytes and mural myocardial layers. The result is a heart with morphological features of cardiomyopathy, and an animal with clinical signs and symptoms of CHF.

Derived from all the above observations, hyperthyroid heart disease results from a combination of direct cellular effects on the heart tissue by the thyroid hormone, hemodynamic effects of the systemic hypermetabolic state, and secondary effects of tachycardia that lead to cardiac remodeling and damage. Together with the known association of cardiomyopathy and sudden malignant ventricular arrhythmias (e.g. ventricular fibrillation), particularly in the setting of increased catecholamine levels, it is not unexpected that a patient such as this one would experience a sudden cardiac arrest leading to anoxic encephalopathy. What is unusual in this modern medical era, is that anyone would experience such severe hyperthyroidism. However, non-adherence with her medical treatment may explain the rarity of this unfortunate complication of hyperthyroid disease.

Suggested Readings

1. Brown CS, Bertolet BD. Peripartum cardiomyopathy: a comprehensive review. Am J Obstet Gynecol. 1998; 178:409-14.
2. Toft AD, Boon NA. Thyroid disease and the heart. Heart. 2000; 84:455-60.
3. Fadel BM, Ellahham S, Ringel MD, Lindsay J Jr, Wartofsky L, Burman KD. Hyperthyroid heart disease. Clin Cardiol. 2000; 23:402-8.
4. Klein I, Ojamaa K. Thyroid hormone and the cardiovascular system. N Engl J Med. 2001; 344:501-9.
5. Gomberg-Maitland M, Frishman WH. Thyroid hormone and cardiovascular disease. Am Heart J. 1998; 135(2 Pt 1):187-96.
6. Borczuk AC, van Hoeven KH, Factor SM. Review and hypothesis: the eosinophil and peripartum heart disease (myocarditis and coronary artery dissection) coincidence or pathogenetic significance? Cardiovasc Res. 1997; 33:527-32.

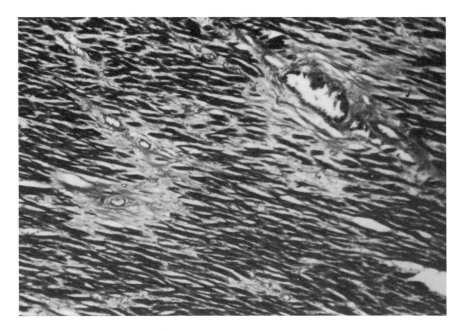

Figure 18. Perivascular and interstitial fibrosis (Trichrome stain, 20X)

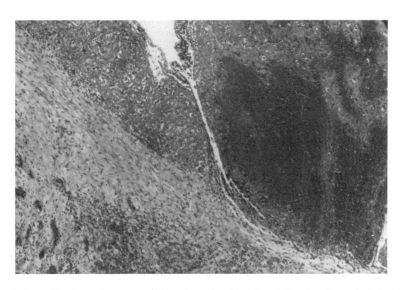

Figure 19. Organizing mural thrombus of right atrium (Hematoxylin and Eosin, 20X)

97

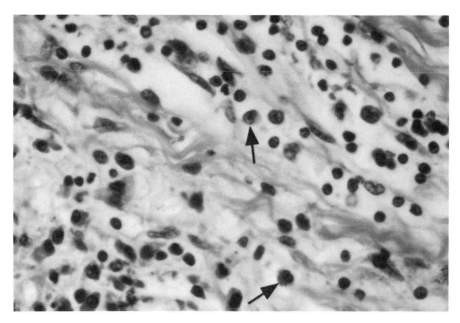

Figure 20. Peripartum cardiomyopathy. The inflammatory infiltrate is composed of numerous eosinophils (arrow)(Hematoxylin and Eosin, 40X)

Case # 11

Clinical Summary

This was the first hospital admission for this 56 year old man, former alcohol abuser, non-diabetic, with history of hypertension; with one week history of shortness of breath, fever, shaking chills, productive cough and pleuritic chest pain. The patient had been a heavy drinker of 8–10 cans of beer a day for many years. He also had been diagnosed with gout, and had a two year history of congestive heart failure treated with digoxin and furosemide. The physical exam on admission was remarkable for a temperature of 40°C, scleral icterus and dull breath sounds in both lung bases. In addition, auscultation of the heart revealed a S3 and S4 gallop. Examination of the abdomen was significant for normal bowel sounds a palpable, moderately tender hepatomegaly (liver span 16 cm midclavicular line), and no splenomegaly. A 1+ bilateral ankle edema was noted. The neurological examination was within normal limits.

Laboratory data and other tests

Laboratory: WBC 8.2; Hb/Hct 14/45; bilirubin T/D 3.4/1.2, SGOT/SGPT 30/29 U/L, AP 75, LD 970, PT/PTT 11.4/18; CK 62. Urine analysis: pH 6, bilirrubin 1+, protein 3+. Urine culture: no growth. Sputum culture: alpha-streptococcus. CXR: bilateral haziness and cardiomegaly. ECG: sinus tachycardia at 140, left bundle branch block. Echocardiogram: diminished ejection fraction and 1+ mitral regurgitation

The patient was admitted with the diagnosis of bronchopneumonia and started on antibiotic therapy. After a week of treatment, even though the pneumonic process was considered resolved, the patient developed progressive pedal edema. On day 12 after admission, he became febrile with a temperature of 39°C, his white count rose to 23,000 and his PT increased to 23. He became hypotensive, the SGOT and SGPT were over 3,000 and the LDH over 6,000. His bilirubin was 2.4 and the uric acid was 17.0. He was diagnosed as having septic shock and transferred to the intensive care unit where he was placed on assisted ventilation. A Swan-Ganz catheter was inserted, revealing a pulmonary artery systolic pressure of 40 and a capillary wedge pressure of 40, with a cardiac output of 4.1 liters. He improved significantly on vasopressor therapy. However, three days later, the patient remained febrile with persistent leukocytosis and began to develop abdominal distension (ileus). Although apparently hemodynamically stable, he continued to depend on vasopressors as his serum BUN/creatinine continued

99

to climb. He also suffered recurrent episodes of tachypnea, tachycardia and diaphoresis interpreted as recurrent pulmonary emboli, so he was started on a short course of anticoagulation therapy. About 1 week after he went into shock, the patient had a major episode of gastrointestinal bleeding, which was eventually stabilized (blood transfusion was required). Thirty six days post-admission and 4 days after the GI bleed, the patient had a cardiopulmonary arrest and expired.

Gross Description

The body measured 194 cm in length and weighed 62 kg. The heart weighed 630 g. The pericardium was smooth without adhesions. The subepicardial fat was present. The epicardium showed areas of fibrous thickening. Both atrial cavities were markedly dilated. The left atrial appendage contained an organized thrombus. The left ventricular wall measured 1.2 cm in thickness and the right ventricle measured 0.4 cm in thickness. The valve leaflets showed focal nonspecific nodularities and a non-bacterial thrombotic vegetation (also known as marantic) in one of the aortic valve cusps. The chordae tendineae were thin and pliable. The papillary muscles of the right and left ventricles appeared moderately hypertrophied. The myocardium had a flabby consistency. There was no evidence of ischemia. The topography of the coronaries revealed a right dominant system with up to 40% occlusion of the lumen by atheromatous plaques. The aorta was of normal caliber. The elasticity of the wall was focally impaired past the aortic arch where two friable and ulcerated, calcific atherosclerotic plaques were present. The lungs weighed 1300 g combined. The pleural surfaces were shiny and the cut surface of the parenchyma revealed bilateral congestion without areas of consolidation. The small bowel and right colon showed segmental discoloration with transmural thinning of the wall. No perforations were noted. The pattern was compatible with chronic ischemic enterocolitis. The liver weighed 1600 g. The capsule showed scattered areas of wrinkling consistent with cyclic episodes of passive congestion and decongestion. The cut surface revealed a preserved lobular sinusoidal pattern with no increased fibrosis, but marked cholestasis as depicted by the yellow-green coloration of the liver.

Microscopic Description

Sections of the right and left ventricle myocardium revealed diffuse myocardial hypertrophy with scattered areas of interstitial and perivascular fibrosis. The subendocardium of the right ventricle displayed myocytolytic changes, and prominent basophilic degeneration of the myofibers was seen in

100

the left ventricle. No areas of coagulative necrosis were noted. Sections of the lungs showed moderate centrilobular emphysema and marked congestion. There was moderate hypertrophy of the walls of small and medium-sized vessels. Examination of both small and large bowel resulted in similar histologic findings. There were areas of acute mucosal ulceration and necrosis alternating with areas of fibrosis of the lamina propria and hypertrophy of the muscular layers and neural elements. Sections of the liver confirmed the macroscopic impression of passive congestion and cholestasis.

Case Analysis

This middle-aged man was admitted to the hospital with pneumonia, and then he developed secondary complications of septicemia due to enterocolitis; however, his underlying heart disease directly led to his demise. In the absence of significant coronary artery disease, in conjunction with the clinical history, the physical findings, and the gross and microscopic pathology of the heart, we can be very confident that this patient had an alcoholic cardiomyopathy. Worldwide, alcoholic cardiomyopathy represents one of the most common causes of secondary (acquired) dilated, congestive cardiomyopathy. In the following discussion we will address the pathogenesis, pathology and clinical findings of alcoholic cardiomyopathy, and attempt to show how this patient had many of the typical features of the condition.

Alcohol in moderation is generally recognized to be beneficial in adults (other than for pregnant women), with apparent protective effects against atherosclerosis. It is only apparent because the scientific evidence for protection is primarily epidemiological and anecdotal. Pathologists have been aware for decades that chronic high dose alcohol abusers tend to have less atherosclerosis than in comparably aged non-alcoholics, but there are also more recent epidemiologic data that suggest benefit (other than mental well-being) from a few drinks of wine or spirits daily. It has also been recognized for decades that chronic alcoholism is associated with heart damage, and congestive heart failure. The absence of an animal model of alcoholic cardiomyopathy has limited our understanding of the syndrome. However, clinical observations have provided significant clues about pathogenesis. There are 3 potential mechanisms that have been proposed for alcoholic cardiomyopathy:
1. nutritional deficiency leading to myocardial damage;
2. direct toxic effect of alcohol or its metabolites on the myocardium;
3. toxic effects of chemicals associated with alcohol.

Nutritional

In the United States, nutritional deficiency has not been a major cause of alcoholic cardiomyopathy since before World War II. Diets deficient in thiamine (vitamin B-1) and protein lead to a particularly virulent form of alcoholic cardiomyopathy, known as beri-beri heart disease. In this syndrome, the heart is markedly dilated and flabby, with very poor contractile function. The affected individual is edematous and in overt congestive heart failure. Malnutrition in the poorer areas of the inner cities, and in the countryside particularly during the Great Depression was associated with nutritional alcoholic heart disease. Today, this entity is rare because intake of adequate calories with a balanced diet is prevalent even among the homeless drinker (e.g. 'wino'). Additionally, commercial foods, such as breads and cereals, are fortified with vitamins, including thiamine, so that sufficient intake is maintained, even when significant caloric substitution is derived from alcohol.

Although beri-beri is hardly ever considered as a diagnostic possibility, it should be considered in another context associated with profound malnutrition: patients with severe chronic bowel disease, either inflammatory or infectious. Malnutrition may affect patients with significant small and large intestinal disease, such as those with Crohn's disease, or those with AIDS-associated bowel disease. Particularly in some patients with AIDS, some of whom may be street people with abuse of alcohol and illicit drugs, malnutrition may contribute to cardiomyopathy. On occasions, the cardiomyopathy that develops may have features of beri-beri, with edema of the myocardial interstitium, and profound heart dysfunction.

Alcohol Toxicity

Direct effects of alcohol on the myocardium may lead to acute depression of ventricular function presumably due to toxicity (e.g. metabolic 'poisoning'). Acute binge drinking may cause mild to moderate depression of ventricular contractility, which is generally reversible following cessation of alcohol intake. Therefore, this reversibility suggests that there has not been damage to myocytes, blood vessels or interstitium. Acute alcohol intoxication also may cause arrhythmia, usually supraventricular tachycardia. On occasions, ventricular arrhythmias may develop. The latter may account for those relatively rare cases of sudden death associated with acute alcohol intoxication. Alcohol withdrawal in chronic alcoholics, often causing neurological symptoms characterized as delirium tremens ('DT's'), is associated with serum electrolyte abnormalities and ventricular arrhythmias causing sudden death, more than in acute alcohol intoxication. However, in neither case is there significant damage to the myocardium. In fact, experimental chronic alcohol use in laboratory animals, as in humans, does not cause major pathological damage to the heart. At most, slight increases in interstitial connective tissue, and myocyte abnormalities characterized as cellular edema and mild mitochondrial swelling have been described. The lack of marked myocardial damage, and the absence of congestive heart failure in animal models, suggests that the duration of experimental alcohol use is insufficient to produce major pathological changes, or that chronic alcoholic cardiomyopathy is species specific. It also raises the question whether there are contributing mechanisms such as hypertension; or whether cigarette smoking (a common associated habit in alcoholics), plays an additive role. Thus, there has been uncertainty over the mechanism(s) of alcoholic damage of the myocardium.

The agent that has been implicated most prominently in chronic alcoholic heart disease is **acetaldehyde**, a chemical that results from alcohol metabolism. Acetaldehyde is toxic, leading to myocellular and vascular damage. Elevated levels of acetaldehyde may directly cause myocellular necrosis, or through intramyocardial blood vessel injury. Thus, there may be a component of intramyocardial, localized ischemia that could lead to foci of myocytolysis. A further contribution to microvascular-induced myocardial necrosis may result from systemic elevation of catecholamine levels, which is common in chronic alcoholics. The elevated catecholamines also cause hypertension, a subject discussed below. The role of acetaldehyde is appealing, but it is still unproven as the primary mechanism leading to cardiomyopathy.

Indirect toxicity

Ethyl alcohol, in all of the forms in which it is imbibed, is not a pure chemical (even vodka, which is the closest to pure distilled spirits, has a number of additives). The possibility that one or multiple chemical additives contribute to cardiac damage is attractive; however, the variety of spirits that are associated with alcoholic cardiomyopathy suggests that this cannot be an all encompassing hypothesis. The only additive that has been directly implicated is cobalt. Cobalt salts were used as a chemical additive in beer to stabilize the foam (head), more than 40 years ago in several areas in North America. The result was an epidemic of 'beer-drinkers cardiomyopathy' in several cities (e.g. Kansas City and Quebec City). The affected individuals had significant myocardial damage, and marked ventricular dysfunction leading to severe congestive heart failure. After an association with beer drinking was proposed, it was demonstrated that the beer involved contained the cobalt additive. Subsequent removal of cobalt, prevented the epidemic form of alcoholic cardiomyopathy, although the sporadic form still exists secondary to excessive beer drinking. The patient in this case drank 8-10 cans of beer daily for many years.

Whether direct or indirect toxicity is the sole pathogenesis of alcoholic cardiomyopathy is unknown; however, it is noteworthy that at least two other mechanisms may contribute. One is hypertension; and the other is the effect of alcohol-induced liver disease, which may lead to the release of other toxic substances into the bloodstream that may secondarily damage the myocardium. As an example, it has been proposed that pulmonary vascular damage in cirrhosis is mediated by either an abnormal liver metabolism, or by the failure of the liver to detoxify potential injurious substances derived from the gut, which are present in the portal circulation. We will briefly discuss these mechanisms below.

Hypertension

The prevalence of hypertension in chronic alcoholics is remarkably high, and even approaches the frequency observed in diabetic patients. The mechanism is probably caused by multiple factors, and is linked to the elevated levels of circulating catecholamines, and fluid retention with increased circulating blood volume.   The hypertension is even more significant in that it occurs despite the marked peripheral vasodilatation induced by alcohol. The combination of alcoholic toxicity and the injurious effects of hypertension could conceivably lead to exacerbated ventricular damage similar to that observed in hypertensive and diabetic cardiomyopathy. The majority of patients with alcoholic cardiomyopathy are hypertensive, as was the case with the patient discussed in this chapter. Hypertension could lead to cardiomegaly, multifocal fibrosis and vascular sclerosis, which are characteristic features of alcoholic cardiomyopathy. However, the alcoholic heart is typically dilated and flabby, whereas the hypertensive heart is typically concentrically hypertrophied with thick ventricular walls.   It is possible that the toxic effects of alcohol contribute to the marked dilatation superimposed on the hypertensive heart.   Whether this combination is a sufficient explanation remains unknown, but it is likely that hypertension does contribute significantly, in at least some patients.

Liver Disease

It is interesting and it remains an unexplained observation, that most patients with alcoholic cardiomyopathy do not have alcoholic cirrhosis. Whether this reflects some unknown genetic protection of one organ versus another, or whether there are some fundamental pathophysiological effects in this relationship, cannot be answered at this time. This is also not to imply that patients with alcoholic cardiomyopathy never have cirrhosis, because some do.   Even patients without cirrhosis have chronic alcoholic liver damage, and perturbed hepatic function.   Therefore, it is possible that the affected liver does not metabolize adequately, leading to indirect toxic damage to the heart.

Pathology and Pathophysiology

The pathology of alcoholic cardiomyopathy does not differ significantly from other types of dilated, congestive cardiomyopathy, although there are some subtle distinct features.   Grossly, there is cardiomegaly, generalized chamber dilatation, and often mural thrombi in any of the chambers.   The left ventricular wall is thinned, in keeping with the profound ventricular dysfunction and remodeling that occurs in late stage cardiomyopathy. The heart tends to be even flabbier that in other types of dilated cardiomyopathy, and it may have a 'greasy' feel due to increased lipid accumulation in myocardial cells. Fibrosis may be visible in the myocardium, and the endocardium is often thickened, focally opaque and gray.   The coronary arteries may or may not have significant atherosclerosis, although as discussed previously there is often a protective affect against atherosclerosis associated with chronic alcohol abuse.   There is an interesting lesion of chordae tendineae first described about a decade ago, apparently related to chronic alcohol intake. Focal individual or several chords of the mitral valve are thickened significantly compared to the adjacent thin, delicate chords. The appearance is different from the chordal involvement in rheumatic heart disease where all of the mitral valve chordae are involved.   The localized chordal thickening is caused by concentric new connective tissue deposited around the normal chord that persists as a core (Figure 21).   Earlier in the process, the chord is involved by mononuclear inflammation. Although the pathogenesis of this process is unknown, it may be related to the proliferative fibrosis associated with chronic alcoholism, which leads to such lesions as Dupuytren's contracture of the hand. There may also be some relationship to the interstitial changes in the alcoholic heart discussed below.

Microscopically, there is myocellular hypertrophy, diffuse interstitial edema and fibrosis, multiple foci of replacement fibrosis, and small vessel disease (Figures 22 and 23).   None of these features are distinct from other forms of dilated cardiomyopathy.   However, as noted above, there is increased neutral fat in the myocardial cell as a consequence of the metabolic injury to the myocyte. This can be demonstrated by staining frozen sections of myocardium (so that the lipid is not dissolved by organic solvents routinely used for processing paraffin-embedded tissue) with special lipid stains (e.g. oil red O). In addition, lipid deposition associated with mitochondria can be demonstrated with electron microscopy. Two relatively characteristic features of alcoholic cardiomyopathy relate to the proliferation of inflammatory cells within the myocardial interstitium, as well as within the surrounding intramyocardial small muscular arteries. The inflammation is not diagnostic of a myocarditis, or vasculitis. The mononuclear infiltrates include lymphocytes, monocytes, mast cells, and most strikingly, Anitschkow cells. The latter are of unknown lineage (for years they were called Anitschkow *myocytes*), but they most likely represent a resident interstitial histiocyte in the myocardium. They proliferate in several types of heart disease; and in rheumatic carditis, these cells become activated and transformed, and participate in the formation of the Aschoff nodule. In alcoholic heart disease they are quite common, often infiltrate the adventitial and medial wall of the small myocardial arteries, and are present in the interstitium, even in areas without fibrosis (Figure 24). The role of the Anitschkow cells and of the proliferative fibrosis and small vessel changes in the pathogenesis of alcoholic cardiomyopathy, remains unknown. Again, as described above, the fibrogenesis and inflammation may be part of a systemic effect of alcohol on multiple tissues.

Pathophysiologically, ventricular dysfunction and congestive heart failure are common features. The failure is often high-output, with increased cardiac output, but diminished tissue perfusion due to decreased peripheral vascular resistance. Late in the course of the disease, the failure leads to reduced cardiac output, with markedly reduced tissue perfusion and shock. This occurred in our patient, with low flow to the bowel causing ischemic enterocolitis, which complicated his course with the development of septic shock. All these combined and superimposed on cardiogenic shock carries virtually a 100% mortality rate. Other pathophysiologic features of alcoholic cardiomyopathy were present in this case: The course of the patient's CHF over 2 years before his death, is comparable to most patients with this illness. He had the expected typical episodes of supraventricular tachycardia, and the commonly seen conduction system abnormality (left bundle branch block). The conduction disorders can be varied, ranging from partial to complete heart block. Finally, his echocardiogram revealed not only severe ventricular dysfunction, with a reduced ejection fraction, but also the presence of mitral valve regurgitation. Again, due to the pronounced ventricular dilatation, with 'stretching' of the valve annulus, regurgitation is common. It can affect the mitral valve and the tricuspid valve, or both, and it may contribute to further compromise of ventricular function.

In summary then, this patient had rather typical alcoholic cardiomyopathy associated with his longstanding drinking history. The pathology of his heart, and the functional defects were characteristic of the diagnosis. His course was one of marked cardiac dysfunction, with subsequent multi-organ failure as a result of inadequate tissue perfusion (shock).

Suggested Readings

1. Patel VB, Why HJ, Richardson PJ, Preedy VR. The effects of alcohol on the heart. Adverse Drug React Toxicol Rev. 1997; 16:15-43.
2. Preedy VR, Richardson PJ. Alcoholic cardiomyopathy: clinical and experimental pathological changes. Herz. 1996; 21:241-7.
3. Maisch B. Alcohol and the heart. Herz. 1996; 21:207-12.
4. Piano MR, Schwertz DW. Alcoholic heart disease: a review. Heart Lung. 1994; 23:3-17.
5. Djoenaidi W, Notermans SL, Dunda G. Beriberi cardiomyopathy. Eur J Clin Nutr. 1992; 46:227-34.

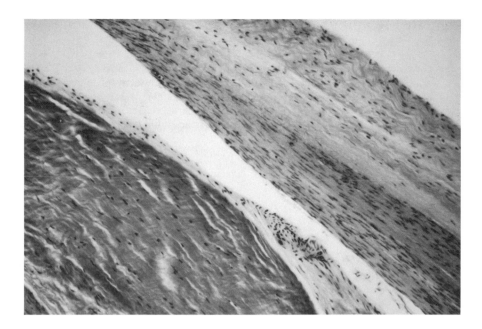

Figure 21. Chordae tendinitis in alcoholic cardiomyopathy, histologic section. There is concentric deposition of loose fibroconnective tissue around the chord accompanied by a mild mononuclear infiltrate (Hematoxylin and Eosin, 10X).

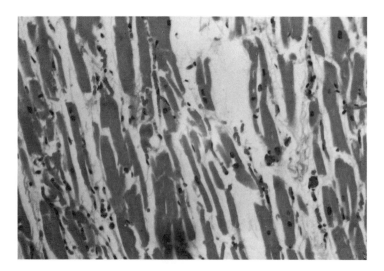

Figure 22. Alcoholic cardiomyopathy, myocardium, histologic section. Interstitial edema, myocyte degeneration and fibrosis are common findings (Hematoxylin and Eosin, 20X).

108

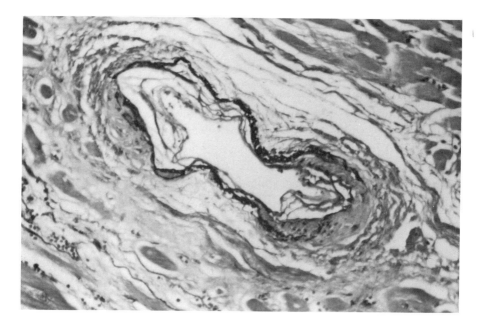

Figure 23. Alcoholic cardiomyopathy, histologic section. Intramyocardial artery showing duplication and disruption of the elastic fibers, and vascular edema (Elastic stain, 40X).

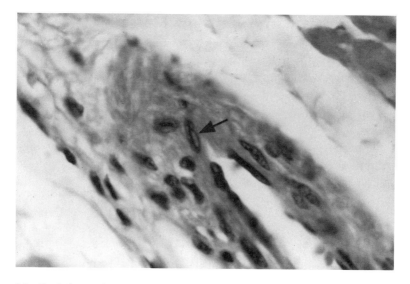

Figure 24. Alcoholic cardiomyopathy, histologic section. Anitschkow-like cells are noted in the wall of a small intramyocardial artery (arrow) (Hematoxylin and Eosin, 60X)

109

Clinical Summary

A 40 year old Hispanic woman, known HIV-infected for the past 3 years and followed by a specialty HIV/AIDS clinic, had a routine chest-x-ray where cardiomegaly was noted. Her most recent CD4 T lymphocyte count was 25 cells/µL, indicating severe immunosuppression. An echocardiogram was performed, which showed a small pericardial effusion, biventricular hypertrophy, mild to moderate mitral regurgitation, moderate to severe tricuspid regurgitation, diffuse left ventricular hypokinesis with diminished left ventricular systolic function, and an ejection fraction of 40%. Four months later she was hospitalized with severe respiratory distress. Heart catheterization revealed right ventricular and pulmonary artery pressures of 58/18 and 38/18 mm Hg, respectively. The pulmonary capillary wedge pressure was 35 mmHg. The diagnosis of cardiogenic shock was made. Renal dysfunction was also present evidenced by a creatinine of 3.3 mg/dL and BUN of 60 mg/dL. She improved and was discharged, but returned to the hospital two months later with shortness of breath, cough and hemoptysis. On this admission her vital signs were: P 120, R 24, T 37°C, BP 78/palpable. Her physical exam was significant for bilateral rales with diminished air entry on the right side, tachycardia and gallop rhythm. The arterial gases were pH 7.17, pCO2 26, pO2 72, O2 sat 87%, BE –18. The chest-x-ray showed bilateral lower lobe consolidation with effusion. The patient was intubated and started on 100% FiO2 and PEEP (>5). Nonetheless, she became severely hypoxic and acidotic, and expired two hours after admission.

Gross Description

The autopsy was performed 3 hours after death. The body length was 160 cm and the body weight was 45 kg. The heart weighed 410 g (heart/body weight ratio of 0.009, normal 0.004-0.005). The pericardium was smooth and glistening. The epicardium was shiny with a moderate amount of subepicardial fat. The atria were of normal size and free of thrombi. The foramen ovale was closed. The right and left ventricular walls were hypertrophied measuring 2.5 and 0.7 cm, respectively (Figure 25). The valve rings measured as follows: TV 10 cm, PV 7 cm, MV 11 cm, AV 7 cm. The valve leaflets were delicate and pliable except for some myxomatous changes. The chordae tendineae were slender. The endocardium was thin and glistening. The myocardium showed multiple foci of myocytolysis. The anterior wall and the interventricular septum had areas of pallor due to ischemia. Subendocardial necrosis was also present. The coronary arteries were unremarkable. The lungs weighed 1550 g, were voluminous, looked essentially identical, and did not collapse upon entering the thoracic cavity. The pleural surfaces had fibrous adhesions. On section, marked pulmonary edema was noted. The left lower lobe showed patchy areas of consolidation and hemorrhage. The right lower lobe showed diffuse acute hemorrhage. Chronic bronchitis was noted. The pulmonary artery and its major branches were unremarkable. The kidneys weighed 200 g combined and had no significant gross abnormalities.

Microscopic Description

Myocardial fibrosis and multifocal myocytolysis were observed (Figure 26). There were focal interstitial and perivascular deposits of a lightly eosinophilic homogeneous material, resembling amyloid. However, Congo-red and crystal violet stains were negative. The elastic stain was only positive in the endocardium and in vessels, but not in the interstitium. Microscopically, sections from both lungs showed extensive interstitial and intraalveolar hemorrhage and a necrotizing intraalveolar exudate. Gram stain revealed clusters of gram negative rods that in culture were identified as Klebsiella pneumoniae. No interstitial amyloid-like material was present in any tissue other than the myocardium.

Sections from the heart were submitted for electron microscopy. The epoxy-resin-embedded sections showed diffuse interstitial and perivascular aggregates of fibrillar materials, which were morphologically distinct from amyloid or collagen fibrils. The fibrils were slightly curvilinear with a diameter of 15-20 nm. A suggestion of helical configurations and periodicity were noted at higher magnifications. These fibrils were loosely distributed in the interstitial space and did not have the close relationship with the myocyte sarcolemma typical of amyloid deposition (Figure 27).

Case Analysis

Diverse pathological manifestations of heart disease have been described in patients with HIV/AIDS. These include a variety of opportunistic infections, drug toxicity, malignancies and idiopathic endocardial and myocardial diseases. Regardless of the etiology, the most common clinical syndromes of cardiac dysfunction seen in these patients include dilated cardiomyopathy, pericardial effusion with or without tamponade, ventricular tachycardia and thromboembolic disease as a result of infectious or non-infectious endocarditis.

Opportunistic infections and malignancies are secondary to immunosuppression, but the ultimate cardiac damage is multifactorial and includes lymphokines and growth factors released by activated lymphocytes and other cellular immune mediators.

Infections

A variety of opportunistic and non-opportunistic infections have been described in the heart of HIV/AIDS patients. These include fungal (Cryptococcus species, Candida species and Aspergillus organisms), bacterial, mycobacterial (tuberculous and atypical mycobacteria), viruses (CMV, HSV), protozoans (Toxoplasma gondii), Pneumocystis carinii infection, and parasitic (Microsporidium, Pentastomiasis). Myocarditis and endocarditis are more often secondary to infection than idiopathic. As in non-AIDS patients, adult myocarditis in an HIV-infected individual may be immunological in origin when it occurs in the absence of an identifiable infectious organism. With the advent of highly active antiretroviral therapy (HAART), the rate of opportunistic infections has decreased significantly compared to those seen previously to the HAART era.

Malignancies

Primary Kaposi sarcoma and lymphomas compromising the heart, have been described, but are extremely rare.

HIV infection of the myocytes

Recognition of HIV-1 DNA sequences by PCR and in-situ hybridization in the heart of HIV/AIDS patients, supports the possibility of selective infection of the myocardium by HIV virions. However, there are several authors that believe that these results are due to HIV contamination of the heart by the patient's infected blood. The proliferation of multilamellar membrane bodies within myocytes with subsequent mitochondrial dysfunction also has been described in HIV infection as a possible explanation of cardiac disturbances, but there is no evidence that these bodies are the result of direct HIV toxicity to the myocyte. CD4 receptors are absent in cardiac myocytes, but their absence does not entirely exclude the possibility of myocardial infection by HIV. Recent studies suggest that perhaps the infection occurs in endothelial cells rather than myocytes, which in this case might explain the multiple foci of chronic ischemia (myocytolysis). If in fact, HIV damages the heart directly, it is not accompanied by a significant inflammatory response.

Dilated Cardiomyopathy

The exact pathogenic mechanism of dilated cardiomyopathy associated with HIV/AIDS is unknown, but diverse factors may play a role. Nutritional deficiencies are known to cause dilated cardiomyopathy (see DCM chapter), and HIV/AIDS wasting syndrome is characterized by persistent poor appetite and generalized cachexia. In addition, gastrointestinal disease with malabsorption and protein loss is a common feature of HIV, but in many cases has no detectable cause. Our patient was thin but not cachectic. In addition, with profound malnutrition and wasting, the adipose tissue deposits are lost, and one of the last ones to disappear is the subepicardial fat (Figure 28). However, in our case, the subepicardial fat was present in normal amounts, indicating that she did not have significant nutritional compromise.

Several drugs such as interferon alpha and nucleoside analogues have been associated with the development of cardiomyopathy. Zidovudine (AZT) in particular is known to cause a striated muscle myopathy that is dose dependent and requires discontinuation for reversal of the effect. The postulated mechanism is through mitochondrial structural and genetic alterations in the myocyte, with abnormal expression of mitochondrial gene products.

Myocardial ischemia due to spasm of the microvasculature, whether associated or not with cocaine use, and excess in catecholamine production have also been described as possible causes of cardiomyopathy in HIV/AIDS patients.

Metabolic alterations

HIV infection and some of its treatment drugs (protease inhibitors), are associated with a decrease in the levels of high density lipoproteins (HDL) and increase levels of LDL and triglycerides; thus increasing susceptibility to atherosclerosis. The benefits of therapy outweigh the risks; however, the risk increases if other factors for cardiovascular disease are present, such as smoking, hypertension, diabetes, and cocaine abuse. Insulin resistance is common in HIV-infected patients, but the prevalence of diabetes is not increased as compared to the general population. There is no known direct association between hypertension and HIV.

Interstitial myocardial disease

Interstitial heart disease, other than myocardial fibrosis, does not appear to be a commonly recognized feature of patients with HIV/AIDS.

The present case is unusual in that it appears to represent a case of microfibrillar cardiomyopathy. This entity is a newly described infiltrative heart disease resembling cardiac amyloidosis. The histology reveals interstitial eosinophilic hyaline material similar to amyloid, but has specific tinctorial properties since it does not stain with crystal violet or Congo red. In addition, distinct ultrastructural features have been described consisting of microfibrillar interstitial deposits loosely organized into bundles, and occasionally associated with elastic matrix. This material was identified by immunoelectron microscopy to be composed of fibrillin, a glycoprotein associated with elastic tissues throughout the body. Furthermore, it represents the matrix protein that is defective in Marfan's syndrome. Clinically, patients with microfibrillar cardiomyopathy present with arrhythmias and/or ventricular dysfunction. It is noteworthy that histopathologic changes of interstitial deposition of fibrils in experimental HIV/AIDS, was initially described in the early 80s in a colony of macaque monkeys.

In this patient, no other specific cause for dysfunction could be identified on either light or electron microscopy. There was no history of diabetes or hypertension, two conditions that could explain a rigid, fibrotic heart. There was evidence of mild atherosclerosis. She was not malnourished and refused treatment with anti-retroviral agents. We are not aware of cocaine or alcohol abuse. The foci of myocardial necrosis were a pre-mortem event due to shock. The ventricular dyskinesis and reduction of ejection fraction were more the result of a restrictive heart disease (diastolic dysfunction), rather than dilated cardiomyopathy. Although she had some degree of cardiac dilatation, she had severe biventricular hypertrophy (wall thickness: LV 2.5 cm and RV 0.7 cm), with extensive fibrosis and collagen deposition, in addition to the microfibrillar changes.

Infiltrative heart disease has not been thoroughly described yet in HIV/AIDS, but remains a likely cause of cardiomyopathy in this case. Recent studies have proven that HIV type 1 protease cleaves the intermediate filament proteins vimentin and desmin, leading to subsequent deposition of these filaments. We wonder if the same mechanism can be applied to increased microfibrillar deposition in a patient infected with HIV.

Regardless of the precise etiology of cardiomyopathy in this case, the ultimate cause of death was diffuse hemorrhagic Klebsiella pneumonia and septic shock. The latter leads to low cardiac output and poor tissue perfusion, even in the absence of previous heart disease. Therefore, is not surprising that she developed myocardial ischemia due to decreased coronary blood flow in an already non-compliant heart. The effects of decreased peripheral vascular resistance on a heart with diastolic dysfunction would further exacerbate the heart failure. It is likely that even with aggressive therapy, she would have not survived.

Suggested Readings

1. Lewis W. Cardiomyopathy in AIDS: a pathophysiological perspective. Prog Cardiovasc Dis. 2000; 43:151-70.
2. Rerkpattanapipat P, Wongpraparut N, Jacobs LE, Kotler MN. Cardiac manifestations of acquired immunodeficiency syndrome. Arch Intern Med. 2000; 160:602-8.
3. Milei J, Grana D, Fernandez Alonso G, Matturri L. Cardiac involvement in acquired immunodeficiency syndrome--a review to push action. The Committee for the Study of Cardiac Involvement in AIDS. Clin Cardiol. 1998; 21:465-72.
4. Yunis NA, Stone VE. Cardiac manifestations of HIV/AIDS: a review of disease spectrum and clinical management. J Acquir Immune Defic Syndr Hum Retrovirol. 1998; 18:145-54.
5. Herskowitz A. Cardiomyopathy and other symptomatic heart diseases associated with HIV infection. Curr Opin Cardiol. 1996; 11:325-31.
6. Flomenbaum M, Soeiro R, Udem SA, Kress Y, Factor SM. Proliferative membranopathy and human immunodeficiency virus in AIDS hearts. J Acq Imm Def Synd. 1989; 2:129-35.
7. van Hoeven KH, Segal B, Factor SM. AIDS cardiomyopathy: first rule out other myocardial risk factors. Int J Cardiol 1990; 67:780-3.
8. Factor SM, Menegus MA, Kress Y, Cho S, Fisher JD, Sakai LY, Goldfischer S. Microfibrillar cardiomyopathy: A new entity resembling cardiac amyloidosis. Cardiovasc Pathol 1992; 1:307-16.

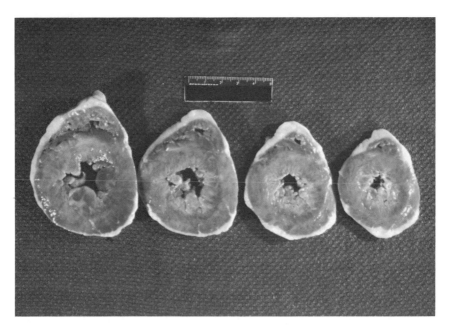

Figure 25. Cross sections of the heart revealing marked concentric hypertrophy of the left ventricle. The right ventricle is also hypertrophied.

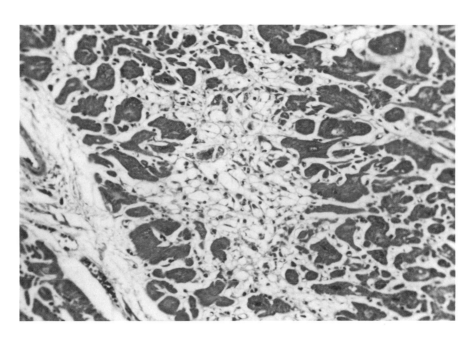

Figure 26. Myocytolysis. The empty spaces represent dead myocytes. Causative factors include localized reperfusion injury due to transient microvascular spasm (Hematoxylin and Eosin, 40X).

116

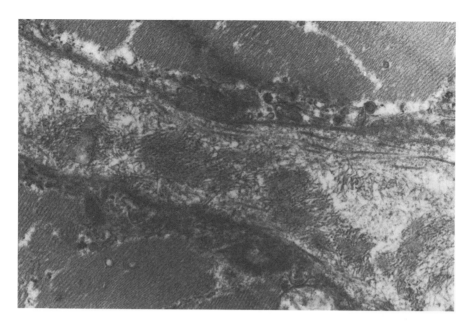

Figure 27. Microfibrillar cardiomyopathy. Loosely tangled, slightly curvilinear fibrils with a diameter of 15 – 20 nm are present in the interstitium between two myocytes (Electron microscopy, magnification 45K).

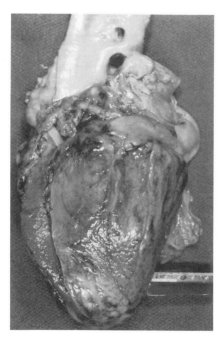

Figure 28. Malnutrition and cachexia. Notice the absence of epicardial adipose tissue.

117

Chapter # 5

VALVULOPATHIES

Case # 13

Clinical Summary

A 78 year old woman was brought to the ER with a 3 day history of respiratory distress. In route to the ER, she was hypertensive, tachycardic and tachypneic (BP 200-220/130 mmHg, P 135, R 28). The ECG showed atrial fibrillation with premature contractions. Upon arrival, she was found to be pale and diaphoretic and she began to experience mild chest pain. Her vital signs at that time were: BP 170/130 mmHg, P 176, R 34 and T 37.8°C. She was placed on a cardiac monitor and on 100% FiO2 by nasal cannula. In addition, sublingual nitroglycerine, aspirin, furosemide, diltiazem, clonidine and digoxin were started. After her admission to the cardiac care unit, her condition improved. There were no complaints of respiratory distress or chest pain, and the cardiac monitor showed occasional premature contractions. Through the day she was occasionally confused, and at one point required hand restraints to prevent her from pulling her IV lines. Her physical exam was significant for scattered bilateral pulmonary rales and lower extremity edema. The chest X ray was suggestive of congestive heart failure and cardiomegaly. The ECG showed atrial fibrillation, left ventricular hypertrophy, right bundle branch block pattern, but no ST-T wave changes. There were no enzymatic changes (CK, LDH or troponin I) consistent with acute myocardial infarction. A repeat chest-x ray was ordered and the patient had a cardiac arrest while in radiology. Resuscitation was unsuccessfully attempted.

Gross Description

The patient weighed 68 kg and measured 147 cm. The heart weighed 430 g. The pericardium was smooth. The left ventricle was hypertrophic (wall thickness 2.7 cm) (Figure 29). The right atrium was also hypertrophic, but the left atrium and right ventricle were unremarkable. The valves had the following measurements: tricuspid 13.5 cm, pulmonic 10.0 cm, mitral 6.5 cm, and aortic 4.0 cm. Stenosis of the mitral valve was mild. The aortic valve was also stenotic with fusion of the cusps (Figure 30). Other findings included valvular and endocardial calcified vegetations, endocardial pseudovalve formation consistent with regurgitation, post-stenotic aortic root dilatation and linear atherosclerotic plaque of the aortic root. Aneurysmal dilatation of the foramen ovale wall was noted. The myocardium of the interventricular septum was scarred with focal myocytolysis. There was diffuse coronary artery disease with 100% occlusion of the right coronary artery, 60% stenosis of the left main artery, left circumflex and left anterior descending arteries. The lungs were heavy (1050 g) and edematous. The liver was congested (1390 g). The kidneys weighed 220 g combined and revealed bilateral stenosis of the renal arteries of up to 80%, and nephrosclerosis. Changes in the brain were consistent with hypertensive atherosclerotic cerebrovascular disease and included lacunar state, fusiform atherosclerotic aneurysm of the basilar artery with remote and recent plaque hemorrhage, small vessel thrombosis and small acute cerebral hemorrhage consistent with thromboembolism.

Case Analysis

Ordinarily, an elderly patient presenting as she did with congestive heart failure and hypertension, would be assumed to have arteriosclerotic cardiovascular disease as the underlying etiology for her symptoms. In fact, she had significant coronary artery disease, with complete occlusion of the right coronary artery, moderately severe stenosis (60%) of the left coronary system, and left ventricular septal scarring consistent with a remote myocardial infarction. She also had bilateral renal artery stenosis, and arterionephrosclerosis consistent with hypertension. The surprising finding at the autopsy, and totally unsuspected clinically, however, was the presence of valvular changes diagnostic of chronic rheumatic heart disease (RHD). A number of questions can be raised about RHD in this 78 year old woman:

1. Why did she survive to her 8th decade, when RHD usually becomes symptomatic before the 3-4th decade?
2. Was the valvular pathology actually RHD? What is RHD?
3. Did the valvular disease contribute to this patient's clinical presentation, and death?
4. Is it possible to determine the pathophysiology of her valvular pathology from the autopsy findings alone, in the absence of diagnostic studies such as echocardiography?

As noted, RHD most often presents in patients in their 20's or 30's, and sometimes even when they are in their teenage years. The explanation for this early onset of a disease acquired usually in childhood (see below), is that RHD invariably affects the mitral valve leading to scarring of the valve apparatus, and hemodynamic stenosis and/or regurgitation. Since the primary valve affected lies between the low pressure left atrium, and the high pressure left ventricle, decreasing the mitral valve orifice (stenosis) or increasing the left atrial volume (regurgitation) leads to an early pressure and/or volume overload of the pulmonary circulation. This configuration does not require much increase in left atrial pressure to affect the pulmonary vessels, since the normal left atrial pressure is only 4-8 mmHg. The scarring of the mitral valve is sufficient to prevent its complete closure, and the resulting regurgitation creates a volume excess that overloads the system. In addition, there's almost always a component of mitral valve stenosis. With overload of the low pressure pulmonary circulation, pulmonary venous hypertension develops along with capillary hypertension in the alveolar septa. With increased pressure, there is capillary congestion and low grade leakage of edema fluid into the alveolar septal interstitium, and even into the alveolar spaces. The relatively thin-walled atrial chambers, which are generally capacitance chambers, cannot hypertrophy sufficiently to counteract the effects of increased atrial pressure and volume. In fact, the atria rapidly undergo degeneration of the thin layers of myocardium in their walls, leading to dilatation and eventual loss of normal contractility. That is why virtually all cases of mitral valve disease due to RHD are associated with the early onset of atrial fibrillation. Thus, patients with RHD and significant mitral valve disease have the early onset of pulmonary vascular congestion that translates clinically into dyspnea, orthopnea, and exercise intolerance. This patient did not present more than 40 years sooner with symptoms because her mitral valve disease was very mild. Her primary valvular damage affected the aortic valve, which presents, as we shall see, with different pathophysiology.

This patient had marked thickening of the aortic valve cusps, with commissural fusion. Although we will come back to the question of whether these features are secondary to rheumatic heart disease, the changes are certainly indicative of aortic valve stenosis. Additionally, there was a *pseudovalve* below the aortic valve, which is secondary to valvular insufficiency. A pseudovalve results from a regurgitant jet of blood crossing an insufficient aortic valve, leading to endocardial damage and subsequent build-up of fibrin and platelet vegetation on the endocardial surface. With time, the vegetation organizes into fibrous tissue, but it is modeled by the direction and pressure of the regurgitant jet. Therefore, the raised fibrous plaque develops a concave surface 'facing' the aortic valve, and a convex surface toward the apex away from the jet. In addition, the jet of blood tends to undermine the concave surface. The end result is a cusp-shaped fibrous endocardial plaque, that resembles a semilunar valve cusp; hence, a *pseudovalve.* Its presence is virtually diagnostic of aortic valve insufficiency (it usually does not occur on the right side below the pulmonary valve, because pulmonary insufficiency is relatively uncommon, and even when present it is generally a low pressure regurgitant jet that does not lead to

121

significant endocardial damage). Two other findings suggest that she had hemodynamically significant aortic valve disease: she had prominent left ventricular hypertrophy (wall thickness 2.7 cm, normal 1.5 cm), and post-stenotic dilatation of the aortic root above the valve. Concentric left ventricular hypertrophy (LVH) could have been partially the result of chronic hypertension, but valvular outflow tract obstruction generally produces a more severe LVH, consistent with the range of what this patient had. The post-stenotic dilatation of the aortic root is a characteristic result of a jet of blood progressing through the narrowed valve orifice, and leading to damage to the aortic root wall, with degeneration of the elastic tissue and secondary aneurysm formation. Thus, this patient had gross morphologic evidence of aortic valve stenosis and insufficiency. Even without an echocardiogram, the diagnosis can be made with absolute certainty. The fact that clinical murmurs were not appreciated (mid-systolic ejection murmur for aortic stenosis, and diastolic murmur for aortic insufficiency heard at the base; diastolic rumble with an opening snap heard at the apex and radiating to the left axilla for mitral stenosis - note that there would be no pre-systolic accentuation due to the atrial fibrillation), can be explained on the basis of her presentation with congestive heart failure with probable decreased stroke volume. There must be adequate flow across the valves in order to produce the fluid turbulence that causes the murmurs.

Aortic valve disease, regardless of etiology, is much better tolerated than mitral valve disease. The latter, as described above, affects the low pressure pulmonary circulation, and may do so early in its course, leading to exercise intolerance and progressive respiratory distress. In contrast, aortic valve disease, particularly stenosis, results in compensatory left ventricular hypertrophy that maintains stroke volume for a prolonged period. Thus, patients with aortic stenosis may have the condition in a well-compensated state well into their 7-8th decade, and sometime even later, with maintenance of their exercise tolerance. Ultimately, there is a cost. There is chronic damage to the subendocardium due to the high end-systolic pressures. Consequently, the newly generated wall stress causes myocyte injury; and the remodeling of the wall and chamber eventually results in elevated end-diastolic pressures. The remodeling is accentuated by aortic insufficiency (volume overload), and coronary ischemia. Although, both were present in this patient, significant remodeling had not yet developed. Regardless, ventricular failure may develop very rapidly in patients with aortic stenosis, leading to the precipitous onset of congestive heart failure, even before remodeling ensues. Thus, in contrast to mitral stenosis, which leads to an early presentation, the course of aortic stenosis is one of prolonged compensation often for many years, and rapid decompensation. The latter, often results in death in weeks or a few months, usually secondary to fatal arrhythmia, or left ventricular failure. This patient's presentation with fulminant congestive heart failure is consistent with decompensated aortic valve disease, even though mitral valve disease, ischemia, and hypertension contributed significantly.

Was this patient's valvular disease rheumatic in origin? It is far more common to have degenerative valve disease affecting patients in their 8th decade, than to have RHD as the etiology. Calcification of the mitral annulus (*mitral annular calcification*), and calcification and fibrosis of the aortic valve (*calcific aortic stenosis of the elderly*) are two degenerative conditions often occurring simultaneously, that can cause mitral regurgitation and aortic stenosis in older patients. Mitral annular calcification, when it affects the valve leaflets, tends to damage the posterior leaflet and focal posterior chordae preferentially, generally sparing the anterior leaflet and chords. Calcific aortic stenosis, by its description, tends to have heavy calcification that often compromises the sinuses of Valsalva. It often affects only mildly the commissures; and, it is usually not associated with aortic insufficiency. In contrast, rheumatic mitral valve disease affects the entire valve, tends to spare the annulus unless very severe, causes commissural fusion, and leads to thickening, shortening and fusion of chordae tendineae (Figures 31 and 32). Rheumatic aortic valve disease causes fibrosis of the cusps (with or without calcification), leads to fusion of commissures, and frequently is associated with insufficiency. Based on these criteria, this patient had rheumatic valvular disease. It is also noteworthy that rheumatic disease always involves the mitral valve, with the aortic valve being the second most affected; however, aortic valve disease without mitral involvement, is not rheumatic in etiology. The relative severity of the two valve lesions may be variable (usually, when there is one valve more affected than another, it is the mitral valve that is more severe; but, on occasion as in this patient, the relationship is inverted).

As a final point, a brief discussion of the pathogenesis of RHD and how it affects the valves, is in order. The clinical manifestations of RHD are virtually always the chronic effects of an inflammatory process that occurred several decades before. The condition results from a childhood infection with rheumatogenic strains of group A, beta-hemolytic streptococcus, often causing pharyngitis ('strep throat'). Then, in a small proportion of susceptible children (less than 3%) an auto-immune reaction develops several weeks after the infection. The auto-immunity is thought to result from cross-reactivity between one or several glycoprotein(s) in the streptococcal capsule (M protein), and antigens expressed in the myocardium, pericardium, and heart valves. During the active inflammatory phase of the disease, a cellular infiltrate involves the interstitium of the heart (myocarditis), the pericardium (fibrinous pericarditis), and the valve tissues including the leaflets, commissures, and chordae tendineae (atrio-ventricular valves). The inflammatory infiltrate, particularly in the myocardium, consists of a granulomatous collection of T lymphocytes, plasma cells, and activated macrophages known as Aschoff cells, often surrounding a focus of fibrinoid collagen necrosis. The entire granuloma is known as an Aschoff body, and it is pathognomonic for rheumatic heart disease (Figures 33 and 34). The Aschoff body may persist for years (its persistence does not necessarily indicate that the inflammatory disease is active), but it often goes on to heal as a fibrous scar. In the valvular tissues, true Aschoff bodies are uncommon, but the inflammatory infiltrate is similar. Scarring then results in fibrous thickening and secondary calcification of the leaflets and cusps with decreased pliability and inability to coapt properly. Furthermore, fusion of commissures leads to narrowing of the valve orifice; and the narrowing, shortening and fusion of chordae, limit the normal excursion of the mitral and less commonly, the tricuspid valves. With time, secondary non-rheumatic vegetations may develop on these valves that organize into additional scar tissue that further distorts and deforms the valve structure. The leaflet and cusp fibrosis, the commissural fusion, and the chordal thickening were the changes identified in this patient, indicating the presence of chronic rheumatic damage that occurred years before. Despite extensive search, no Aschoff bodies were identified, but the diagnosis of chronic rheumatic valvulitis does not require their presence.

Suggested Readings

1. Feldman T. Rheumatic heart disease. Curr Opin Cardiol. 1996; 11:126-30.
2. Shulman ST. Complications of streptococcal pharyngitis. Pediatr Infect Dis J. 1994; 13(1 Suppl 1):S70-4; discussion S78-9.
3. Veasy LG, Hill HR. Immunologic and clinical correlations in rheumatic fever and rheumatic heart disease. Pediatr Infect Dis J. 1997; 16:400-7.
4. Rose AG. Etiology of valvular heart disease. Curr Opin Cardiol. 1996; 11:98-113.
5. Baxley WA. Aortic valve disease. Curr Opin Cardiol. 1994; 9:152-7.
6. Stollerman GH. Rheumatogenic streptococci and autoimmunity. Clin Immunol Immunopathol. 1991; 61:131-42.
7. Adler Y, Fink N, Spector D, Wiser I, Sagie A. Mitral annulus calcification- - a window to diffuse atherosclerosis of the vascular system. Atherosclerosis. 2001; 155:1-8.

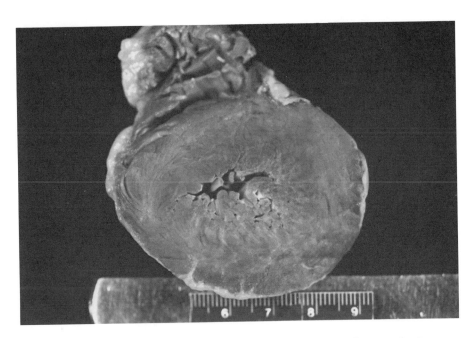

Figure 29. Cross section of the heart revealing severe left ventricular hypertrophy due to aortic valve stenosis.

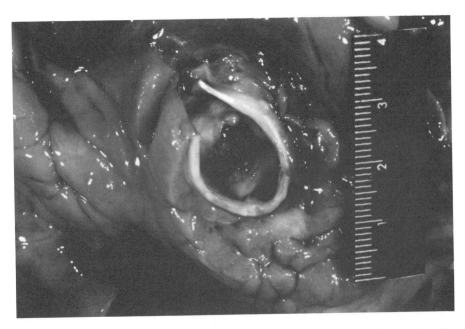

Figure 30. Rheumatic heart disease involving the aortic valve (viewed from the aorta) with a superimposed fresh thrombus.

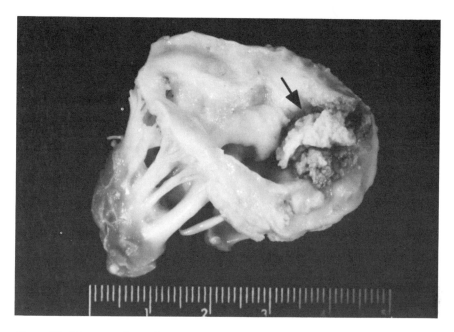

Figure 31. Rheumatic heart disease. Resected mitral valve with thickened chordae and leaflets, and superimposed adherent, calcified vegetations (arrow).

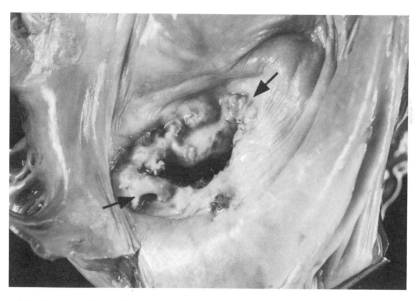

Figure 32. Rheumatic heart disease. In this example the mitral valve shows thickened and calcified leaflets with commissural fusion (arrows). The patient had symptoms of mitral stenosis and insufficiency.

127

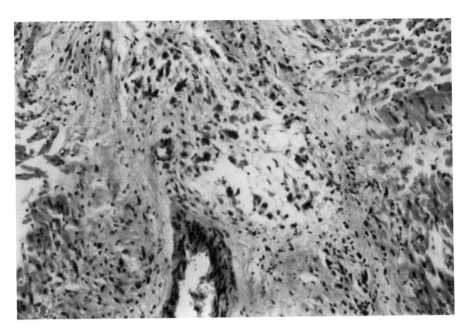

Figure 33. Rheumatic heart disease, histologic section. Aschoff body (center)(Hematoxylin and Eosin, 20X).

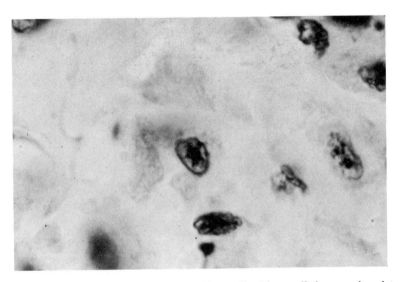

Figure 34. Rheumatic heart disease with Anitschkow cells. These cells have oval nuclei and centrally condensed chromatin. Due to the pattern of nuclear chromatin, these cells are also known as caterpillar cells in longitudinal section and owls' eye in cross section (Hematoxylin and Eosin, 100X)

128

Case # 14

Clinical Summary

This is the case of a 60 year old Hispanic man who presented to the hospital with complaints of shortness of breath. A few months earlier, a mid-systolic click and a late systolic murmur III/VI, radiating to the axilla, were discovered on a routine physical exam. An echocardiogram was done revealing significant mitral regurgitation. Catheterization showed severe mitral valve regurgitation with flaring posterior leaflet, normal ejection fraction and 50% right coronary artery stenosis. Mitral valvuloplasty was performed with the post-surgical complication of atrial fibrillation and flutter for which the patient was started on the anticoagulant coumadin. Ten days post-surgery, the patient was found at home unconscious with agonal respiration. CPR was performed to no avail and the patient was pronounced dead on arrival to the emergency room.

Gross Description

The patient measured 176 cm and weighed 81 kg. A healing 14 cm long sternotomy scar was seen on the right sternal border. The heart weighed 575 g. The pericardial surfaces had a fibrinous exudate consistent with pericarditis, and the sac contained 500 cc of sero-sanguineous fluid. Both atria showed well healed surgical incisions. The left atrium was dilated. The right atrium was of normal size. Mitral valve annuloplasty was evident, and the cusps and leaflets showed fibromyxomatous degeneration. Excess tissue was present, and the chordae tendineae were thickened and elongated (Figure 35). The remaining valves were unremarkable. The left ventricle was mildly hypertrophied (wall thickness 1.6 cm). The right ventricle had a normal chamber size. The lungs weighed 900 g combined, and were congested. Intimal plaques were noted in the pulmonary vasculature. The other significant post-mortem finding was the presence of multiple subacute and remote infarcts affecting cerebral cortex, subcortical white matter and thalamus.

Microscopic Description

Sections from the pericardium revealed extensive granulation tissue with thick deposits of fibrin, focal hemorrhage and giant cell proliferation. Myocyte hypertrophy with interstitial fibrosis and adipose tissue infiltration was noted in the myocardium. The mitral valve showed fibromyxomatous

129

changes (Figure 36). Coronary arteriosclerosis was moderate with no evidence of plaque, hemorrhage or thrombotic occlusions. The aorta exhibited thickening of the wall with proliferation of the intima and extensive deposition of cholesterol with focal ulceration in the areas of calcification. Sections from the central nervous system confirmed the gross impression of multiple infarcts.

Case Analysis

Mitral valve regurgitation has multiple etiologies. The most common is chronic rheumatic heart disease (see previous chapter) followed by ischemia, congenital valve anomalies (endocardial cushion defects), endocarditis, mitral valve prolapse, fibroelastosis, calcification of the mitral annulus, chamber dilatation and remodeling in myocarditis and dilated cardiomyopathy. In this patient, the diagnosis of chronic rheumatic heart disease is unlikely. Rheumatic valvulopathy usually affects the aortic valve as well, and is often symptomatic early in the course of the disease due to elevated left atrial pressure, secondary pulmonary hypertension and right-sided heart failure. This patient was 60 years old by the time he presented with shortness of breath, and he had no evidence of aortic valve changes. Rheumatic heart disease not only causes mitral regurgitation, but also mitral stenosis with fibrosis of the leaflets and fusion of the commissure and chordae tendineae. Mitral regurgitation as the sole manifestation of rheumatic disease is rare and more common in males than in females.

Mitral annular calcification is rarely associated with regurgitation or stenosis, and seldom produces symptomatic valvular dysfunction. Regurgitation is secondary to deformity of the mitral valve ring by the presence of calcium deposits. These deposits impair the motion of the annulus and cause traction and elevation of the leaflets. It affects patients over 60 years of age, mostly women. Grumous degeneration may occur within the calcifications with accompanying foreign body giant cell reaction (Figure 37).

Ischemic heart disease may also cause mitral regurgitation, either acutely or chronically. The acute form is due to rupture of the papillary muscle or chordae tendineae. As a consequence, a sudden increase in volume and pressure occurs in the left atrium with no time for compensatory hypertrophy of the atrial wall. The end result is acute pulmonary edema and death, unless immediate surgical intervention ensues. Infarction of a portion of the papillary muscle with subsequent fibrosis may also lead to retraction of the valve and secondary insufficiency. Our patient had only moderate coronary atherosclerosis and no evidence of acute or remote myocardial infarction. Which disease then, may cause chronic mitral valve regurgitation that is often asymptomatic for years, and incidentally discovered during physical exam? The answer is mitral valve prolapse or MVP.

MVP, also known as Barlow's syndrome or "floppy" valve disease, occurs in 3-5% of the general population. It affects females more than males and may be associated with connective tissue disorders such as Marfan and Ehlers-Danlos syndromes. MVP may also be inherited as an autosomal dominant condition with variable penetrance. Occasionally, MVP may lead to severe mitral regurgitation with elevation of the mean left atrial pressure and resultant dilatation of the left atrium. This pathologic dilatation is a predisposing factor for the development of atrial fibrillation and flutter.

In order to understand the pathophysiology of this type of valvulopathy, it is necessary that we review the physiology of the normal valve. The mitral valve consists of the following structures: the annulus, 2 leaflets (anterior and posterior), the chordae tendineae and 2 papillary muscle groups, one antero-medial and the other postero-lateral. The annulus is an asymmetric ring where the leaflets attach. The posterior leaflet, despite the fact that it is the smaller of the two, occupies most of the annulus circumference. Both leaflets are composed of fibrous tissue lined by endothelium. They are attached to the anterior and posterior papillary muscles by delicate thin bands of tissue known as chordae tendineae. There are a total of 24 main chordae and 120 branches that insert not only at the free edge of the leaflets, but also at the undersurface (rough zone). The nature of this insertion assures proper closure and prevents eversion of the leaflets into the atrium during systole. Abnormal valvular movements are also prevented by overlapping of the leaflets during their closed position and by the fact that the anterior leaflet runs parallel to the blood flow. During diastole, the valve's leaflets are forced into a semi-closed position by the passive stretching of the papillary muscles during ventricular filling. In mitral valve prolapse, regurgitation occurs when the valvular tissue protrudes into the left atrium during systole. The leaflets prolapse due to two main reasons: 1) the tissue is excessive and 2) the leaflets are no longer fibrous, but rather myxomatous (rich in mucopolysaccharides) which makes them thin, soft and highly mobile. In addition, the chordae tendineae may be thin and elongated.

The heart murmur of this patient was characteristic of MVP. The midsystolic click occurs when the redundant leaflet enters into the left atrium and is suddenly pulled back to its original position. The murmur is the result of turbulence caused by the regurgitant blood flow. In our case, despite the annuloplasty, the post-mortem mitral valve findings are consistent with the diagnosis of MVP. The leaflets had marked fibromyxomatous degeneration and the chordae tendineae were long and only mildly thickened. Following surgery, this patient developed arrhythmia and was anticoagulated to avoid microthrombi that could embolize in the systemic circulation. However, the autopsy revealed subacute and remote infarcts that occurred prior to surgery.

The thrombi originated either in the dilated atrium or beneath the redundant leaflets of the mitral valve. In some cases, superimposed bacterial infection (e.g. endocarditis) may develop. MVP is managed clinically unless it progresses to severe mitral regurgitation; and when that happens, as in this case, surgical repair is required. Valve replacement for this condition is not as common, and carries a higher risk of post-surgical complications. Furthermore, patients who undergo cardiac surgery are always at risk for thromboembolic events, bleeding, infections and arrhythmias.

A well described complication of open heart surgery is the post-cardiotomy syndrome. This entity develops a week to ten days after the procedure and is clinically undistinguishable from Dressler's syndrome, a complication of myocardial infarction. Dressler's syndrome is an idiopathic form of acute pericarditis manifested as chest pain, pleural and pericardial effusion, fever and increased white blood cell count. A pericardial friction rub is present on auscultation. Possible causes include activation of a latent viral infection and/or an immunologic response with the formation of anti-heart antibodies. As in Dressler's, post-cardiotomy syndrome has also been associated with viral illness.

Post-cardiotomy syndrome may present as cardiac tamponade, as in this case, with significant accumulation of sero-sanguineous fluid and associated fibrinous pericarditis. Presumably, the blood comes from the numerous new vessels that comprise the granulation tissue that is part of the healing process of the pericardium. Increased vascular permeability added to the effects of coumadin therapy (anticoagulant), contributed to the continuous bleeding into the pericardial sac, leading to compression of the heart (tamponade) and the patient's death. The microscopic exam of the pericardium revealed extensive granulation tissue and hemorrhage in both visceral and parietal layers. The lungs had evidence of pleuritis with adhesions, chronic congestion with numerous intraalveolar hemosiderin-laden macrophages and thickened vessels consistent with pulmonary hypertension. It appears that the mitral regurgitation had just recently become severe. The changes in the pulmonary vasculature were mild and focal, the left atrium was only slightly dilated, the ejection fraction was normal and significant changes in the right side of the heart were absent. Interestingly, the ring of the tricuspid valve was dilated (13 cm) and similar histologic changes to those seen in the mitral valve were noted in the tricuspid leaflets (myxomatous degeneration). These findings suggest a mild form of tricuspid valve prolapse that can be seen in approximately 40% of patients with mitral valve prolapse. Similar changes can affect the pulmonic and aortic valves, but less frequently (10% of cases). Unfortunately, the patient's clinical course deteriorated so rapidly that treatment could not be instituted. Patients with cardiac tamponade may experience pulsus paradoxus (decline in systemic arterial pressure of more than 10mm of Hg during inspiration). Pulsus paradoxus is an exaggeration of what occurs normally when a person inhales. During inspiration, the arterial pressure diminishes and the venous pressure increases. Increased venous return produces a septal shift from the right ventricle into the left ventricle that is restored when the patient exhales. These changes are enhanced by the external, mainly atrial compression exerted by the fluid in the pericardial sac with severe compromise of the cardiac output. The diagnosis can be made by examining the jugular vein pulsations. Echocardiography is confirmatory. Pulsus paradoxus does not occur in the setting of significant left ventricular hypertrophy. When the left ventricle is hypertrophic with no associated dilatation, the rigidity of the wall precludes the inspiratory effect of septal displacement.

Treatment of cardiac tamponade varies and includes pericardio-centesis and open surgical drainage. In cases of post-cardiotomy syndrome, less severe than in the present case, anti-inflammatory treatment appears to be effective, which further supports the notion that this entity has an immunologic basis.

In addition to surgical trauma and anticoagulant therapy, other conditions should be considered as etiologic or precipitating factors of cardiac tamponade such as ruptured myocardial infarction, ruptured aortic dissection, renal failure, metastatic malignancies and sepsis.

Suggested Readings

1. Chambers J. The clinical and diagnostic features of mitral valve disease. Hosp Med. 2001; 62:72-8.
2. Carabello BA. The pathophysiology of mitral regurgitation. J Heart Valve Dis. 2000; 9:600-8.
3. Kronick-Mest C. Postpericardiotomy syndrome: etiology, manifestations, and interventions. Heart Lung. 1989; 18:192-8
4. Engle MA. Humoral immunity and heart disease: postpericardiotomy syndrome. Adv Exp Med Biol. 1983; 161:471-8

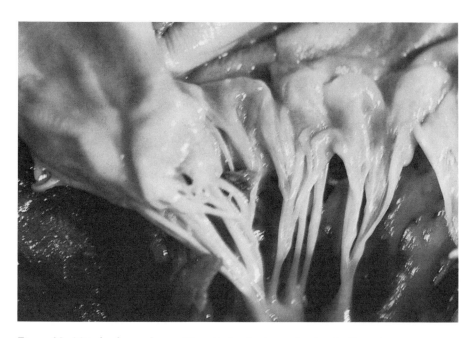

Figure 35. Mitral valve prolapse. The mitral valve has redundant leaflets and the chordae tendineae are long and mildly thickened.

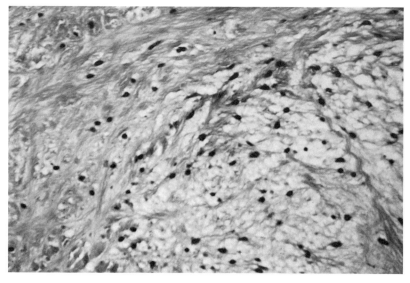

Figure 36. Mitral valve prolapse, histologic section. Fibromyxomatous degeneration of the mitral valve is characterized by loose connective tissue and deposition of myxoid material (Hematoxylin and Eosin, 40X)

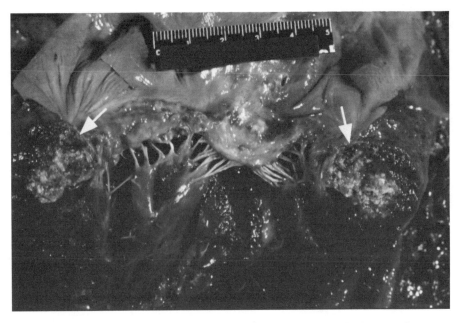

Figure 37. Mitral valve annular calcification. There is a diffuse ring of calcium with grumous degeneration involving the annulus and extending into the myocardium (arrows).

Chapter 6

CONGENITAL HEART DISEASE

Case # 15

Clinical Summary

The patient was a 28 year old Hispanic woman with mild mental retardation, and a known congenital heart defect. She lived with a foster family and always had decreased activity or exercise intolerance with episodes of dyspnea.

The current illness began a few days prior to her admission with the development of diarrhea, vomiting, abdominal pain and fever. Her foster family took her to the hospital, where she was rehydrated and sent home with the diagnosis of a viral syndrome. At home she had a seizure manifested by stiffness, turning of the head and cyanosis. The next morning she was lethargic, had poor respiration and weak pulses. The paramedics were called and on their arrival they found the patient pulseless, without detectable blood pressure or respiration. She was immediately intubated and CPR was started. Her post-resuscitation physical exam revealed BP 70/palpable, P 134/min, T 37°C; evident peripheral cyanosis and clubbing. There was no lymphadenopathy, or edema. Neurologically her pupils were dilated, fixed, and non-reactive. There were no doll's eyes or caloric and pain responses. The cardiovascular exam showed no jugular distension; an S1 present, diminished S2 and no murmurs; peripheral pulses were present. The lungs had equal breath sounds bilaterally.

Laboratory data and other tests

Laboratory: WBC 11, Hb/Hct 22/65, Plt 203; BUN/creat 6/1.2, Na 133, K 3.3, Cl 98, CO2 16, glucose 505, lactate (nl 0.3-1.3) 2.6, bilirubin T 0.2, SGOT/SGPT 48/50, Protein T/alb 4.2/2.5, AP 64, LD 316, CK 260; PT/PTT 14.7/41.5. Arterial blood gases (pre/post-resuscitation): pH 6.83/7.24, pCO2 83/31, pO2 54/41, O2 sat % 60/68. CXR: right middle lobe consolidation and congestive heart failure. ECG: normal sinus rhythm, right ventricular hypertrophy, and T-wave inversion in III.

The patient was admitted in the intensive care unit where she was persistently hypotensive. An echocardiogram was done showing right ventricular hypertrophy, overriding aorta and a ventricular septal defect. The patient became ventilator dependent and died the day after admission.

Gross Description

The body measured 160 cm and weighed 55 kg. The external exam was significant for clubbing of fingers and toes. There was no evidence of past thoracic surgery.

The heart weighed 460 g and had right ventricular prominence with a double apex. The pericardium was smooth and glistening. There was a moderate amount of subepicardial fat. The right atrium was hypertrophied, but the left was normal in size and free of thrombi. The foramen ovale was closed. The right and left ventricular wall thickness was 1.1 and 1.5 cm, respectively. Both ventricles were hypertrophied and the right ventricle was dilated as well. The membranous interventricular septum was absent, and thus there was a large high ventricular septal defect measuring 2 x 1.5 cm (Figure 38). The aortic valve, which had three normal cusps, was shifted to the right and opened over the right ventricle, with a small area overriding the ventricular septal defect. Therefore, the left ventricular outflow was through the ventricular septal defect and into the aorta. The ductus arteriosus was closed. The pulmonary artery trunk and left and right pulmonary artery branches were atrophic and fibrotic with no identifiable lumen (Figure 39). There was no associated identifiable pulmonary valve. The lungs received their arterial supply from two large bronchial arteries arising from the descending aorta. These arteries arose at the level of the aortic valve. The lungs drained via four normal pulmonary veins into the left atrium (two from each lung). The valve leaflets were delicate and pliable except for mild myxomatous change of the mitral valve. The chordae tendineae were slender. The endocardium was thin and glistening. The myocardium was brown-red of average consistency. The coronary arteries were of normal caliber and distribution with right dominance. There were no occlusions. The superior and inferior caval veins were unremarkable. The aorta showed extensive fatty streaking, especially in the abdominal portion. A non-adherent thrombus was present in the right carotid artery.

The lungs weighed 1360 g combined. The visceral and parietal pleural surfaces were adherent. Dilated pleural lymphatic vessels were seen. On section, the parenchyma showed confluent areas of firmness in the upper lobes, apices of the lower lobes and to a lesser extent in the lung bases. Within the upper lobes there were foci of necrosis.

The brain weighed 1120 g. The calvarium was unremarkable. The dural sinuses were free of thrombi. The leptomeninges over the base of the brain were focally opaque and contained exudate consistent with basal meningitis. The cerebral hemispheres were asymmetrical. The right frontal lobe was soft and replaced by an abscess (Figure 40). There was evidence of cerebral herniation with bilateral uncal grooving and necrotic tonsils. The pons was soft. The spinal cord was grossly normal.

Microscopic Description

Sections of the heart showed bilateral myocyte hypertrophy. The aorta had focal fibrous plaque and subendothelial degeneration with increased basophilic ground substance. All lobes of the lungs showed extensive bronchopneumonia with hemorrhage and associated bronchiolitis. Fungal stain revealed pseudohyphal forms in the upper lobes consistent with Candida species. The most significant finding was present in the pulmonary arteries. The small pulmonary arteries showed variable degrees of intimal hyperplasia with thickening of the media. Some vessels had evidence of complete luminal occlusion with recanalization (Figure 41). Many vessels had reduplication of their elastic lamellae making it very difficult to distinguish bronchial and pulmonary arteries. No bronchopulmonary anastomoses were identified on the sections examined.

The brain abscess showed necrotic tissue surrounded by mild gliosis. No capsule was present. Within the areas of necrosis, many gram positive cocci, some in chains, were seen associated with neutrophils and macrophages. The hippocampus had many hypoxic-ischemic neurons. In the area of the temporal horn, there was focal ventriculitis. In addition, the choroid plexus was denuded of epithelium and revealed numerous bacterial colonies as well as focal necrosis.

Case Analysis

In 1888, Professor Etienne-Louis Arthur Fallot authored a paper entitled, "Contribution 'a L'Anatomie Pathologique de la Maladie Bleue (Cyanose Cardiaque)". It is the blue sickness, or cyanotic heart disease, that is the crux of this case; the particular entity known as **Tetralogy of Fallot** (TOF), which represents the most common of the cyanotic congenital heart diseases. Although Fallot's paper followed prior descriptions of the syndrome by more than 200 years, it is his name that has been associated with the condition. One does not always have to be first to win the battle of the eponyms! It helps to write well and to provide a detailed report; it also helps to have your predecessors forgotten in obscurity.

Fallot detailed all of the characteristics of the syndrome at a period in medical history when interest in heart disease was attaining a new level of sophistication. He described four components (hence, **tetralogy**): 1.

pulmonary outflow tract obstruction; 2. ventricular septal defect; 3. dextroposition of the aorta (or aorta over-riding the ventricular septal defect); and, 4. right ventricular hypertrophy. The TOF has far more complex features than indicated by a simple listing. It also is a syndrome that is virtually never encountered today in adults, except in Third World countries that do not have easy access to open heart surgery. Early surgical repair is common and has a high level of success. Despite the rarity of the disease in adults, a case such as this is instructive at many levels. The following discussion will address many of the embryological, pathophysiological, pathological and clinical issues.

TOF is the most common of the cyanotic congenital heart diseases. This may be in part because it does not lead to intra-uterine fetal demise. There are no significant hemodynamic effects to the fetus, and the disease only becomes manifest after birth. The reasons for this will become obvious as we discuss the pathology and pathophysiology. The primary abnormality in TOF is **obstruction to pulmonary outflow**. The lungs are essentially non-functional *in utero*. There is high pulmonary vascular resistance with shunting of oxygenated blood returning from the placenta through the patent foramen ovale and patent ductus arteriosus into the systemic circulation. Thus, obstruction to right ventricular outflow has no effect. It is only after birth, with a fall in pulmonary vascular resistance and closure of the foramen ovale and the ductus arteriosus that symptoms may develop. Their severity and rapidity of onset depend on several factors to be described. Before we address them, however, we should discuss the embryology to better understand why the tetralogy has four components.

TOF develops as a result of a defective **bulbus cordis**, which is the most cranial portion of the primitive cardiac tube. It participates in separation of the aorta and pulmonary arteries, the formation of the ventricular septum, and the organization of the right ventricular outflow tract. An abnormal bulbus cordis at 5-7 weeks of fetal development leads to inappropriate septation of the **truncus arteriosus**, the common artery leading from the cardiac tube. If the spiral septum in the truncus is shifted toward the right, the pulmonary artery may be hypoplastic (if the shift is partial) or atretic (if the shift is complete). At the same time, since the bulbus is involved with the development of the membranous septum, its failure leads to a high ventricular septal defect. With the aorta now shifted rightward, it results in the dextroposition of the aorta over the interventricular septum immediately superior to the membranous septal defect, with blood from both right and left ventricular chambers mixing and entering the aorta. Thus, after birth, there is a venous-arterial shunt with oxygen de-saturated blood mixing with oxygenated blood. If the pulmonary artery is atretic, then the only exodus for right ventricular blood is through the ventricular septum. The bulbus also affects the development of the infundibulum (the region below the pulmonic

140

valve), and the pulmonary valve itself. Accordingly, defects associated with tetralogy may include infundibular stenosis, valvular stenosis or atresia, pulmonary artery hypoplasia or atresia, or combinations. In the case being discussed, there was pulmonic valve and pulmonary artery atresia. Finally, the fourth component of the tetralogy is right ventricular hypertrophy. This results from increased right ventricular work secondary to increased resistance at the level of the outflow tract (if it is stenotic), and pumping against systemic pressure in the left ventricle. Characteristically, since the left ventricular volume is decreased due to less blood returning from the lungs (see below), the left ventricle is generally not hypertrophied. The total mass of the lungs may be normal, or at most moderately increased; however, most of the increase is from the right ventricle.

The question arises as to how blood reaches the lungs post-natally? If there is stenosis and/or hypoplasia of the infundibulum, valve, or artery, a decreased volume of blood will be ejected into the pulmonary artery. With time, the stenosis may remain static, or as the heart grows disproportionately to the stenotic outflow tract, it may increase in relative severity. A progressive, but slower course of obstruction may permit collateral circulation to develop to partially compensate for the decreasing flow of blood through the outflow tract. If the ductus arteriosus remains patent, this serves as a conduit. In most cases, however, the ductus closes over weeks to months after birth. If that occurs, then flow to the lungs is entirely dependent on collateral supply. The bronchial arteries arising in the aorta rapidly enlarge. The bronchial vessels in the pulmonary parenchyma anastomose with the pulmonary vessels, thus permitting some flow to reach the lungs for oxygenation. Other collaterals may also participate, including intercostal arteries and the internal mammary arteries. If the ductus arteriosus closes rapidly after birth in the setting of complete outflow tract obstruction, then either collaterals open rapidly, or death occurs. In this patient, since the ductus was closed and with complete valvular and pulmonary artery atresia, all blood supply to the lungs was through large bronchial arteries from the descending aorta. In some cases, because pressure in the right atrium may be higher than that in the left atrium, the foramen ovale remains open, thereby providing another pathway for de-oxygenated blood to reach the systemic circulation. If there is either a true atrial septal defect due to a defective formation of the atrial septum, or an acquired type of defect through a patent foramen ovale, the addition of an atrial septal defect to the four components of the tetralogy has been called Pentalogy of Fallot.

The first surgery performed for the palliation of TOF in 1945, the Blalock-Taussig operation, was an attempt to artificially create a collateral blood supply to the lungs by anastomosing the left subclavian artery to the pulmonary artery. Another early collateralization approach was the Potts anastomosis, with a surgical window between the aorta and pulmonary artery.

Until the advent of open heart surgery in the 1950's, these procedures permitted prolonged survival until the 3rd and 4th decades. These operations are still employed as temporizing measures until the baby reaches a sufficient size to allow for definitive surgical repair without significant increasing operative mortality. Alternatively, in cases where there is only partial outflow tract obstruction, immediate definitive repair can be undertaken.

The signs and symptoms of TOF are dependent on the severity of the anatomical outflow tract obstruction. There are 3 groups of patients:

1. Babies who are cyanotic at birth, usually associated with the most severe obstruction of the right ventricular outflow. Because there is generally complete atresia or marked hypoplasia of the valve and/or artery, there is no systolic murmur, or if there is one, it is of low intensity. These babies suffer anoxic spells, and they die within a short time, unless the ductus arteriosus remains open and/or collateral circulation develops rapidly, or there is surgical intervention. As collateral flow increases, there may be a continuous murmur auscultated over the left chest.

2. The most common type of TOF is the one in which cyanosis develops after one month of age, and increases in intensity during the first year of life. These babies generally have outflow tract stenosis. Accordingly, they have a loud systolic murmur, and they may not have continuous murmur of collateral flow. Anoxic spells may not occur until months after birth. Other signs and symptoms develop as they begin to ambulate. Without surgery, these infants survived until the 2nd or 3rd decades, and their death was usually secondary to stroke or congestive heart failure. Today, the natural history has been markedly improved with surgical intervention. However, with increasing numbers of adults living into their 4th and 5th decades and beyond, after TOF surgical repair in infancy or childhood; there have been reports of significant late cardiac dysfunction secondary to a cardiomyopathy. The cardiomyopathy may even occur at an early age. Late deaths and cardiac transplantations for ventricular failure have occurred.

3. The 3rd type of tetralogy generally does not become cyanotic until after one year of age. These have been referred to as 'acyanotic or pink TOF'. They have less severe stenosis of the outflow tract, and with reduced pulmonary vascular resistance the pulmonary blood flow is adequate to prevent immediate cyanosis. They may not have anoxic episodes. Symptoms, however, do increase with age, and particularly with exercise. At rest they may not be dyspneic, but with exercise they may develop shortness of breath and cyanosis. This may also be exacerbated with cold weather. They do not have

significant polycythemia. Without surgery they may survive until the 2nd to the 4th decade of life.

The general signs and symptoms include paroxysmal episodes of **dyspnea on exertion**, and **syncope** particularly associated with exercise. The infants and children have **central cyanosis**. They characteristically often **squat**, following minimal exercise. This posture is spontaneous; and it is thought to result from an attempt to maximize central blood flow to the lungs by decreasing blood flow to the legs and increasing venous return to the heart. With age and more severe cyanosis, the red blood cell mass increases, leading to **secondary polycythemia**. Hematocrits of 65 to 70 vol.% or higher are possible, although there are consequences to this compensatory mechanism (discussed below). Also secondary to the oxygen de-saturation (and possibly the intra-pulmonary collateral circulation) is the development of **clubbing**. Clubbing is a growth of connective tissue and thickening of periosteal bone at the junction between the nail and soft tissue of the fingers and toes. It is not unique to TOF, but occurs in other cyanotic heart diseases, as well as in association with lung disease (particularly carcinoma) and cirrhosis. Although hormonal stimulation and blood flow phenomena have been implicated, the etiology remains unknown.

There are signs of the condition that may be evident. Today, the diagnosis is easily made with echocardiogram. In the past, clinicians depended on chest X-ray, electrocardiogram, and ultimately ventricular angiography. The chest X-ray typically demonstrates hypoperfused lung fields. The heart may not be enlarged, but if so it is the right ventricle that increases the cardiac silhouette. The pulmonary artery segment, below the aortic knob, is either absent or decreased in prominence; depending on whether the artery is hypoplastic or atretic. The result of a prominent right ventricle and an absent pulmonary artery segment gives rise to a **boot-shaped heart**, or **coeur en sabot**. The ECG shows right axis deviation, and enlarged R waves in the right precordial leads. The degree of right ventricular hypertrophy is dependent on the degree of stenosis. On auscultation, in addition to the murmurs described above, there is a decreased second heart sound without splitting.

An unusual physical finding, virtually never seen any more because of surgical intervention, is the development of hemi-atrophy of the body. The atrophy occurs opposite the side in which the aorta arches. In other words, the normal side would be the left, if there were a normal left-sided aortic arch. Since another associated finding seen in TOF, which we have not discussed, is the presence of a right aortic arch (up to 30% of cases), the hemi-atrophy would be on the left side, with the right side normal. The condition can be diagnosed clinically with this finding alone. Obviously, on chest X-ray or echocardiography the anomaly can be confirmed. The etiology is not understood.

The complications of tetralogy have been altered by surgical intervention, but now include the late-onset cardiomyopathy and heart failure as described above. Complications include sudden death secondary to prolonged anoxic spells. Other complications are directly related to the flow across the ventricular septal defect, and flow across a stenotic pulmonary outflow tract. Thus, endocarditis may occur, particularly in regions of turbulent high velocity flow. A particular complication associated with right to left shunt, characteristic of tetralogy but not unique, is the development of cerebral abscess. This was the cause of death in our patient. Cerebral abscess is a result of flow from the right-sided circulation with organisms from the intestinal tract and elsewhere, which cross the membranous septum and gain access to the systemic circulation. It has been suggested that the decreased filtering of organisms by the hypoperfused lungs contributes to this complication. It is also possible that infected emboli may pass paradoxically across the septum and directly travel to the brain. Cerebral infection may also occur as a result of secondary bacterial seeding of bland cerebral thrombi.

Cerebral and other organ thrombi are common in tetralogy as a result of the polycythemia. Thus, thrombotic, non-infectious strokes may occur. The increased red blood cell mass enhances thrombogenesis, particularly when the hematocrit is greater than 70 vol.%. At this level, there is sludging of flow, and also decreased capillary flow with secondary local tissue ischemia. It is also important to recognize that there may be relative anemia in these children, even with hematocrits of 40 vol.%, and hemoglobin of 10-13 g/dL. These levels, though normal for children without cyanotic heart disease, are distinctly abnormal for children with TOF. Iron deficiency may be an important contributing factor.

As discussed earlier, this case is extremely unusual in this era of aggressive surgical intervention. It is unknown why she was not surgically repaired, although there was speculation that it had to do with her mental retardation and placement in foster homes. She had severe pulmonary outflow tract obstruction with atresia of the valve and the artery. The ductus arteriosus was closed. Thus, the only blood supply to her lungs was through the very large bronchial arteries that extended to both sides. She did not have a murmur upon admission, although admittedly since she was in a terminal state secondary to her cerebral infection and septicemia, the cardiac contraction may not have been sufficient to generate one. She had no splitting of the second heart sound. She had clubbing, cyanosis, and polycythemia. There was moderate cardiac hypertrophy, with both right ventricular hypertrophy and mild dilatation. She died secondary to a cerebral abscess, with changes that were subacute consistent with a duration of days to several weeks. The abscess demonstrated gram-positive cocci that eventually grew

144

gamma-hemolytic streptococcus. In addition, she had ventriculitis and meningitis, and the extensive cerebral infection led to cerebral edema and herniation. She also had bronchopneumonia. The lungs demonstrated multiple thrombi, with organization and recanalization. The latter, is another common finding in tetralogy that may contribute to late deterioration of right ventricular function due to increasing pulmonary vascular resistance, even in those patients without severe obstruction. Her survival to age 28 is fairly characteristic of TOF as an overall group (without surgery), but distinctly rare with the type of complete outflow obstruction she had. The survival can only be attributed to the large size of the bronchial collateral vessels that produced a spontaneous shunt comparable to a Blalock-Taussig anastomosis.

Suggested Readings

1. Friedman WF, Silverman N. "Congenital Heart Disease in Infancy and Childhood". In Braunwald: Heart Disease: A Textbook of Cardiovascular Medicine. Sixth ed. Braunwald E, Zipes DP, and Libby P eds. W. B. Saunders Company, 2001

2. Deanfield JE, Gersh BJ, Warnes CA, Mair DD. "Congenital heart disease in adults". In Hurt's The Heart. Ninth Edition. Alexander WR, Schlant RC, and Fuster V eds. McGraw-Hill Co, Inc., 1998

3. Hokanson JS, Moller JH. Adults with tetralogy of Fallot: long-term follow-up. Cardiol Rev. 1999; 7:149-55.

4. McNamara DG. The adult with congenital heart disease. Curr Probl Cardiol. 1989; 14:57-114.

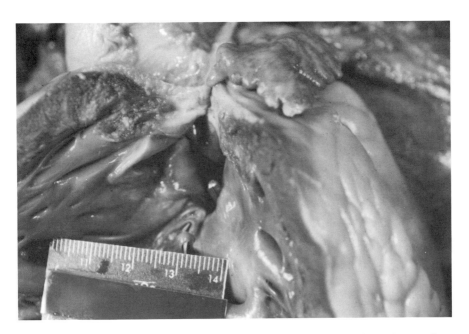

Figure 38. Tetralogy of Fallot. Large ventricular septal defect (VSD). The probe is peeking through the VSD and the aortic valve.

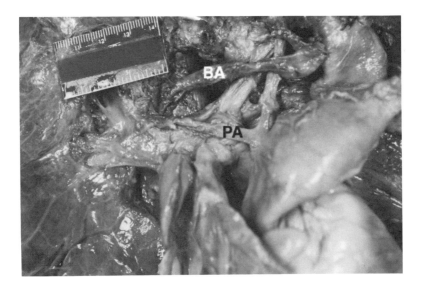

Figure 39. Tetralogy of Fallot. Hypolastic pulmonary arteries (pa) and prominent bronchial arteries (ba) originating from descending aorta.

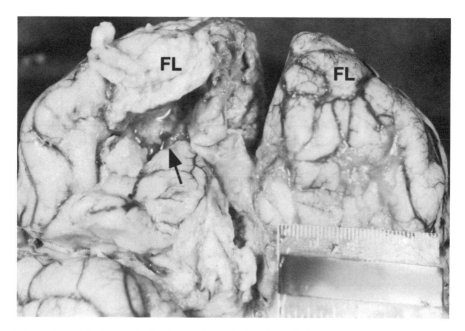

Figure 40. Right frontal brain abscess (arrow) (FL frontal lobes)

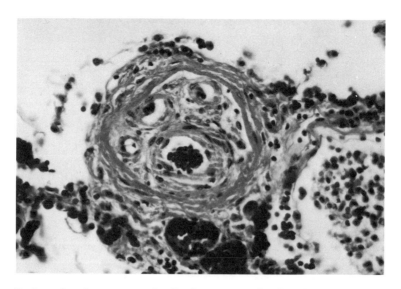

Figure 41. Lung, histologic section. Small pulmonary vessel with evidence of organized thrombosis with recanalization (Hematoxylin and Eosin, 40X)

Case # 16

Clinical Summary

This was a 74 year old female with several medical problems including adult onset diabetes mellitus, hypothyroidism treated with thyroxine, congestive hear failure and one transient cerebral ischemic attack without residual deficit. She was partially deaf and required a left hearing aid. Her body habitus and primary amenorrhea suggested Turner's syndrome, and a buccal smear performed several years before demonstrated 4% Barr bodies consistent with Turner's mosaicism. The patient was admitted to the hospital with signs and symptoms of CHF. She experienced somnolence, increasing dyspnea and pedal edema for several weeks. On admission, her vital signs were BP 100/86mm Hg, P 80, irregular; RR 20, and T 37°C. Significant findings on her physical exam included webbed neck, jugular venous distension, bilateral carotid bruits and delayed upstroke of the carotid pulsations, fullness in the anterior neck; wide-spaced nipples; normal S1 and S2, S4, a III/VI systolic ejection murmur at the aortic area, and a III/VI holosystolic murmur at the apex and left sternal border radiating to the axilla. The extremities showed 3+ edema and 2+ pulses throughout. The abdominal and neurologic exams were normal.

Laboratory data and other tests

Laboratory: WBC 14.1, Hb/Hct 13/38, Plt 240. CXR: cardiomegaly, bilateral pleural effusions and congestive changes. ECG: 120/min, paroxysmal atrial tachycardia (PAT), axis at 90°, right bundle branch block (RBBB).

The patient was treated with furosemide and digoxin, and remained relatively stable until the fourth day post-admission, when she developed agonal respirations and died.

Gross Description

The body measured 122 cm in length and weighed 52 kg. In addition to short stature, the external exam revealed webbed neck, wide spaced nipples, underdeveloped clitoris, sacral and lower extremity edema and kyphoscoliosis. The pleural cavities contained 1.0 L each of straw-colored fluid. The pericardial sac contained also 30 cc of clear yellow fluid. The heart weighed 400 g with concentric hypertrophy and dilatation of the left ventricle (wall thickness 1.8 cm, normal up to 1.5 cm). The right ventricle wall measured 0.5 cm. The papillary muscles were hypertrophied and the myocardium showed fibrosis of the left ventricular wall with no acute changes. The aortic valve was bicuspid, and the aortic cusps were thickened with calcifications (Figure 42). The chordae tendineae were slightly thickened in the mitral valve. The coronary arteries showed focal atherosclerosis with less than 50% luminal narrowing. There was a circumferential ridge in the aortic wall, just distal to the ligamentum arteriosus, with a large ulcerative plaque distal to the ridge. The intercostal arteries were not dilated. The lungs and liver were congested. The only other significant autopsy finding was the absence of normal thyroid tissue. A curved band of fibrous tissue was in the normal position of the gland with the major portion occupying the midline (isthmus) region.

Microscopic Description

The left ventricle showed marked myocellular hypertrophy, focal myocardial fibrosis and myocytolysis. Sections from the lungs and liver confirmed the presence of acute and chronic congestive changes. The thyroid was markedly fibrotic with scattered nests of atrophic follicles and a prominent interstitial lymphocytic infiltrate.

Case Analysis

This complex patient presented with what appeared to be fairly rapidly progressive congestive heart failure (CHF) over several months, of unclear etiology. She was admitted to the hospital, but then suffered a sudden and unexpected cardiac arrest. The questions are: 1. Based on the clinical findings, can we develop a list of differential diagnoses, any one or a combination that might explain her course?; and 2. With the addition of the pathology results, can we pin down a specific etiology for her CHF and demise?

What do we know objectively? She was an older woman who had presented initially with dyspnea and pulmonary congestion. Dyspnea, or an increased sense of discomfort breathing (likely associated with exercise), and pulmonary congestion (either rales or radiographic findings of increased vascular markings), are signs and symptoms of left-sided heart failure. To cause pulmonary venous and capillary congestion, she probably had increased end-diastolic pressure in the left ventricle, and elevated filling pressures in the left atrium. If this was the result of ischemic heart disease, which would be the most likely etiology in a woman in her 8th decade of life? Although she did not have any complaints that might suggest ischemia, she also was diabetic and may have had 'silent' ischemia. In addition, there was a history of one event 4 years prior consistent with a transient cerebral ischemic attack

(TIA), which often is associated with platelet aggregates developing in the carotid or cerebral vessels, generally secondary to atherosclerosis. Thus, she almost certainly had some element of systemic atherosclerotic disease, possibly affecting the coronary arteries. On the other hand, a relatively rapid progression of congestive symptoms, in the absence of an acute myocardial infarction, would not be explained entirely by coronary artery ischemia. Moreover, we have no evidence of such an event; however, she might have had prior myocardial damage with decompensation of an ischemic heart. Yet, we do not know what her cardiac function was, and specifically as to whether she had a poorly contracting dilated heart. But certainly, cardiomyopathy with decompensation, and coronary artery disease with atherosclerosis, must be considered in the differential diagnosis.

In regard to cardiomyopathy, she progressed from apparent left-sided to right-sided heart failure, when pedal edema developed. The most frequent cause of right-sided heart failure is left-sided compromise. A dysfunctional and poorly contracting left heart, leads to pulmonary congestion, and volume and pressure overload of the right ventricle. In spite of this, cardiomyopathy of various etiologies may directly affect right heart function, secondary to the generalized damage of the right ventricular myocardium, and right atrial wall. Ischemia is usually not a common cause of such damage. Based on the patient's history, are there other possible causes for cardiomyopathy? There are at least two. She was diabetic, and she was hypothyroid.

Diabetic cardiomyopathy must be considered, but it does not appear to be a likely explanation. It has been discussed in case #7. For one thing, she had had adult-onset Type II diabetes for only 6 years, and she was not even being treated with medication. Secondly, cardiomyopathy usually develops in diabetic patients of more than 10 years, and generally in those who are not controlled solely by diet. Lastly, it is most commonly seen in diabetics who are also hypertensive, and there was no evidence of hypertension during her prior evaluations. Therefore, diabetic cardiomyopathy should not be a diagnosis high on our list.

What about hypothyroidism? Does it cause cardiomyopathy? The answer is yes. In fact, both hyperthyroidism and hypothyroidism can cause cardiac dysfunction and congestive heart failure, although through two distinctly different mechanisms. Hyperthyroid disease is associated with tachycardia and elevated catecholamines, which may lead to multiple foci of myocardial cell necrosis (e.g. myocytolysis). Clinically, hyperthyroidism may cause high-output heart failure, but mostly in patients with pre-existing heart disease. Atrial fibrillation is common, usually with a rapid ventricular response. The high-output state is secondary to the tachycardia, which together with peripheral vasodilatation and decreased afterload, increases stroke volume but results in poor organ perfusion (similar to an arteriovenous fistula). Tachycardia may reduce diastolic filling time, and compromise

151

coronary blood flow, thus leading to angina pectoris. Furthermore, persistent tachycardia can lead to a remodeling of the left ventricle, with mural thinning and ventricular cavity dilation. However, hyperthyroid patients usually present because of the rapid heart rate or chest pain, before the left ventricle changes occur. An additional effect of increased thyroid hormone, is its function as a protein synthesis promoter that may stimulate myocyte hypertrophy, and ultimately ventricular hypertrophy, independent of hypertension. However, this effect alone is not sufficient to account for the development of heart failure.

Hypothyroidism leads to cardiomyopathy through different mechanisms. There is often associated hypertension and left ventricular hypertrophy. The hypothyroid state elevates low density lipoproteins (LDL) cholesterol, and may lead to accelerated atherosclerosis. Thus, in addition to the metabolic effects of hypothyroidism, there may be an element of coronary artery ischemia. The hypothyroid heart has increased sensitivity to catecholamines, which may lead to small areas of myocyte necrosis and subsequent fibrosis. The pathogenesis of hypothyroid cardiomyopathy is the result of leakage of myxoid glycoprotein into vessel walls and into the interstitium of the heart, similar to the development of myxedema in the skin and subcutaneous tissue. There is also a metabolic intracellular effect, with the accumulation of myocyte sarcoplasmic inclusions. This condition has been termed 'basophilic degeneration of the heart', because the material stains blue with hematoxylin (Figure 43). The inclusions are a glycoprotein, identical to the interstitial and cutaneous material. It stains strongly with periodic acid-Schiff (PAS stain), but it is not digested with diastase, thereby indicating that it is not glycogen. Although its metabolic effects are unknown, it is thought to damage the contractile apparatus of the cell. One additional non-cardiomyopathic consequence of hypothyroidism that may lead to heart failure, is the leakage of proteinaceous fluid into the pericardial sac which may progress to tamponade. The fluid leaks as a result of altered permeability of lymphatic and venular vessels, and increased venous pressure secondary to heart failure. The pericardial effusion is unique, and post-percardiocentesis, its gross examination can be used to diagnose hypothyroidism: The fluid has gold flecks floating in it, which represent cholesterol crystals. This is one of those increasingly rare situations in medicine, where a complex disease can be diagnosed by simple observation (with no requirement for CT scan, MRI, or echocardiogram!!).

This patient was hypothyroid, a common association with Turner's syndrome (a subject to which we will return shortly), as a result of autoimmune thyroiditis (Hashimoto's disease), present in up to 20% of affected individuals. Although she was chronically treated with thyroid replacement hormone (thyroxine), she may have been non-adherent and stopped taking her thyroid medication along with diuretic and digitalis. Also, her requirements for the hormone may have changed. If hypothyroid patients become increasingly out of control, there may be infiltration of glycoprotein into the intestinal wall, which may impair drug absorption, thus setting up a vicious circle. We certainly should consider a metabolic etiology for this woman's progressive and acute heart failure; on the other hand, except for the presence of somnolence for several days prior to admission, there were no obvious findings referable to hypothyroidism (e.g. thin and fragile hair, myxedema, enlarged tongue, etc.). Since somnolence may be related itself to CHF, another etiology besides hypothyroidism should be considered.

This woman had Turner's syndrome, a relatively rare (1/2500) condition, with 25% of Turner's patients having mosaicism (46XX/45X). This results from chromosome loss during gametogenesis in either parent, or from a mitotic error during early zygote division. This woman's 4% Barr bodies on buccal smear, together with the phenotypic features of Turner's syndrome, is indicative of a mosaic genotype. Barr bodies derive from inactivation of one of the two X chromosomes (so-called lyonization, after Dr. Mary Lyon who described the phenomenon); therefore a genotypic Turner's syndrome individual with 45X would have no Barr bodies. Though the phenotype of mosaic Turner's syndrome is variable, this patient had many characteristic features of the condition. She had primary amenorrhea, short stature, webbed neck, wide-spaced nipples, deafness, and hypothyroidism. She also had cardiovascular disease; the question is whether any of her cardiac findings were related to Turner's syndrome.

There are a number of cardiovascular anomalies associated with Turner's syndrome (see Table 2). Although coarctation of the aorta is the most common defect, it may variably narrow the aortic lumen (Figure 44). Slight narrowing produces no hemodynamic changes. More significant stenosis may be associated with upper extremity hypertension, lower extremity hypotension, weak femoral pulses, and rib-notching (secondary to enlarged intercostal arteries that serve as collateral supply around the obstruction, and lead to erosion of costal bone along its inferior surface) (Figure 45). She had no clinical findings consistent with a marked coarctation. She did have an aortic murmur (III/VI systolic ejection murmur at the base) consistent with aortic stenosis, which may be secondary to degeneration of a bicuspid aortic valve associated with Turner's syndrome (described below). The III/VI holosystolic murmur was most likely due to mitral or tricuspid valve regurgitation, secondary to ventricular failure and annular dilatation, rather than a structural valve lesion. With ventricular dilatation and remodeling, the coaptation of the mitral and/or tricuspid valve leaflets is affected. The leaflets are separated, and the papillary muscles are splayed outward. Thus, during systole, the leaflets no longer close completely, and there is leakage of blood into the atria ("incompetency vs. insufficiency").

153

Aortic stenosis can arise as a result of a bicuspid aortic valve (Figure 46). This is a condition that can occur as an isolated anomaly, or one associated with coarctation of the aorta. As we have seen, patients with Turner's syndrome may have coarctation of the aorta and bicuspid valve along with a number of other skeletal and cardiovascular anomalies. The role of the X chromosome, and hormonal stimulation leading to development of the aorta and aortic valve is unknown. Additionally, since coarctation and bicuspid valve can occur in either sex, hormonal or X chromosomal determination may only be incidental.

Bicuspid aortic valve may become stenotic and clinically symptomatic at a much earlier age, than stenosis occurring secondary to calcification and degeneration of the normal 3 cuspid valves. The latter, generally termed calcific aortic stenosis (of the elderly), usually presents in the 7th decade or later. It has been considered to be a complication of atherosclerosis, but there is little to support that suggestion. It is of unknown etiology and pathogenesis. There is some recent interest in the possibility that it represents the results of a chronic infection of the valve tissues; but the evidence is controversial and not very strong. For one thing, it is not just the valve that is damaged; the initial site of calcification and degeneration occurs within the sinuses of Valsalva. It presents as nodular accumulations of calcium apatite and debris, which then may progressively spread to the aortic surfaces of the cusps. In contrast, most inflammatory and infectious valvular complications affect the ventricular surfaces of the cusps and then spread to the commissures that insert in the aortic wall. The stenosis associated with calcific aortic valve disease tends to be less severe than stenosis secondary to rheumatic inflammation, which invariably leads to scarring and fusion of the commissures. The pathophysiologic reason for the former condition, is that the primary degeneration is in the sinus of Valsalva and along the aortic surface of the valve, with some sparing of the commissures. Therefore, relative lack of commissural fusion allows for greater cusp excursion and less obstruction to outflow.

Aortic disease associated with bicuspid valve often presents as early as the 2nd or 3rd decades, and may be significantly symptomatic. The bicuspid valve is anatomically and hemodynamically abnormal. There is asymmetry of the two cusps, with a longer one, often partially divided by an incomplete commissure (known as a raphe), which may extend from the cusp free edge towards the aortic wall. The asymmetry of the cusps leads to inappropriate coaptation (e.g. the cusps close irregularly with buckling at the closing edges of the cusps), and outflow tract turbulence. It has been suggested that the abnormal closure and turbulence leads to endocardial cell injury, small vegetations on the cusp surfaces, and connective tissue breakdown. With time, there is dystrophic calcification of the vegetations and the cuspal tissue. Eventually, the cusps become stiff and calcified, with inadequate opening

154

during systole, or closure during diastole. Following the development of aortic stenosis and insufficiency, these valves require replacement with a prosthesis at a relatively young age. Alternatively, they may lead to ventricular failure (both diastolic and systolic, due to left ventricular hypertrophy, and strain on the ventricle with significant remodeling, hypertrophy and fibrosis), angina pectoris (due to increased left ventricular wall strain associated with left ventricular hypertrophy, and inadequate coronary perfusion), or sudden death (due to lethal arrhythmia).

This woman's presentation is consistent with relatively rapid ventricular decompensation due to aortic stenosis. In contrast to mitral valve disease, which presents early and is poorly tolerated, aortic stenosis is well tolerated for prolonged periods. The explanation is related to the ability of the left ventricle to hypertrophy to compensate for outflow tract narrowing. Although aortic stenosis may present in young patients when associated with bicuspid valve, it can be delayed until the 7th or 8th decade, similar to aortic stenosis occurring with a 3 cuspid valve (calcific aortic stenosis of the elderly). Of course, her other medical conditions including diabetes mellitus and hypothyroidism, may have contributed to her presentation with CHF, but a relatively sudden ventricular decompensation is more likely. Unfortunately, once such a decompensation occurs, the ability to stabilize or reverse the condition with drug therapy is very limited. Furthermore, the development of a sudden fatal cardiac arrhythmia is a common outcome. It is for this reason, that early evidence of ventricular decompensation due to aortic stenosis is considered by some cardiologists to be a surgical emergency. By the time this patient presented to the hospital, however, she had already progressed too far, and she was not a surgical candidate.

Thus, the cause of death in this patient with multiple medical problems, appears to be secondary to her genetic condition, with phenotypic manifestation of a bicuspid aortic valve and aortic valve stenosis. The autopsy was, in fact, confirmatory. She had an enlarged heart, bicuspid aortic valve, aortic stenosis, and ventricular dilatation consistent with remodeling and decompensation. She had evidence of congestive heart failure with pleural effusions, hepatic and pulmonary congestion, both acute and chronic, and peripheral edema. She had chronic thyroiditis. A minimal pre-ductal coarctation was present, but it was of no significance. Microscopic examination revealed evidence of myocardial fibrosis, but no changes consistent with hypothyroid heart disease.

Table 2: Cardiovascular Anomalies in Turner's Syndrome

1.   Coarctation of the aorta, with or without bicuspid aortic valve
2.   Bicuspid aortic valve with aortic stenosis
3.   Ventricular septal defect
4.   Atrial septal defect
5.   Partial anomalous pulmonary venous drainage without ASD
6.   Dextrocardia

Suggested Readings

1. Elsheikh M, Conway GS, Wass JA. Medical problems in adult women with Turner's syndrome. Ann Med. 1999; 31:99-105.
2. Ward C. Clinical significance of the bicuspid aortic valve. Heart. 2000; 83:81-5.
3. Saenger P. Turner's syndrome. N Engl J Med. 1996; 335:1749-54.
4. Van der Hauwaert LG, Fryns JM, Dumoulin M, Logghe N. Cardiovascular Malformations in Turner's and Noonan's Syndrome. Br Heart J. 1978; 40:500-9.

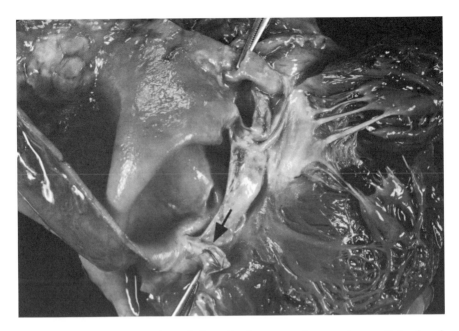

Figure 42. Bicuspid aortic valve. The heart has been opened to reveal two well developed aortic cusps. The third cusp is rudimentary (arrow).

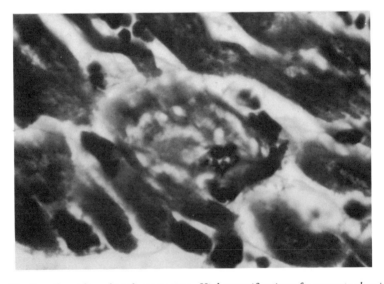

Figure 43. Hypothyroidism, histologic section. High magnification of a myocyte showing basophilic degeneration of the cytoplasm (Hematoxylin and Eosin, 100X).

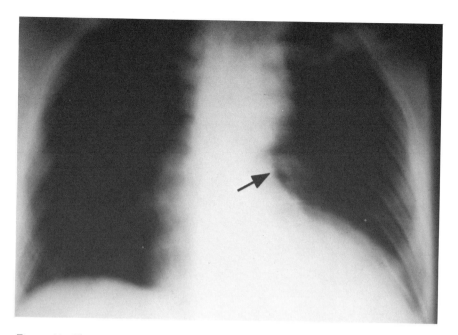

Figure 44. Chest-x-ray, frontal view, showing post-ductal coarctation of the aorta (arrow).

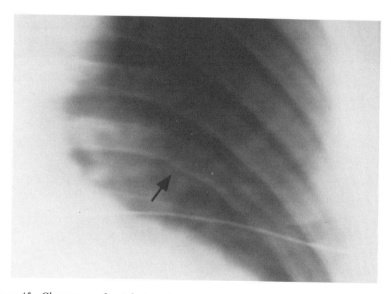

Figure 45. Chest-x-ray, frontal view, showing rib notching (arrow) in a patient with coarctation of the aorta.

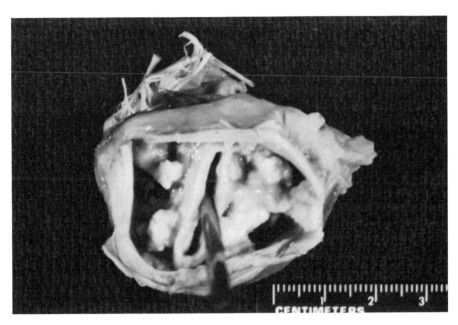

Figure 46. Resected biscuspid aortic valve with calcifications of the cusps and within the sinuses of Valsalva..

160

Case # 17

Clinical Summary

The patient was a 52 year old woman with past medical history significant for morbid obesity (205 kg), cigarette smoking with chronic obstructive pulmonary disease (COPD), and cor pulmonale. She was on oxygen therapy at home for the past 7 months. She presented to the hospital with complaints of increasing weight gain, abdominal and lower extremity edema with pruritus and skin ulcers. She had no fever, chills, cough, dysuria, chest pain or palpitations. She denied any trauma to her legs. Her breathing was at baseline and she denied any acute shortness of breath.

Her physical exam on admission revealed vital signs: BP 100/70, HR 72, RR 16, T 37°C. Morbidly obese woman, with oxygen, resting comfortably in bed. Skin: bilateral lower extremities erythema with multiple vesicular lesions (<1 cm in diameter). HEENT: unremarkable, no evidence of jaundice or conjunctival pallor. Neck: jugular venous distension (JVD), but no bruit. Heart: regular rhythm, S1S2 no S3 or S4, no murmurs appreciated. Lungs: expiratory wheeze without crackles or rales. Abdomen: globulous, positive bowel sounds, abdominal wall edema, skin dimpling, soft, and non-tender. Extremities: bilateral pitting edema (+++).

Laboratory data and other tests

Laboratory: WBC 7.7, Hb/Hct 17/55, Plt 186; bilirubin T/D 9.1/5.5, LD 378, BUN/creat 20/1.3, glucose 88, cholesterol 173, CO_2 37, Ca 9.7; PT/PTT 14/29. ECG: NSR, right axis deviation, tachycardia (107), and RVH. CXR: cardiomegaly. An echocardiogram showed no pericardial effusion, normal LV systolic function, moderate to severe tricuspid regurgitation, severe pulmonary hypertension (RSVP 70 mmHg), dilated RV and RA.

She was aggressively diuresed with IV furosemide to treat her right heart failure. She was also treated for skin and soft tissue infection with IV antibiotics. Despite the therapy, the patient continued to have signs of worsening cor pulmonale with increased shortness of breath and lethargy. Ten days after admission, she was found apneic and pulseless.

Gross Description

The body weighed 205 kg, and measured 2 m (BMI > 50, indicating massive obesity). The heart weighed 760 g. The pericardium was smooth and contained 100 cc of serous fluid. The right atrium was significantly dilated. Both right and left ventricles were dilated and hypertrophied (wall thickness 0.7 and 1.3 cm, respectively). The valve ring measurements were as follows: tricuspid 13, mitral 10, pulmonic 8.5, and aortic 7 cm. The cusps and chordae tendineae were slender and pliable. The myocardium was not discolored or scarred. The coronaries showed mild atherosclerosis. The most significant finding in the heart was the presence of a **patent ductus arteriosus** (Figures 47 and 48)

Each of the pleural cavities contained 200 cc of serous fluid. The lungs weighed 1600 g combined. Their cut surfaces showed diffuse congestion but no discrete lesions were noted. Intimal plaques were seen in the pulmonary vessels. Upon entering the abdominal cavity, 4 L of serous ascitic fluid were obtained. The liver was congested and fatty (2800 g). The kidneys weighed 400 g combined, with no identifiable lesions. The brain was unremarkable.

Microscopic Description

H&E stained sections from the cardiovascular system revealed perivascular fibrosis, fat infiltration of the myocardium, myocyte hypertrophy, and mild atherosclerosis of the aorta and coronary arteries. Severe plexogenic arteriopathy was noted in the pulmonary vessels. Numerous hemosiderin-laden macrophages consistent with chronic alveolar hemorrhage, were present in association with the damaged vessels. The plexogenic changes were better appreciated with the elastin stain. These changes included medial hypertrophy, intimal proliferation and fibrosis, obliteration of the lumen and branching of the vessels (Figures 49 and 50).

Case Analysis

This is a complex clinical presentation, with several differential diagnoses to consider as the etiology of this patient's severe pulmonary hypertension and right ventricular heart failure. This middle-aged woman was massively obese, and a cigarette smoker with chronic obstructive pulmonary disease (COPD) and oxygen dependence. She had signs of severe hypoxia (pO2 60 mmHg and O2 saturation 85%), hypercapnia (pCO2 60 mmHg), and polycythemia (Hgb 17.4, Hct 55 vol%) indicating that the arterial blood gas findings were chronic. There was no description of cyanosis or peripheral clubbing, but both findings may have been prevented by chronic oxygen therapy. She had elevation of bilirubin and LDH, possibly secondary to liver congestion. There were no findings of pleural effusion or ascites during life, but these may have been obscured by her massive obesity. The latter, and the thickened chest wall, could also have accounted for the

162

lack of appreciation of any cardiac murmurs, as well as the expansion of the chest cavity due to COPD. The question to be addressed is whether either COPD and/or obesity are sufficient explanation for pulmonary hypertension of such severity (mean systolic pressure 70 mmHg), which ultimately led to a sudden cardiac arrhythmia and death.

COPD can certainly cause cor pulmonale, which is right heart failure secondary to pulmonary hypertension. In general, chronic bronchitis, which is associated with bronchiolar and pulmonary vascular sclerosis, leads to pulmonary hypertension more than emphysema. However, since patients with COPD typically have both emphysema and chronic bronchitis, this distinction is not that meaningful. The pulmonary hypertension secondary to COPD is generally moderate in severity. However, it would be very unusual to have pulmonary pressures above 30-40 mmHg, independent of any other condition. Pathologically, this would generally be associated with vascular sclerosis no more than grade II-III in the Heath and Edwards classification (see table 3 and below for a further discussion). We know from the clinical presentation that this patient had virtually systemic levels of pulmonary artery pressure, which makes it very unlikely to be secondary to COPD alone.

Could the massive obesity have been the additional contributing factor to cause such marked pulmonary hypertension? Although it is possible, it is unlikely. Furthermore, the subsequent post-mortem finding of plexogenic lesions in the pulmonary circulation virtually rules out obesity as the etiology. Obesity may have several effects on the cardiovascular system. It has been associated with a dilated congestive cardiomyopathy of uncertain etiology. Partly, the chronic stress of supplying an increased body mass, together with the known association with hypertension, may lead to pathological hypertrophy, and eventual remodeling of the ventricular wall. Contributions from chronic tissue hypoxia may also result in tissue damage. The morbidly obese patient is chronically hypoxic, a condition known as "Pickwickian syndrome", derived from an obese and somnolent character in Dickens' "Pickwick Papers." Due to the massive panniculus there is difficulty in expanding the chest wall, leading to inadequate lung volumes. Moreover, there is increased pulmonary vascular resistance due to localized areas of atelectasis, and eventual pathologic damage to blood vessels with sclerosis. Again, the changes are rarely more than grade II-III, and the pulmonary artery pressures generally do not reach systemic levels. With time, these stresses can progress into marked pressure overload of the right ventricle, with the development of right ventricular hypertrophy, eventual dilatation and right-sided heart failure. However, even with severe COPD combined with morbid obesity, it would be extremely unusual to find pulmonary artery pressures to the level attained by this patient.

The autopsy, unexpectedly, revealed the etiology of the severe pulmonary hypertension. This patient had a patent ductus arteriosus (PDA), which accounted for the plexogenic pulmonary hypertension (PPH, see table 4). This congenital heart defect is a primary cause of pulmonary hypertension at systemic levels. Moreover, plexogenic lesions in the pulmonary vasculature occur in small to medium size vessels, often in association with atherosclerosis in larger vessels (the pulmonary artery is virtually immune from atherosclerosis, except in the presence of severe pulmonary hypertension). The plexogenic lesion is a cluster or conglomeration of small vascular channels, connective tissue, and smooth muscle cell proliferation, which develops in an area of vascular wall damage leading to a psuedoaneurysm. The latter, is an area of vessel wall destruction partially walled-off by surrounding tissue, or by reactive fibrosis if it develops slowly over time. In contrast, a true aneurysm represents a bulge in the actual vessel wall. The plexogenic lesions are often associated with localized tissue hemorrhage (as a result of vessel wall disruption), and they also can be adjacent to diffuse angiomatous dilatation of surrounding thin-walled blood vessels. In the Heath and Edwards classification of pulmonary vascular injury, they represent lesions ranging from grade IV to VI (Table 3).

There are multiple etiologies of plexogenic lesions (Table 4); however, COPD and morbid obesity, even combined, are not usual causes. Of course, one must consider the possibility that a morbidly obese patient may have taken anorexigenic drugs such as fenfluramine-phentermine (Fen-Phen). However, in the presence of a known cause of PPH, such as a PDA, it is not necessary to postulate another etiology: Left-to-right shunts (systemic to pulmonary) are known causes of PPH, due to an increased volume and pressure overloads on the pulmonary vasculature. These lead to increased pulmonary vascular constriction, and eventual damage to the vessel wall. Early in childhood, the functional constriction of the vasculature is transformed into anatomic constriction, with sclerosis and plexogenic lesion formation. The degree and extent of the pathologic damage to the vessels is determined by the size of the left-to-right shunt. Once the plexogenic lesions develop, the condition is irreversible, and it will result in marked right ventricular hypertrophy, and eventually right ventricular failure (e.g. cor pulmonale). With time, the hemodynamic load on the right heart progresses, and a reversal of the shunt may occur, either intermittently or continually. This takes place when the right-sided pressures in the pulmonary artery are equal to or higher than the left-sided pressures in the aorta. This condition is known as "Eisenmenger's syndrome". It is a cyanotic heart condition due to the reversal of blood flow, mixing de-oxygenated blood in the systemic circulation, and is often associated with clubbing (bulbous overgrowth and deformation of the distal phalangeal bone associated with marked chronic de-oxygenation). Based on the absence of cyanosis and clubbing in this patient, it is likely that she had not yet developed the reversed flow through her PDA. She probably had a balanced shunt, where the actual flow through the PDA

164

was limited by the equalization of pressures in the aorta and pulmonary artery, possibly explaining the absence of a murmur. When this occurs, demonstration of a PDA may be difficult by auscultation, since the continuous murmur disappears, and it may be non-visualized with diagnostic techniques such as echocardiogram with Doppler flow evaluation. Altering thoracic vascular resistance through techniques such as the Valsalva maneuver, may elicit a change in flow through the PDA.

The autopsy certainly revealed the severity of her cardiac and pulmonary disease. She had marked cardiomegaly (760 g, normal 350-400 g maximum, even with her obesity), right ventricular hypertrophy, and left ventricular dilatation. In fact, both ventricles were described as dilated and hypertrophied, consistent with the chronic pathology, as well as with the ventricular failure. As a sign of right-sided failure, she had pleural effusions, ascites, and liver congestion. The gross examination of the lungs revealed atherosclerotic plaques in the large pulmonary vessels; however, microscopic examination demonstrated plexogenic lesions in small vessels (these can only be demonstrated microscopically; thus, in suspected clinical cases of PPH, open lung biopsy is required for diagnosis). These lesions are almost certainly the result of the PDA and right-to-left shunt, although there may have been a contribution from her COPD and morbid obesity. It is noteworthy, that PPH is virtually only seen at levels of mean arterial pulmonary pressure of 60-70 mmHg or above. Her sudden death should not have been unexpected; particularly if her physicians knew that she had PPH, which can be an extremely lethal condition with a high prevalence of sudden ventricular arrhythmia. Unfortunately, there is no long-term treatment as vascular dilating agents (e.g. calcium channel blocking drugs and nitric oxide) have only been used to decrease pulmonary vascular resistance acutely. The single accepted therapy when there is severe pulmonary hypertension and cor pulmonale is a heart-lung transplant. Mean survival after this transplant is approximately 2-3 years, although longer survivals are becoming more frequent. The transplantation was not available to the patient because of her morbid obesity, nor was any medical therapy likely to prevent her sudden fatal outcome.

Table 3. Heath and Edwards Classification of Pulmonary Hypertension

I.   Hypertrophy of the media of small muscular pulmonary arteries and arterioles
II   Intimal cellular proliferation and medial smooth muscle hypertrophy
III Advanced medial thickening with hypertrophy and hyperplasia, with luminal narrowing
IV   Focal vascular wall damage of the muscular pulmonary arteries and arterioles with plexiform and angiomatous lesions
V   Widespread occlusive plexiform lesions and angiomatous lesions and hyalinization of intimal fibrosis
VI   Changes as in IV and V with necrotizing vasculitis

Table 4. Etiology of Plexogenic Pulmonary Hypertension

1   Primary pulmonary hypertension (e.g. idiopathic)
2   Congenital heart disease with left-to-right shunts (patent ductus arteriosus, ventricular septal defect, and less frequently atrial septal defect)
3   Cirrhosis
4   HIV/AIDS
5   Anorexigenic drugs (e.g. Fen-Phen)
6   Anti-migraine headache drugs (e.g. methysergide)
7   Chronic residence at high altitude

Suggested Readings

1. Rich S. Pulmonary Hypertension. In Braunwald: Heart Disease: A Textbook of Cardiovascular Medicine. Sixth ed. Braunwald E, Zipes DP, and Libby P eds. W. B. Saunders Company, 2001.
2. Voelkel NF, Tuder RM. Severe pulmonary hypertensive diseases: a perspective. Eur Respir J. 1999; 14:1246-50.
3. Brickner ME, Hillis LD, Lange RA. Congenital heart disease in adults. First of two parts. N Engl J Med. 2000; 342:256-63.
4. Hang CL, Sullebarger JT. Patent ductus arteriosus presenting in old age. Cathet Cardiovasc Diagn. 1993; 28:228-30.
5. Alpert MA. Obesity cardiomyopathy: pathophysiology and evolution of the clinical syndrome. Am J Med Sci. 2001; 321:225-36.
6. Anderson RC, Fagan MJ, Sebastian J. Teaching students the art and science of physical diagnosis. Am J Med. 2001; 110:419-23.
7. Kopelman PG. Obesity as a medical problem. Nature. 2000; 404:635-43.
8. Heath D, Edwards JE: The pathology of hypertensive pulmonary vascular disease: A description of six grades of structural changes in the pulmonary arteries with special reference to congenital cardiac septal defects. Circulation 18:533-547, 1958.

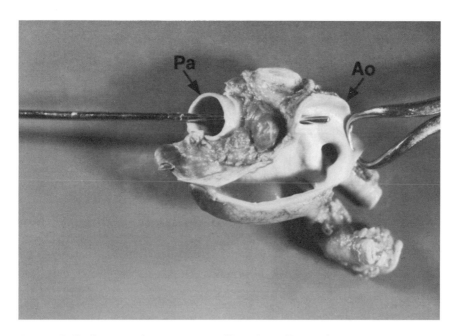

Figure 47. Probe-patent ductus arteriosus (Ao = Aorta, Pa = pulmonary artery).

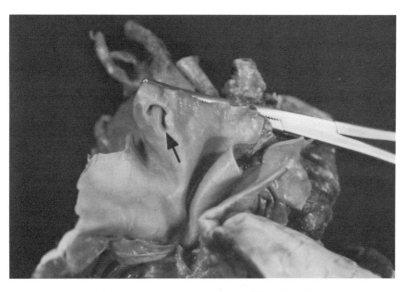

Figure 48. Patent ductus arteriosus (arrow) viewed fom the pulmonary artery.

168

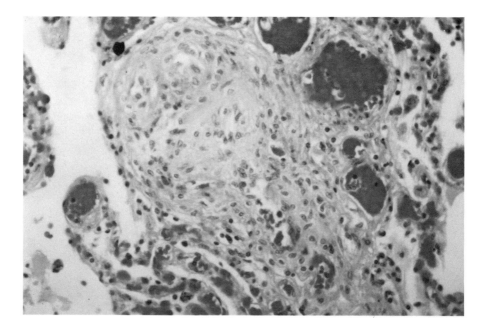

Figure 49. Lung, histologic section. Plexogenic arteriopathy in pulmonary hypertension (Hematoxylin and Eosin, 40X)

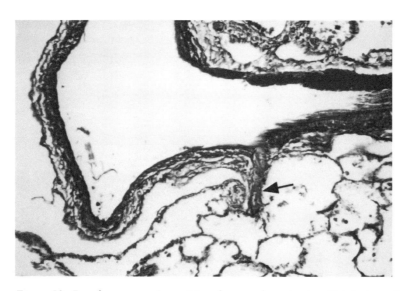

Figure 50. Pseudoaneurysm (arrow) in pulmonary hypertension, histologic section. The internal elastic lamina is disrupted (Elastic stain, 40X).

Chapter 7

ENDOCARDITIS

Case # 18

Clinical Summary

This patient was a 60 year old man with a history of cigarette smoking and alcohol use, who visited his internist with complaints of shortness of breath, intermittent fever, fatigue and weight loss. The physical exam revealed splenomegaly (4 cm below the left costal margin), a holosystolic murmur, and bilateral pulmonary rales. His laboratory tests were significant only for "mild pancytopenia" and hematuria. His liver chemistry was within normal limits. A bone marrow exam was done and reported as reactive. An abdominal CT scan was considered unremarkable except for splenomegaly. The echocardiogram showed mild to moderate mitral valve regurgitation. He was given antibiotics and was referred to a pulmonary specialist and an oncologist with the diagnoses of chronic obstructive pulmonary disease and probable lymphoma.

A few months later, the patient called the paramedics with complaints of severe dyspnea. He was found agitated and in respiratory distress. During transportation to the hospital, the patient became apneic and was intubated. He arrived to the emergency room without vital signs. Defibrillation was attempted several times without success and the patient was pronounced dead.

Gross Description

The body measured 195 cm and weighed 85 kg. The thoracic cavity was unremarkable except for bilateral pleural adhesions. No fluid accumulation was present in the pleural cavities. The heart weighed 610 g. The left atrium was dilated, but free of thrombus. The right and left ventricles measured 0.6 and 1.8 cm in thickness, respectively. The valve leaflets were translucent except those of the mitral valve, which were thick and contained large vegetations. The largest vegetation, located on the anterior leaflet, showed evidence of re-endothelialization on the closing edge along with ulceration and hemorrhage (Figures 51 and 52). The chordae tendineae were short and focally fused. The myocardium was brown-red and of average consistency. The epicardium had multiple small abscesses, but the pericardium was smooth and shiny. The coronary arteries showed up to 70% stenosis by atheromatous plaques. There were no complete occlusions. The aorta and its branches were also affected by severe atherosclerosis with plaque ulceration and hemorrhage. The lungs were edematous and had a combined weight of 1700 g. Bilateral apical bullous emphysema was evident, and the rest of the parenchyma failed to show areas of consolidation. The liver showed signs of passive congestion with a weight of 2400 g. The spleen weighed 750 g and was significantly enlarged (20 cm in length). A 3.5 x 3 cm defect and a subcapsular hematoma were located on the posterior surface compatible with acute splenic rupture (Figure 53). In addition, there were multiple acute and subacute splenic infarcts, the largest of which measured 4.0 cm in its greatest dimension. There was evidence of retroperitoneal hemorrhage with approximately 500 g of clotted blood and 2 L of ascites. The kidneys weighed 460 g combined, and were grossly unremarkable except for a healed infarct in the cortex of the right kidney and a left cyst at the corticomedullary junction measuring 0.8 cm in diameter. The cervical, mediastinal and abdominal lymph nodes were not enlarged. The brain did not show any pathologic changes.

Microscopic Description

Sections of the heart, stained with H&E, showed active infective endocarditis of the mitral valve with septic vasculitis and acute epicarditis with microabscess formation. The lungs and liver had changes of chronic passive congestion. The lungs were also affected by centrilobular emphysema. Sections from the spleen revealed multiple infarcts with cavitation, as well as hemorrhage in the area of rupture and acute inflammation. The kidneys showed interstitial chronic nephritis, but no recent infarcts. The bone marrow and lymph nodes were reactive with no evidence of malignancy.

Case Analysis

This case represents another example of cardiovascular sudden death. However, in contrast to the common fatal ventricular arrhythmia discussed previously; the cause of death in this case was directly related to a sudden but unexpected, non-arrhythmic complication of infectious endocarditis (IE). It is reasonable to say that IE virtually never causes sudden death, with the rare exception of septic embolization of a coronary or cerebral artery, arising from an infected vegetation. This case represents a rare event, but one that is instructive regarding the often subtle and difficult diagnosis of IE.

The clinical and pathological features are a classic example of what previously was called subacute bacterial endocarditis, or SBE. Today, for reasons outlined below, the generally accepted designation is *infectious endocarditis.* This is an unusual patient because it illustrates so clearly how elusive the diagnosis of IE can be since it may mimic an indolent systemic disease of many different etiologies. The '*take home message*' from this case is that if the possibility of IE is not considered, reaching the correct diagnosis will be very unlikely. The consequences of such an oversight, as exemplified here, can be devastating.

What is the difference between subacute bacterial endocarditis (SBE) and acute bacterial endocarditis (ABE), and why has there been a trend away from these designations? Historically, both SBE and ABE were described in the pre-antibiotic and pre-cardiac surgery era, at a time when there was no treatment for the valvular infection(s). Thus, the natural history was dependent on the virulence of the infective organism, and the underlying valvular pathology. SBE was usually a slow, progressive, indolent infection of a valve. Most often it involved the mitral and/or aortic valves. The right-sided disease was uncommon. The mitral valve was the most frequently affected, since pre-existing chronic rheumatic mitral valvulitis with scarring and calcification was highly prevalent. The valvular damage allowed for infection by organisms that ordinarily could not colonize 'healthy' valvular tissues. These organisms include Streptococcus viridans (normal mouth flora), and Staphylococcus epidermidis (normal skin colonizer). Healthy valve tissue covered by endothelium (endocardium), does not routinely permit adherence of non-pathogenic organisms. In contrast, scarred and distorted valves with turbulent blood flow over the valve surface, serve as anchor areas for the development of pathological infectious vegetations. Even non-pathogenic organisms can adhere to sub-endocardial connective tissue; and colonize small platelet and fibrin vegetations that may develop on denuded valve linings. The bacteria, particularly S. viridans, circulate in the bloodstream following oral manipulation as common as brushing teeth. With more vigorous dental work there may be a more significant bacteremia, which explains why patients with known valvular disease, must have antibiotic prophylaxis before and after dental procedures.

Infection of valvular tissue with a non-virulent organism leads to a smoldering infection, and a prolonged clinical course. Patients with such infections could often live for many months even before antibiotics were available. The causes of death were usually valve destruction, non-cardiac tissue damage, or systemic complications of sepsis. This was the classic SBE: **infection of an (almost always) abnormal heart valve persisting for more than 6-8 weeks**. With the persistent, often low-grade infection, patients have indolent symptoms of chronic disease. These may include variable weight loss, anorexia, fatigue, intermittent fever, chills, and night sweats. These are symptoms remarkably similar to those seen with occult cancers, collagen-vascular disease, and tuberculosis (today, we should also consider HIV/AIDS). The weight loss, anorexia, and fatigue could also be ascribed

173

among others, to depression, diabetes mellitus, and adrenal cortical insufficiency. The clinical presentation might suggest SBE if there were typical findings of a heart murmur that was changing in intensity at different times. Additionally, patients with SBE may have small mucocutaneous hemorrhages peripherally, particularly in their nail beds or the so-called 'splinter hemorrhages', and cutaneous petechiae. These lesions are generally thought to be secondary to small non-infected emboli from the valve vegetation, although infected material or immune mediation may play a role. Since the spleen is frequently enlarged, patients may present with left upper quadrant pain and tenderness. Splenic involvement includes changes associated with sepsis ('acute splenitis'), infarction and/or abscess formation (septic emboli). Moreover, when the infection has persisted for some time, the valves leaflets or cusps are destroyed, which results in valvular insufficiency, and ultimately in ventricular failure. Often, patients succumb secondary to systemic embolization, particularly to the brain, where they might develop cerebral infarctions, abscesses, and meningitis. Patients may also develop systemic disease related to the prolonged indolent course of their infection. Specifically, the subacute infection may lead to the development of antigen-antibody complexes, with the antigen being bacterial membrane protein. These complexes can circulate in the bloodstream, and ultimately deposit in small skeletal muscle and skin vessels, and in glomerular capillaries of the kidney. In the former sites, they may lead to a necrotizing vasculitis, with tissue inflammation and necrosis. When present in the palms, finger pulp, or soles of the feet, they are known as Osler's nodes. In the kidney, a focal, necrotizing glomerulonephritis may develop, which is not secondary to embolism of vegetations (even though classically it has been called focal embolic glomerulonephritis). Other manifestations of immune complex disease include arthralgias and arthritis.

Despite the relative ease with which the diagnosis of SBE should be made in patients who present with these clinical signs and symptoms; the fact remains that, even in this modern era of echocardiography, it is still a disease associated with a high number of mis-diagnoses. The primary reason, other than physicians not considering it, is that many patients do not present with all of these classic features. Since the infection is often a subtle one, and given the intermittent nature of active bacterial release into the blood stream, negative blood cultures may be common, unless taken frequently. Furthermore, once the bacteria extend into the valve tissue, or into the peri-valvular annulus, they are not released into the bloodstream. Clinically, there may be no changing murmur; petechiae may not be present, or in dark-skinned patients, may be difficult to appreciate; and complications associated with immune complexes may not develop. However, non-specific clinical symptoms may suggest cancer, or systemic diseases like lupus erythematosus. Laboratory signs such as low-grade leukocytosis (with white blood cell counts between 10,000-15,000), and elevated erythrocyte sedimentation rate (ESR) are relatively non-specific, and may not be present. So again, as stated previously, if you don't think of the diagnosis, you won't make it!

In contrast to SBE, acute bacterial endocarditis (ABE) has different features and pathogenesis. It is generally associated with infection by virulent organisms, particularly Staphylococcus aureus, Streptococcus pneumoniae (pneumococcus), enterococci, and a number of Gram-negative bacilli. As a result of the virulence of these or other pathogens, pre-existing valve damage may or may not be present. With aggressive, rapidly growing, and destructive organisms, there is an acute and progressive tissue disruption associated with collagenolysis of valvular and annular connective tissue. Intra-valvular and annular abscesses may occur. Large platelet and fibrin vegetations develop, which are very susceptible to fragmentation and embolization. The time course of the disease is rapid, often measured in days or few weeks. Moreover, signs and symptoms of valvular insufficiency are frequent and occur early. Systemic embolization to other organs, with tissue infarction and abscess formation, is common. Because of the acuteness of the disease, there is generally not sufficient time for the immune complexes to develop. Thus, the immune complications characteristic of SBE are usually absent. Historically, death ensues in a relatively short time, usually secondary to cardiac failure with valve destruction, or septicemia. With these features, ABE has been defined as: **infection of a normal or abnormal heart valve by a virulent organism, with disease generally less than 4 weeks in duration.**

With such a clear distinction between SBE and ABE, why are these designations inappropriate today? Why is the preferred terminology: **active infectious endocarditis?** The simple answer is because antibiotics, and earlier diagnoses with the advent of echocardiography, have modified the natural history of the disease. In addition, surgical intervention has had a major impact in the course of this disease. Prolonged survival is now possible with non-virulent **and** virulent organisms, allowing for the possibility of immune-mediated complications to develop. Finally, as a result of intravenous drug use and the HIV/AIDS epidemic, infections with fungi (aspergillus and candida species, in particular), rather than bacteria, have gained tremendous attention. Although it is still true, that infection with Staphylococcus aureus and pneumococcus is more severe and more destructive than infection with S. viridans, medical intervention has changed the classic features of SBE and ABE.

This patient presented in a terminal state, and had a cardio-pulmonary arrest during transportation to the hospital. Death was a result of septicemia, cardiac failure, and acute splenic rupture. It is unlikely that he had hypovolemia, as only 500 cc of blood were found in the retroperitoneal space. The presence of 2 liters of ascites in the peritoneum was most probably from congestive heart failure (there was no evidence of cirrhosis). His heart was almost twice normal size (610 g), with a dilated and hypertrophied left ventricle, as a result of prolonged mitral valve regurgitation. The regurgitation was secondary to active and healed vegetations of his mitral valve, with ulceration, and actual partial destruction of the anterior leaflet. Vegetations, infected and bland, embolized to distant organs like the spleen, where they produced septic infarctions, and infected vasculitis. The latter, is referred to as a mycotic aneurysm. They are called mycotic even though they are usually not the result of a fungal infection. They represent an infection of the vessel wall, with eventual arterial destruction, and the development of a pseudo-aneurysm, which has the potential to rupture. This patient's partial valvular healing was most certainly due to the antibiotics he was given for intermittent fever during his lengthy clinical course (in retrospect, at least 3-4 months in duration). Unfortunately, though gram-positive cocci were found in the valve tissues, no culture was performed. It is most likely that the organism was one of the saprophytic ones, such as S. viridans. Even though the valve was significantly distorted by the infection, it appeared to have non-specific leaflet thickening, and focal fusion of several chordae tendineae. The latter finding may result from chronic alcohol abuse. Prior valve damage may have predisposed this man to infection with S. viridans.

As a final point, it would be instructive to consider why he was followed for months with a diagnosis of probable lymphoma, or some other type of hematologic malignancy. A local physician, based on symptoms of fatigue, weight loss, and intermittent fever made this diagnosis. He was referred to an oncologist at the same hospital where his wife was employed. In contrast to the leukocytosis one would expect from a persistent infection, this patient was pancytopenic. However, chronic or overwhelming infection may, on occasions, have bone marrow suppression. The symptoms, the peripheral blood findings, and the splenomegaly are all consistent with a diagnosis of leukemia/lymphoma. Unfortunately, the presence of a holosystolic murmur, and the confirmation of mitral valve regurgitation, was disregarded. Since the vegetations on the mitral valve were not large, they were not identified on the echocardiogram. His bone marrow showed reactive changes, which are benign findings and not confirmatory of lymphoma or leukemia. He was short of breath, and this was thought to be due to COPD, rather than CHF. Thus, he was referred to a pulmonologist for consultation, rather than a cardiologist. The diagnosis of active infectious endocarditis was never entertained prior to his death several months later. Again, the lesson from this case is: *if you do not think of the diagnosis, you will not make it.*

Suggested Readings

1. Hoesley CJ, Cobbs CG. Endocarditis at the millennium. J Infect Dis. 1999; 179 (Suppl 2):S360-5.
2. Farmer JA, Torre G. Endocarditis. Curr Opin Cardiol. 1997; 12:123-30.
3. Cunha BA, Gill MV, Lazar JM. Acute infective endocarditis. Diagnostic and therapeutic approach. Infect Dis Clin North Am. 1996; 10:811-34.
4. Harris PS, Cobbs CG. Cardiac, cerebral, and vascular complications of infective endocarditis. Cardiol Clin. 1996; 14:437-50.
5. Keys TF. Infective endocarditis: prevention, diagnosis, treatment, referral. Cleve Clin J Med. 2000; 67:353-60.
6. Burke AP, Kalra P, Li L, Smialek J, Virmani R. Infectious endocarditis and sudden unexpected death: incidence and morphology of lesions in intravenous addicts and non-drug abusers. J Heart Valve Dis. 1997; 6:198-203.

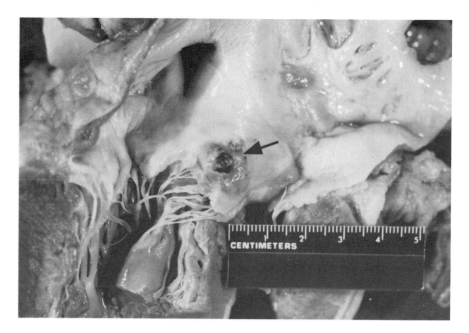

Figure 51. Infective endocarditis, mitral valve. A large vegetation is present on the atrial surface of the leaflet (arrow). There is associated hemorrhage and ulceration.

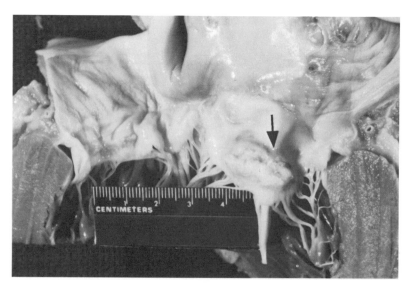

Figure 52. Infective endocarditis. The anterior leaflet of the mitral valve has a vegetation with evidence of re-endothelialization (arrow).

178

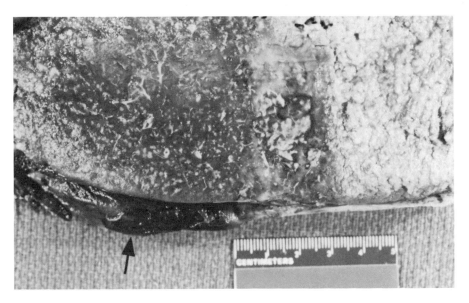

Figure 53. Section of the spleen showing a subcapsular hematoma (arrow). There is also softening of the parenchyma due to septic splenitis.

Case # 19

Clinical Summary

This 51 year old African American homosexual man, with a history of intravenous drug abuse, was admitted to the hospital with a chief complaint of increasing dyspnea on exertion, fever and left facial droop. He also had a history of non-productive cough and a 23 kg weight loss over the past few months. He had been seen by a cardiologist who performed an echocardiogram, told the patient he had congestive heart failure (CHF), and started him on furosemide and digoxin.

On admission his vital signs were T 39.4°C, Pulse 105/min, R 20/min, BP 140/60 mmHg. His physical exam was remarkable for anterior cervical and inguinal lymphadenopathy. His cardiac exam revealed a split S1, a grade II/VI holosystolic murmur best heard at the apex and radiating to the axilla, and another II/VI systolic murmur best heard along the lower left sternal border. Pistol shot pulses with strong upstrokes and fast downstrokes were noted. Pedal edema was present bilaterally. The neurologic exam revealed left facial weakness, confusion, weaker left grip, and left pronator drift. Asterixis was noted on the left.

Laboratory data and other tests

Laboratory: WBC 13.2, Hb/Hct 8.6/26, Plt 320; bilirubin T/D 9.1/5.5, LD 378, BUN/creat 26/1.6, glucose 89, CO2 20. ECG: Sinus tachycardia, Q waves and decreased T waves in lead III. CXR: bilateral interstitial infiltrates. Head CT: remote left temporal lobe infarct.

The patient was admitted with the presumptive diagnosis of endocarditis and AIDS-related pneumonia, and was started on ampicillin, nafcillin, cefoxitin and trimethoprim-sulfamethoxazole (TMP/SMX). Blood cultures grew pneumococci and enterococci. The antibiotics were changed to penicillin, and gentamicin. A lumbar puncture was performed which demonstrated RBC 690, WBC 170 (90% polymorphonuclear leukocytes), protein 14, and glucose 41 (serum glucose 87). India ink and gram stains of the cerebrospinal fluid were negative. Echocardiography revealed prominent aortic insufficiency, with aortic and mitral valve vegetations. During his hospital stay he developed left hemiparesis with flat affect. A repeat head CT with contrast demonstrated no ring enhancement of his existent left fronto-temporal lobe lesion. During his 5th hospital day, he developed a pericardial friction rub and was started on captopril to reduce his cardiac afterload. On day 9 post-admission he was found in the bathroom pulseless and unresponsive. Resuscitation efforts, which included pacemaker insertion, were unsuccessful.

Gross Description

The body was that of a well-developed, well nourished black man measuring 162 cm in length and weighing 63 kg. The heart weighed 490 g and was of the expected shape. The atria were normal in size and free of thrombi. The foramen ovale was closed. The right and left ventricular walls measured 0.6 cm and 1.8 cm in thickness, respectively. There were multiple large vegetations on the aortic, mitral and tricuspid valves with hyperemic margins. The aortic valve vegetations hung free in the ventricle (Figures 54 and 55). Just distal to the coronary arteria ostia and above the non coronary cusp there was a pseudo-aneurysm with rupture into the pericardium causing hemopericardium (200 cc). The pericardium showed fibrinous pericarditis. The endocardium was thin and glistening. The chordae tendineae were thickened. The myocardium was grossly unremarkable. The aorta and its branches showed moderate calcific atherosclerosis, especially in the abdominal portion. The lungs weighed 1800 g combined and were affected by centrilobular emphysema. The kidneys weighed 400 g combined. The renal parenchyma showed multiple small abscesses (<0.5 cm diameter). The spleen was grossly unremarkable (weight 250 g). The brain weighed 1480 g and had evidence of an old left fronto-temporal lobe and recent right fronto-parietal and insular cortex infarcts.

Microscopic Description

Sections from the heart stained with hematoxylin and eosin revealed mild myocellular hypertrophy with scattered areas of old myocytolysis. The mitral and aortic valves showed active infective endocarditis. In addition, sections from the aortic tear and pericardium showed acute and chronic aortitis and fibrinous pericarditis, respectively. The kidneys demonstrated acute necrotizing glomerulitis. Sections from the upper lobe of the right lung revealed a solitary infiltrating moderately differentiated adenocarcinoma with a bronchioalveolar pattern. The non-neoplastic lung parenchyma showed acute and organizing interstitial pneumonitis. Sections of the right fronto-parietal area of the brain confirmed the presence of subacute infarcts. The middle cerebral artery had an occluded branch containing a septic thromboembolus with colonies of bacteria and numerous neutrophils and mononuclear cells within and around the vessel.

Case Analysis

Fulminant, acute bacterial endocarditis (ABE) or subacute endocarditis (SBE)? This case illustrates the confusion in the terminology discussed previously. A rapidly progressive disease leading to death within one week involving virulent organisms (pneumococcus and enterococcus), no obvious pre-existing valve pathology, extensive valvular and blood vessel destruction, and widespread systemic complications of embolization. It certainly fits with the features of ABE, yet he also had significant weight loss over several months, and glomerular inflammation (e.g. glomerulitis), which indicated an immune complication of a more indolent disease. Of course, with his history of continuing intravenous drug abuse, and homosexual contact, one could explain at least the weight loss as HIV/AIDS-related. It was only at autopsy, however, that his HIV status became known as negative. It was also evident that the glomerular inflammation resulted from microscopic emboli of infected vegetations, and not from the development of antigen-antibody complexes in the glomerular basement membranes. With the uncertainty, it is preferable to designate cases such as this as active IE. But as discussed previously, such designation should not be used to obscure the unique features of someone with a fulminant, aggressive infection superimposed on normal heart valves.

The other important lesson in this case, as in the previous discussion of endocarditis, is the failure of several clinicians to consider the diagnosis of active IE, even in the face of some very obvious clues. A local physician had seen this patient, probably for complaints of shortness of breath and exercise intolerance. He had an echocardiogram, which led to a diagnosis of CHF. Presumably, even though we do not have access to this echocardiogram, it most likely showed ventricular contractile dysfunction, and possibly mitral valvular insufficiency. As we have seen previously in patients with dilated cardiomyopathy, ventricular dysfunction and valvular insufficiency may result from ventricular remodeling and annular dilatation. If vegetations are not appreciated or looked for on the valves, the etiology may be missed, and ascribed to myocardial disease. Certainly, with his personal history and his weight loss, the assumption that he had HIV/AIDS cardiomyopathy, or cocaine-induced cardiomyopathy, is not unreasonable. On the other hand, with intravenous drug use and acute onset CHF, it is equally reasonable to include IE in the list of possible differential diagnoses. Regardless, this patient was diagnosed as having CHF, and he was started on diuretic and digitalis therapy. Shortly after the initial visit with a local physician, the patient presented to an affiliated hospital complaining of weakness. Unfortunately, the work-up did not demonstrate a cause, and he was discharged.

The failure to diagnose this patient with IE in the days before his final presentation to our hospital had devastating consequences. By the time he was admitted with fever, increasing dyspnea on exertion, and a left facial droop, his disease was already advanced. He had signs and symptoms of at least two compromised valves, even before confirmation by echocardiography. Specifically, he had aortic insufficiency, with a wide pulse pressure (140/60 mmHg), and a low diastolic pressure secondary to the rapid diastolic backflow into the left ventricle through an incompetent aortic valve. Normally, the diastolic pressure results at least partially from the recoil of the aorta as it are distended during systole. With stretching of the elastic fibers in the aortic media, the vessel normally 'snaps-back', providing the coronary arteries with blood flow during diastole. If the aortic valve is insufficient, the elastic recoil is attenuated, and the diastolic pressure falls. This also accounts for the II/VI diastolic murmur heard along the left sternal border, although one would expect such a murmur to be heard loudest at the heart base. As a correlate of the aortic insufficiency, he also had pistol-shot pulses (strong upstroke followed by a rapid downstroke). The upstroke is a sign of a vigorous ventricular contraction, while the rapid downstroke is a result of the valve being anatomically open during diastole, comparable to the low diastolic pressure. The pistol-shot sound, which can be auscultated, also occurs because of the diastolic collapse. It is typically a loud sound that can be heard over the femoral arteries. It is one of classical pulsation abnormalities reported in aortic insufficiency (these physical examination findings were all described by physicians in the 19th century, during a period in medicine when aortic insufficiency due to infectious endocarditis, chronic rheumatic heart disease, and syphilitic aortic valve disease were common). Other signs include: 1. Corrigan's pulse, a 'water-hammer' sound due to a rapid collapse of pressure late in systole and during diastole. This sound is the banging in pipes associated with rapid sudden flow, or gas bubbles in the fluid; 2. Duroziez's sign, a to-and-fro sound heard over the femoral arteries; and, 3. Quincke's pulse, which refers to the filling and emptying of nail-bed capillaries, seen when firm pressure is applied to the fingertip. All of these phenomena result from the movement of blood back through an insufficient valve, and its association with diastolic collapse.

This patient also had evidence of mitral valve disease. He was noted to have a grade II/VI holosystolic murmur at the apex radiating to the left axilla. This is a typical location of a mitral valve murmur, and the holosystolic nature of the murmur is consistent with mitral regurgitation. The II/VI systolic murmur heard along the left sternal border is less easily characterized as to site of origin. It may represent turbulent flow across a distorted and damaged aortic valve, or ventricular cavity turbulence resulting from the aortic and mitral valve insufficiency. Ultimately, specific aortic valve and mitral valve disease was confirmed on echocardiography, with large vegetations on both valves, and prominent aortic insufficiency. It is noteworthy that the intensity of the murmurs was not as loud as one would expect from the degree of damage appreciated on echocardiography, or eventually found at autopsy. This is not an unusual observation, as the intensity of the murmur may vary with cardiac function, size of vegetation, and degree of valvular pathology. If, for instance, there is a perforation of the leaflet or cusp, this may intermittently be covered by vegetation with no flow through the hole. In the case of a torn cusp or ruptured group of chordae tendineae, the flail tissue may not move consistently with each cardiac cycle, thereby making the murmur variable in intensity. This anatomical variability is the explanation for the so-called 'changing murmur', which can occur in IE. Other manifestations of anatomic distortion of valvular tissues includes the musical or high-pitched cooing murmurs due to rapidly vibrating loose tissue or ruptured chordae; and the Austin Flint murmur (mid-diastolic rumbling), which is thought to result from the impingement of blood coming through an insufficient aortic valve, striking the ventricular surface of the mitral valve, and causing it to vibrate. At this point, you have probably realized that no other area in medicine is as rife with eponyms as valvular heart disease and endocarditis.

As noted above, the failure to diagnosis this patient earlier had major consequences that contributed to his death. By the time of presentation, he not only had fever and CHF, but also dysarthria, a left facial droop, and drooling. These findings were presumptive evidence of intracerebral emboli, and the presence of brain infarction or abscess. Confirmation came from the lumbar puncture, which demonstrated pleocytosis with polymorphonuclear predominance and decreased CSF glucose (CSF to blood ratio less than 2/3), suggesting meningitis. Cerebral abscess from embolized fragments of vegetation can often extend to the meningeal surface with the development of meningitis. Small fragments of vegetation preferentially embolize to the microcirculation at the cortico-medullary junction in the brain; then a micro-abscess develops and extends to the brain surface, where it secondarily infects the meninges. Alternatively, there may be direct seeding of meningeal blood vessels by the infective material. Cerebral abscess and meningitis are particularly common with pneumococcal endocarditis, which was one of the two organisms isolated from his blood culture (another eponym associated with endocarditis is the Austrian's triad: pneumococcal endocarditis, pneumonia, and meningitis). Often, by the time IE embolizes systemically, the process is too far advanced for any meaningful intervention. In this case, shortly after confirmation by echocardiography of the aortic and mitral valve involvement, the patient developed left hemiparesis, and mental status changes. Despite CT scan findings of an old left temporal lobe infarction with no new lesions (it may take several days for new cerebral infarctions to become visible), clinically, he had obvious findings consistent with acute

184

cerebral embolization. Although surgical intervention was considered, the clinicians caring for this patient considered his cardiac function stable, and before attempting valve replacement surgery, wanted to sterilize his valves with antibiotics.

Several days before his death he developed a new, and potentially ominous complication: a pericardial friction rub. This new physical finding should have led to additional diagnostic work-up, including a repeat echocardiogram and possibly a pericardiocentesis with culture of the aspirated material. No such studies were carried out. This finding should have been considered a serious new complication because it almost certainly represented spread of infection to the pericardial sac, with the development of fibrinopurulent exudate on the parietal and visceral pericardial surfaces. It is the contact of these surfaces during the cardiac cycle that leads to the auscultatory finding of friction rub (similar to the sound of two sheets of fine sandpaper rubbed together). If there is sufficient fluid or pus in the pericardial sac to separate the two layers of pericardium, the friction rub may not occur, or it may disappear if it was previously heard. There are multiple mechanisms leading to a pericardial friction rub in IE. None of them is benign:

1. There may be spread of infection from the valve surface to the fibrous annulus of the valve, where it produces an annular (or valve ring) abscess. This is a very difficult lesion to treat, because the annulus is virtually avascular, and bactericidal levels of antibiotic may not reach this tissue. Annular abscess is often a cause of a smoldering, persistent infection. It is also difficult to diagnose because blood cultures may not be positive. Additionally, it is common in patients with infection of prosthetic heart valves, particularly mechanical valves, which rarely become infected on the surface components of the valve, but are susceptible to bacterial growth in the area of the cloth-covered sewing ring (where it can spread to the annulus). The valve annulus is immediately adjacent to epicardial adipose tissue, and the epicardial surface. Thus, infection can easily spread to the pericardial sac.

2. Other mechanisms for purulent pericarditis include direct spread from the vegetation to epicardial blood vessels through the blood stream. There may also be embolization of coronary vessels leading to myocardial abscess. The abscesses that develop in the heart tend to be preferentially located in the subepicardium and mid-wall myocardium due to the anatomical organization of the microcirculation (similar to the anatomy of the cerebral microcirculation, which predominantly leads to the development of abscesses at the cortico-medullary junction). A subepicardial abscess can extend directly to the epicardium, where it causes infective pericarditis.

3. A final pathogenic mechanism is the one that affected the patient in this case. There was spread of infection from the aortic valve cusps to the aortic wall immediately superior to the valve, in the aortic root. Aggressive

organisms can adhere to endothelial tissue triggering a local vascular infection (infective vasculitis). They can also spread from the annulus to the adventitia of the aorta where external invasion of the vessel may occur. In this case, the virulent infection resulted in the formation of a vascular abscess, and vessel wall destruction. A pseudo-aneurysm developed in the region, known as a mycotic aneurysm. With spread of infection through the vessel into the adventitia and beyond, pericarditis developed, since the pericardium envelops not just the heart but extends around the ascending aorta up to the aortic arch. Ultimately, the pseudo-aneurysm ruptured leading to hemopericardium. The blood in the pericardial sac (200 cc), together with the fibrinous pericarditis, was sufficient to cause pericardial tamponade, and his sudden death. Clinical recognition of fibrinous pericarditis in a patient with aortic and mitral valve endocarditis, might have led to urgent surgical intervention with valve replacement, and a vascular graft repair of the aortic root. On the other hand, at the time when patients have such widespread embolization, with cerebral and meningeal involvement, surgical cure is extremely unlikely.

Several closing remarks are worth mentioning. The renal findings were, in fact, infective glomerulitis due to micro-emboli, and not immune-complex glomerulonephritis. In addition, multiple micro-abscesses, secondary to embolization, were evident. Surprisingly, there were no infarctions or abscesses in the spleen, an organ that is commonly involved in patients with active IE. Moreover, neuropathology examination revealed infected thromboemboli associated with organizing right fronto-parietal and insular infarcts. The valvular involvement (e.g. more than one valve) is often observed in patients with fulminant endocarditis. Vegetations can spread relatively easily from the aortic valve to the anterior leaflet of the mitral valve. If there is extension into the aortic valve annulus, or to the sinuses of Valsalva above the valve, infection can cross to the tricuspid valve, which lies adjacent to these structures. In our case, the severe damage to the aortic and the mitral valves did spread secondarily to the tricuspid valve. However, as is usually the case, the pulmonic valve was not involved (the aortic, mitral, and tricuspid valve annuli are anatomically adjacent, and potentially at risk for infectious spread; the pulmonic valve is embryologically and anatomically separate). Furthermore, the pulmonic valve is relatively resistant to endocarditis because of the low-pressure flow across it, and the closure of the valve with pulmonary diastolic pressure. In contrast, the tricuspid valve, which is also affected by low pressure flow, closes with higher right ventricular systolic pressure.

The partial destruction of aortic and mitral valve tissues led to the valvular insufficiency, which is characteristic of IE. The bacterial organisms coupled with the inflammatory response, triggers the synthesis and release of local collagenases that destroy the collagen framework of the cusps and leaflets, along with the chordae tendineae. Even when endocarditis heals, it

186

generally leaves evidence of tissue loss, with perforations, irregular tears, and flail leaflets associated with chordal rupture. Valve stenosis virtually never occurs, except when vegetations obstruct the function of a mechanical valve, or form very bulky vegetations that occlude the orifice of a native valve.

As an incidental finding, this patient had a moderately large, previously undiagnosed, adenocarcinoma of the right upper lobe of the lung. As it extended to the pleural surface, it was potentially a fatal neoplasm.

Suggested Readings.

1. Alestig K, Hogevik H, Olaison L. Infective endocarditis: a diagnostic and therapeutic challenge for the new millennium. Scand J Infect Dis. 2000; 32:343-56.
2. Murphy JG, Steckelberg JM. New developments in infective endocarditis. Curr Opin Cardiol. 1995; 10:150-4.
3. Bayer AS, Bolger AF, Taubert KA, Wilson W, Steckelberg J, Karchmer AW, Levison M, Chambers HF, Dajani AS, Gewitz MH, Newburger JW, Gerber MA, Shulman ST, Pallasch TJ, Gage TW, Ferrieri P. Diagnosis and management of infective endocarditis and its complications. Circulation. 1998; 98:2936-48.
4. Pawsat DE. Inflammatory disorders of the heart. Pericarditis, myocarditis, and endocarditis. Emerg Med Clin North Am. 1998; 16: 665-81.
5. Taylor SN, Sanders CV. Unusual manifestations of invasive pneumococcal infection. Am J Med. 1999; 107(1A):12S-27S.

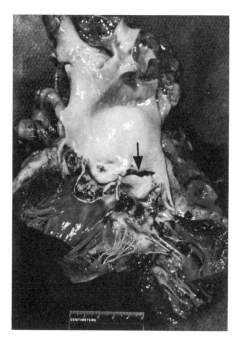

Figure 54. Infective endocarditis. The aortic valve has been destroyed by large vegetations. An aortic tear is evident (arrow), that resulted from infection of the aortic root.

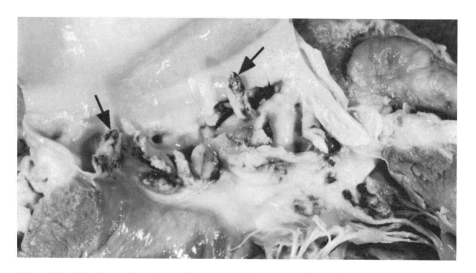

Figure 55. Infective endocarditis. The aortic valve contains large, hemorrhagic vegetations.

189

Chapter 8

MYOCARDITIS

Case # 20

Clinical Summary

A 38-year-old African American man presented to the emergency room with shortness of breath, chest and abdominal pains of 4 days duration. An electrocardiogram (ECG) revealed acute antero-lateral myocardial infarction and a conduction delay with A-V dissociation. He was in shock with low cardiac output and renal insufficiency. His physical exam on admission was significant for tachycardia (100-110 ppm), hypotension (80/50 mmHg), an S3 gallop and bilateral rales up to mid-lung fields.

Laboratory data and other tests

Laboratory: WBC 16, Hb/Hct 12.5/38, Plt 210; BUN/creat 30/1.5, glucose 148; CK 900 (MB 7.8), LD 1790. Combined M mode and 2-D echocardiograms demonstrated normal valves, decreased cardiac output, enlarged left atrium and ventricle, moderate mitral regurgitation, right-sided chambers of normal size and severe antero-lateral left ventricular wall hypokinesis. A small posterior pericardial effusion was also noted. Blood and sputum cultures were negative.

The diagnosis of acute CHF secondary to an acute myocardial infarction was made. He was treated with dobutamine, furosemide and oxygen. Shortly after endotracheal intubation he developed cardiac tachyarrhythmias with subsequent electromechanical dissociation. Resuscitation was unsuccessful.

Gross Description

The body was that of a well-developed, well-nourished 38-year-old man measuring 1.70 m and weighing 80 kg. The heart weighed 480 g. Both right and left chambers were dilated (Figure 56). The epicardial surface was mildly roughened. There were no other significant findings except for areas of yellow discoloration in the myocardium and moderate atherosclerosis involving the left anterior descending coronary artery. The lungs were congested, edematous and weighed 2150 g.

Microscopic Description

H&E stained sections of the heart revealed extensive diffuse myocarditis. The infiltrate was predominantly lymphocytic and involved all chambers including the conduction system at the base of the heart, as well as the papillary muscles. The lymphocytes appeared reactive with enlarged irregular nuclei (Figure 57). Extensive confluent and focal transmural myocardial necrosis was noted. Inflammation and necrosis were seen adjacent to the atrio-ventricular conduction system, which explains the conduction block on presentation. Histologic features of organization and granulation tissue formation were consistent with an interval of 10-14 days. Other areas were less than a week old and many foci showed acute active inflammation (24 hours). Active inflammatory pericarditis was also noted. Additional findings included congestion of the lungs, spleen and liver, consistent with the clinical diagnosis of acute congestive heart failure.

Case Analysis

Inflammation of the human myocardium due to infectious and non-infectious agents is collectively termed as myocarditis. This case represents an atypical presentation of myocarditis in an adult, but would be the commonest one in children. The fulminant presentation is usually secondary to a viral infection of the cardiac tissues, and with appropriate cultures the virus may be grown. The onset and progression tend to be relatively rapid and the outcome is usually fatal over a period of days to weeks. The atypical lymphocytes infiltrating this patient's heart are consistent with an acute reaction to a viral agent. The adult often presents with a more indolent course and the pathogenesis is invariably immunologic.

The extensive multifocal, and in some areas, confluent myocardial damage seen in this patient, can resemble clinically a transmural myocardial infarction. Both the ECG and the cardiac enzyme elevations were indicative of myocardial necrosis. However, in contrast to the global injury seen in fulminant myocarditis, the damage seen in a myocardial infarction is generally limited to the territory of a coronary artery. Although the autopsy revealed moderate atherosclerosis of the left anterior descending coronary artery, ischemia played no role in the myocardial damage.

The histology demonstrated that extensive damage was at least 2 weeks old at the time of the patient's demise, although he allegedly was not symptomatic until 4 days prior to admission. It is not unusual for myocarditis to be clinically "silent" until sufficient myocardium is damaged to lead to the development of CHF, arrhythmia, chest pain, or sudden death. In this case, even if the patient had been admitted several days prior to the onset of his symptoms, the outcome would have probably been the same. The damage was so extensive that supportive therapy with vasopressors and/or intra-aortic balloon pump, would have been only of short term benefit.

Other non-infectious etiologies to consider in this patient include immune-mediated diseases, and toxic and drug related injury. Although, there is no clinical history to support either of these possibilities, they may have fulminant presentations as well. However, the pathology in such acute cases may be of significant value, since it can identify features associated with specific etiologies (e.g. rheumatoid nodules in rheumatoid arthritis involving the conduction system).

In Europe and the United States of America the most important infectious cause of myocarditis are viruses, of which Coxsackie A and B, ECHO and Influenza A and B are the major types. In this patient, even if the viral agent had been identified, specific antiviral treatments are not currently available. In addition, immunosuppressive therapy is of no value in fulminant myocarditis, and may even exacerbate the already severe condition. In South and Central America parasitic infections of the heart account for a significant number of myocarditis cases with Chaga's disease one of its main causes, along with chronic cardiomyopathy. Furthermore, with increasing numbers of immunocompromised patients, disseminated infections (HIV/AIDS, toxoplasmosis, aspergillosis, candidiasis) will continue to be associated with myocardial damage and dysfunction.

The clinical course of myocarditis depends not only in the causative agent, but also in the type, degree and duration of the damage. The host plays a pivotal role because of the genetic determinants that define its inherent susceptibility and the response to the injury. The various infectious agents may directly affect the myocytes, exert a cytotoxic effect (toxin-mediated), cause injury via an immune-mediated mechanism or cause myocardial dysfunction as it spreads from adjacent inflammatory foci. In addition, these agents can induce a vascular damage that in turn will affect the myocardium.

The specific immune alterations associated with myocarditis are unknown. The expression of major histocompatibility complex (MHC) antigens class I and II during the course of human viral myocarditis supports the possibility of this process having an autoimmune component. Messenger ribonucleic acid of perforin, the pore-forming protein that mediates cytotoxicity, has been identified in the cytoplasmic granules of inflammatory cells. Interleukins 1, 6 and 8 as well as tumor necrosis factor also appear to play a role in myocardial damage. Recently, myosin-specific antibodies have been identified in the serum of a large percentage of adult patients with myocarditis. These antibodies may arise as a result of tissue injury or may

193

induce actual tissue damage. Cytomegalovirus (CMV) induced cross-reacting antibodies to myosin have also been described. In certain mouse strains (DBA/2) there is an increased susceptibility to myocarditis following in vivo administration of myosin-specific antibodies. It appears that autoimmune myocarditis mediated by myosin-specific antibodies has a genetic basis, which is complex and has yet to be defined.

Endomyocardial biopsies to evaluate the presence of myocarditis are obtained from the right side of the ventricular septum. The Dallas Classification was developed to standardize the histopathological diagnosis of active and chronic myocarditis. In the acute cases, in addition to the inflammatory infiltrate, there is necrosis and degeneration of myocytes. However, clinical improvement usually precedes histologic recovery. In chronic myocarditis, necrosis is not a required feature, but interstitial fibrosis and loss of myofibers will indicate the degree of severity of the injury. Other terms such as ongoing, resolving and healed myocarditis can be used in subsequent biopsies.

In this case, the outcome was determined by the diffuse and extensive acute inflammatory damage to the myocardium. Although some authors have proposed that fulminant myocarditis can have a good long-term prognosis, the majority of patients die as a result of severe hemodynamic alterations.

Suggested Readings

1. Feldman AM, McNamara D. Myocarditis. N Engl J Med. 2000; 343:1388-98.
2. Mason JW. Myocarditis. Adv Intern Med. 1999; 44:293-310.
3. Kearney MT, Cotton JM, Richardson PJ, Shah AM. Viral myocarditis and dilated cardiomyopathy: mechanisms, manifestations, and management. Postgrad Med J. 2001; 77:4-10.
4. Klingel K, Selinka HC, Huber M, Sauter M, Leube M, Kandolf R. Molecular pathology and structural features of enteroviral replication. Toward understanding the pathogenesis of viral heart disease. Herz. 2000; 25:216-20.
5. Aretz HT, Billingham ME, Edwards WD, Factor SM, Fallon JT, Fenoglio JJ Jr, Olsen EG, Schoen FJ. Myocarditis. A histopathologic definition and classification. Am J Cardiovasc Pathol. 1987; 1:3-14.
6. Liao L, Sindhwani R, Leinwand L, Diamond B, Factor SM. Cardiac alpha-myosin heavy chains differ in their induction of myocarditis. Identification of pathogenic epitopes. J Clin Invest 1993; 90:2877-82.
7. Liao L, Sindhwani R, Rojkind M, Factor SM, Leinwand L, Diamond B. Antibody-mediated autoimmune myocarditis depends on genetically determined target organ sensitivity. J Exp Med 1996; 181:1123-31.
8. Kuan AP, Chamberlain W, Malkiel S, Lieu HD, Factor SM, Diamond B, Kotzin BL. Genetic control of autoimmune myocarditis mediated by myosin-specific antibodies. Immunogenet 1999; 49:79-85.

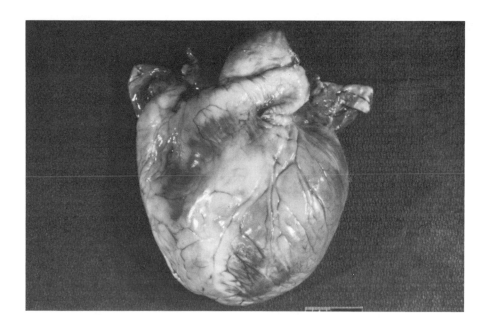

Figure 56. Myocarditis. Globular dilatation of the heart as a result of remodeling.

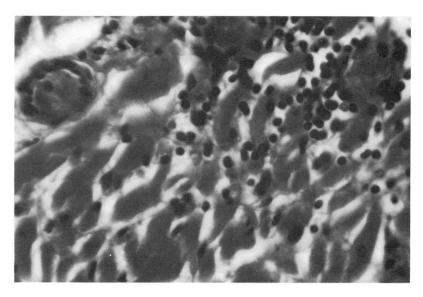

Figure 57. Myocarditis, histologic section. Lymphocytes infiltrate around necrotic myocytes (Hematoxylin and Eosin, 40X).

196

Case # 21

Clinical Summary

This is the case of a 2 year old girl who was taken to the emergency room by her parents with vomiting and difficulty breathing. The child had a several week history of intermittent fever and vomiting diagnosed as a viral syndrome by her pediatrician. On initial evaluation she was tachycardic (160 ppm), and tachypneic (50 rpm). On auscultation there were coarse rales. A chest-x ray revealed a left lower lobe infiltrate. She was hydrated and given oxygen. However, a few hours later, she had a cardiorespiratory arrest with initial ventricular fibrillation followed by asystole. Resuscitation was unsuccessful and she was pronounced dead.

Gross Description

The autopsy revealed significant pleural, pericardial and peritoneal fluid accumulation (60cc right, 5cc left, 15cc and 50cc, respectively). The heart weighed 55 g (normal for age 58 ± 11 g), with no discrete lesions noted. The lungs weighed 120 g combined, (normal for age 160 g), and showed no focal lesions. The liver was mildly enlarged and congested.

Microscopic Description

Sections of the left ventricular septum and right ventricle revealed a diffuse band-like infiltrate involving predominantly the outer and inner third of the ventricular wall, with focal transmural extension. The infiltrate was composed of enlarged mononuclear cells, eosinophils, occasional mast cells, histiocytes and fibroblasts (Figure 58). There were areas of organization and active necrosis, with myocyte damage directly associated with the inflammatory cells, along with myocytolysis. Segments of interstitial and replacement fibrosis were also present. The inflammation and organizing necrosis were acute to 3 weeks duration, but areas of more mature scarring were 4-5 weeks old representing an on-going process. Only rare foci of myocardium were spared in the septum. A section of the left ventricular free wall had similar inflammatory infiltrates, necrosis, and fibrosis. A section of the annulus (the tissue supporting the atrio-ventricular valves, and also adjacent to the AV node) was also heavily infiltrated by inflammatory cells. The attached atrium was uninvolved. The right ventricle connected to the septal section was markedly affected as well. The coronary arteries showed no inflammation, but there was edema in the inner lining.

A section of a cervical lymph node revealed follicular hyperplasia with reactive germinal centers. The thymus had expansion of the medullary tissue into the cortex with reactive and atypical lymphocytes. Both lungs showed peribronchial and interstitial aggregates of mononuclear cells associated with eosinophils. Intranuclear viral inclusions consistent with adenovirus were noted in the bronchial epithelium. Additionally, there was bronchial epithelial hyperplasia and mucosal necrosis. Alveolar spaces were filled with histiocytes and numerous inflammatory cells infiltrated the interstitium. A section of the liver had centrilobular acute and chronic congestive changes consistent with cardiac failure. The central veins were dilated and fibrosed indicating longstanding congestive heart failure (CHF).

Case Analysis

The cause of death in this case was overwhelming viral pneumonitis and fulminant viral myocarditis, causing CHF and terminal fatal arrhythmia. The damage in the heart had been present for at least a month prior to this child's demise, as indicated by the extensive fibrosis in areas of persistent active inflammation. The signs of CHF were evident from the fluid accumulation in the pleural spaces, pericardial and abdominal cavities, and the acute and chronic dilatation of the central veins in the liver. The presence of large atypical mononuclear cells in the heart and lung, as well as the adenoviral intranuclear inclusions, confirms the viral etiology of this illness.

Myocarditis in infants and young children is almost always due to a specific viral infection of the heart, which leads to inflammatory injury and myocardial cell necrosis. In, contrast myocarditis in older immunocompetent children and adults, is frequently an immune-mediated disease. Myocarditis is usually suspected in cases of unexplained onset of CHF and arrhythmia, after a respiratory (upper respiratory infection or URI) or systemic febrile illness. The viral etiology may be suggested by epidemiologic clustering of cases during seasonal epidemics of certain viruses (enteroviruses), diagnostic serologic studies, and the application of molecular techniques, like in situ hibridization and polymerase chain reaction (PCR), to detect genomic sequences in tissue samples such as endomyocardial biopsies. Other rare causes of myocarditis include, bacterial infections of the heart, which result from direct extension to myocardial tissue with microabscesses, or from toxin-mediated injury (e.g. diphtheria). Occasionally, contiguous spread from the endocardium or pericardium can occur, most commonly from pneumonic foci.

This girl presented with fever, episodes of vomiting and respiratory distress. Her pediatrician ascribed these non-specific symptoms to a viral syndrome, and decided just to follow her clinically. This approach is fairly common in pediatric medicine. Even if a child is symptomatic, but is overall stable with adequate cardiovascular and neurologic function, he or she will be monitored over time. Still, consideration of several facts may be warranted. First, the issue of intermittent fevers may be of importance. Fever represents a non-specific host response to an on-going process, which can be significant or trivial. What define the importance of the fever are concomitant symptoms and their progression and/or resolution. In this case, if the fever had been daily or frequent, it should have prompted a more thorough physical exam and laboratory analyses to detect potentially treatable conditions. The crucial elements to evaluate include the height of the fever, associated signs and symptoms (particularly rashes, change in mental status, respiratory signs and hemodynamic stability), and response to therapy (e.g. antibiotics, antipyretic drugs).

In the beginning of the illness, her main symptom was vomiting (there is no mention of change in bowel habits, or rashes). Enteroviruses predominantly cause fever, gastrointestinal, respiratory and skin manifestations. Therefore, it is conceivable that her symptoms were due to an enteroviral infection. The turning point came when she began developing respiratory complaints, and on physical exam she had signs of pulmonary compromise characterized by coarse breath sounds and rales. Clues that this illness perhaps represented more than a self-limited viral syndrome include the progressive involvement of new organ systems. Other diagnoses to consider are progressive lung involvement such as significant pneumonia with or without effusion, diffuse interstitial lung disease, sepsis syndrome, hereditary cardiomyopathies or congenital heart disease.

The clinical history, physical examination and pathologic findings of the heart definitely excluded the possibility of a common pediatric illness of unknown etiology, Kawasaki's disease. This entity is a non-infectious, immune-mediated disorder, which afflicts infants and young children. It is a systemic vasculitis that affects the small and medium muscular arteries, resulting in fever, rash, mucositis, lymphadenopathy, and the hallmark coronary artery inflammation. Other potential fatal conditions in children, that may present subacutely, are those related to toxic ingestions or toxin-mediated illnesses. Again, in the absence of epidemiologic and clinical history, and with the strong pathologic evidence of myocarditis, it is very unlikely that there was a different cause that may have resulted in this child's death.

Even though the majority of myocarditis episodes end up being idiopathic, of those identified with a specific etiology, viruses account for a significant number of cases. Coxsackie B viruses, are small stranded RNA viruses, which have a natural affinity for the myocardium by interacting with specific receptors on the myocardial cell surface, and can be identified in 25-40% of acute cases (mostly types B2-B5). The determinant for host susceptibility is the lack of serotype-specific antibodies. Neonates are particularly prone to viral myocarditis due to both Coxsackie B and ECHO (enteric cytopathogenic human orphan) viruses. Clusters of neonatal cases may occur when mothers lack specific antibodies to the prevalent strains. Affected neonates will present with feeding difficulty, listlessness, and respiratory distress. Cyanosis, fever and hepatosplenomegaly may occur in 50-75% of babies. The mortality rate may reach 75%, and is associated with multiorgan failure.

Cardiac scarring occurs over a fixed period of time, with at least 2 weeks required for collagen to deposit in the tissues. The estimation that the girl's disease had been on-going for at least a month prior to her death was predicated on the findings of organizing inflammation, necrosis, and fibrosis in the heart. Additionally, the enlargement of the heart requires weeks to develop. Thus, well before this child presented to the emergency room, she already had extensive cardiac involvement. Because it often is a silent condition, it is of no surprise that there were no specific features suggesting the diagnosis of myocarditis in this girl. The initial clinical presentation is often a vague flu-like or gastrointestinal illness. In this case, there was a respiratory infection (pneumonitis), in addition to the cardiac inflammation. By the time she was brought to the emergency room, the severity of the damage to the heart was so overwhelming, that her chances for survival were negligible. Since viral myocarditis is a generalized disease, the extent of the lesion can be extrapolated from the massive injury in the sections examined. These sections were obtained at random, and the diffuse and extensive involvement is a statistical confirmation that the remainder of the heart was equally affected.

Finally, it is likely that in our case, the initial infection was respiratory, given the typical adenoviral nuclear inclusions in the bronchial epithelium; and then the virus spread to the heart via the blood stream. Although, adenoviral myocarditis is uncommon, co-infection with other pathologic agents cannot be excluded.

Suggested Readings

1 Penninger JM, Bachmaier K. Review of microbial infections and the immune response to cardiac antigens. J Infect Dis. 2000; 181 Suppl 3:S498-504.

2 Huber SA, Gauntt CJ, Sakkinen P. Enteroviruses and myocarditis: viral pathogenesis through replication, cytokine induction, and immunopathogenicity. Adv Virus Res. 1998; 51:35-80.

3 Bowles NE, Towbin JA. Molecular aspects of myocarditis. Curr Opin Cardiol. 1998; 13:179-84.

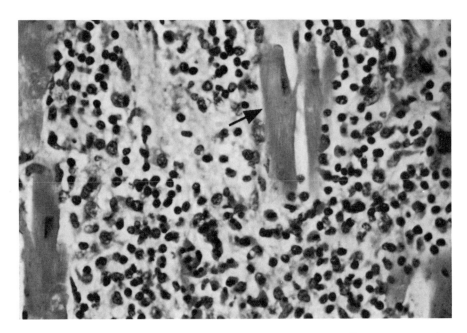

Figure 58. Myocarditis, histologic section. Numerous inflammatory cells are present in the myocardium. Viable myocytes and striations are still present (arrow) (Hematoxylin and Eosin, 40X)

Chapter 9

CARDIAC TUMORS

Case # 22

Clinical Summary

The patient was a 34 year old African American woman, HIV negative, smoker (one pack per day for 20 years), asthmatic, with a history of positive PPD and tuberculous infection, treated with 4 antituberculous medications. As part of the work-up a CT scan of the chest was done, which revealed a large mass involving the middle and lower lobes of the right lung. In addition, a bronchial washing was reported positive for adenocarcinoma, and subsequently she underwent right pneumonectomy. The right lung as well as the mediastinal lymph nodes were involved by a moderately to poorly differentiated adenocarcinoma. Moreover, the lung showed focal emphysematous changes and several 0.5 cm arteriovenous malformations. After the operation she returned to work, but came back to the ER twice complaining of dyspnea and productive cough with yellow sputum. Jugular venous distension was absent and left breath sounds were clear. She was treated with albuterol and discharged on prednisone (20mg qd x 5 days). She then experienced increasing shortness of breath and the emergency medical service was called. The paramedics found her able to talk, but soon thereafter, she lost consciousness, suffered a cardiac arrest and died on her way to the hospital.

Gross Description

The body was that of a thin, well-developed woman measuring 168 cm and weighing 62 kg. The skin was unremarkable except for a right thoracotomy scar. Upon opening the chest, the mediastinum was noted shifted to the right side. The right border of the heart was 10 cm from the right lateral chest wall. The posterior aspect of the right thoracic cavity was occupied by scar tissue, and the anterior portion was filled with clotted blood and fibrin. The left lung was expanded. Multiple lymph nodes were present in the mediastinum, the largest being 3 cm in maximal dimension. The left lung weighed 500 g. The pleural surfaces were smooth and shiny. On section, the parenchyma revealed an area of increased firmness and hemorrhage in the lower lobe, measuring 5 cm in greatest dimension, extending to the visceral pleura. In addition, there was a moderate loss of parenchyma with formation of smooth-lined cysts of up to 0.5 cm in diameter. These cysts were present in both lobes throughout. The larynx, trachea, major and segmental bronchi were of average caliber. Organizing emboli measuring up to 3 mm occluded small branches of the pulmonary artery.

The heart was 240 g and of the expected shape. The parietal pericardium was smooth and glistening. The sac contained approximately 500 cc of serosanguineous fluid. The epicardium was thickened, dull, firm and white in a few areas with multiple hemorrhagic foci of up to 0.2 cm (Figure 59). The atria were normal and free of thrombi. The foramen ovale was closed. The right and left ventricular walls measured 0.4 cm and 1.2 cm in thickness, respectively. The valve rings measured as follows: tricuspid valve 12 cm, pulmonic valve 7 cm, mitral valve 8.5 cm, and aortic valve 6 cm. The valve leaflets were pliable and the chordae tendineae were thin and slender. The myocardium and endocardium were unremarkable. The coronary arteries were of normal caliber and distribution. The aorta showed mild atherosclerosis in the abdominal portion.

The liver weighed 1400 g and was of normal size and shape. The cut surface showed marked acute centrilobular congestion and multiple tan, firm nodules measuring 0.2 to 0.4 cm. The lobular pattern was preserved otherwise. The remaining organs had no significant pathologic changes.

Microscopic Description

Sections from the epicardium showed many single and small clusters of poorly differentiated carcinoma cells, near the epicardial surface. Some of these cells contained vacuoles consistent with mucin droplets of adenocarcinoma. The malignant cells were large with pleomorphic nuclei and prominent nucleoli. Some were present within lymphatics. Metastatic carcinoma was present bilaterally in hilar lymph nodes. The firm, hemorrhagic areas in both lobes of the left lung corresponded to foci of hemorrhagic infarcts. Surrounding arteries contained numerous acute, organizing and recanalized thrombi. The tan nodules present in the liver did not represent metastatic adenocarcinoma but rather foci of adenomatosis. They were composed of thickened cords of hepatocytes separated by sinusoids and devoid of portal tracts, bile ductules or scars.

Case Analysis

The heart can be involved by primary as well as metastatic tumors. Primary tumors of the heart are rare (< 0.3 % in postmortem series), with myxoma the most frequent. Metastases from neoplasms arising in other organs are far more common and include carcinomas, sarcomas, hematologic malignancies and melanoma. Nonetheless, cardiac metastases are infrequent. Why is the heart relatively protected from metastasis? Possible explanations include the continuous forceful stroke of the heart, rapid blood flow and afferent lymphatic circulation. If these hypotheses were true, cardiac tumors would be present almost invariably in patients with previous cardiac damage with reduced pump action and blood flow, but there is no such confirmatory data in the literature. Regarding afferent lymphatics, metastatic dissemination in the heart occurs most commonly through lymphatic invasion. Overall, the heart is probably protected as a result of the combination of all these and other unknown factors. Moreover, tumor type, metabolic properties of the heart, and adhesion molecules among others, are under consideration and require further investigation.

Secondary tumors may involve the heart by direct extension, hematogenous spread or lymphatic dissemination. Direct extension occurs from tumors arising in the lungs or mediastinum (i.e. bronchogenic and esophageal carcinoma, malignant thymoma, thymic carcinoma). Hematogenous spread is often seen with sarcomas (e.g. uterine. leiomyosarcomas can reach the heart through the inferior vena cava), leukemia, multiple myeloma, and with certain types of carcinoma (e.g. hepatocellular carcinoma). However, the lymphatic pathway appears to be the most significant. This is demonstrated by the frequent metastatic involvement of the pericardium, richly supplied by lymphatic channels that drain in the anterior and posterior mediastinum. In the present case, the patient had a history of adenocarcinoma of the lung involving mediastinal lymph nodes; therefore, it is not surprising that she presented with a pericardial effusion and associated cardiac tamponade. Pericardial involvement in a patient with a known primary malignancy, should be suspected in the setting of pericardial effusion, intractable heart failure or hepatomegaly in the absence of metastatic lesions. The differential diagnosis includes congestive heart failure in a patient with a cardiomyopathy, and non-malignant pericardial effusions (infectious and non-infectious). This patient was young, with no history of heart disease. Although she had asthma in the past and evidence of chronic obstructive pulmonary disease as per the autopsy exam, she did not have pulmonary hypertension or cor-pulmonale.

Tuberculous (TB) pericarditis is a consideration based on her prior history of PPD positivity and antituberculous treatment. TB pericarditis may develop insidiously, or acutely with a large effusion and cardiac tamponade, particularly in immunosuppressed patients. She was HIV negative and had not been treated with chemotherapeutic agents. If she had lived, the diagnosis of malignant pericardial effusion could have been made with a pericardiocentesis and cytologic examination of the fluid. Adenocarcinoma cells are readily identified in pericardial fluid by their tri-dimensional arrangement, distinct cell borders, high nuclear-cytoplasmic ratio and prominent nucleoli (Figure 60). They must be differentiated from reactive mesothelial cells, which is not often easy. Reactive mesothelial cells, especially in long-standing effusions can also exhibit a glandular arrangement, prominent nucleoli, mitotic figures and even vacuolization that mimic adenocarcinoma. Immunohistochemistry is useful in distinguishing the two. Both cell types are immunoreactive to cytokeratin, but only adenocarcinoma stains with the adenocarcinoma marker B72.3 and carcinoembryonic antigen (CEA).

Pulmonary adenocarcinoma arises preferentially in the periphery of the lung parenchyma. Central lesions may occur, but are less frequent. This type of tumor can develop in smokers as well as in non–smokers, de novo or in areas of pre-existing scarring. Our patient was a smoker for 20 years. Although she had a risk factor for lung cancer, the aggressive behavior of this tumor (stage T2, N2 at initial diagnosis) suggests a genetic predisposition.

The advent of cardiovascular imaging studies has improved the diagnosis of cardiac involvement by metastatic disease, but the prognosis remains poor. In a recent study done at the Tottori University School of Medicine in Japan, 46 of 161 patients had secondary cardiac tumors diagnosed by echocardiography. The most common primary site was the lung followed by mediastinum, liver, uterus and testis. Forty seven percent of the cases had pericardial involvement, 32% involved the right side of the heart and 14 % involved the left. Metastases on both sides of the heart were noted in 7% of cases. It is unknown why intracavitary lesions are less common, but there is evidence that certain tumors have predilection for this pattern of growth (Figures 61 and 62). In our experience, squamous carcinoma arising in different sites has the tendency to invade and seed cardiac valves, endocardium and myocardium. Prior valve damage or endothelial damage appears to be a *sine qua non* in such cases. As a result, death can occur due to arrhythmia with or without conduction system involvement and embolization. Changes in the electrocardiogram such as prolonged elevation of the ST segment are indicative of myocardial invasion.

In the present case, the patient died of cardiac tamponade due to a malignant pericardial effusion. In addition, she was in a hypercoagulable state with numerous acute and organizing pulmonary emboli leading to areas of hemorrhagic infarction. Her symptoms of dyspnea and shortness of breath were related to both the pulmonary embolism and evolving cardiac tamponade. Of note, dyspnea is the most common manifestation of cardiac tumors in general, and is suggestive of cardiac decompensation. Treatment is palliative, aimed at controlling effusions, arrhythmia and heart failure. Radiotherapy is the treatment of choice to manage malignant effusions. In some instances, a pericardial window is required to treat tamponade. Chemotherapy has been used to prevent further cardiac involvement, but its use is limited by its cardiotoxicity. In rare instances, surgical debulking is indicated to alleviate obstructive cardiac masses.

Suggested Readings

1. Ghosh K, Dusenbery KE, Twiggs LB. Cardiac metastasis of cloacagenic carcinoma of the vagina: a case and review of gynecologic malignancies with cardiac metastasis. Gynecol Oncol. 2000; 76:208-12.
2. Majano-Lainez RA. Cardiac tumors: a current clinical and pathological perspective. Crit Rev Oncog. 1997; 8:293-303.
3. Raaf HN, Raaf JH. Sarcomas related to the heart and vasculature. Semin Surg Oncol. 1994; 10:374-82.
4. Vohra A, Saiz E, Davila E, Burkle J. Metastatic germ cell tumor to the heart presenting with syncope. Clin Cardiol. 1999; 22:429-33.

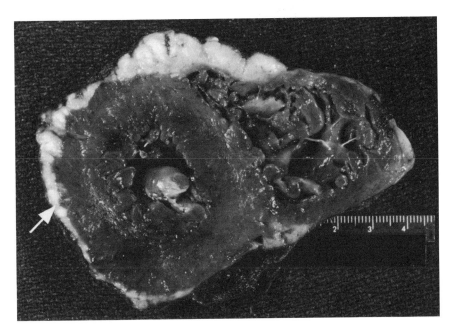

Figure 59. Cross section of the heart showing metastatic carcinoma involving the epicardium with focal invasion of the myocardium (arrow).

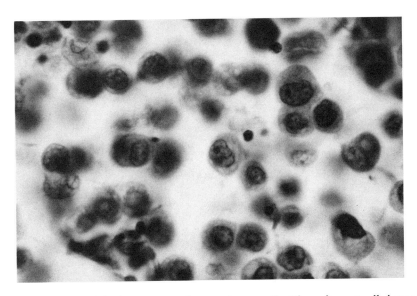

Figure 60. Pericardial fluid containing adenocarcinoma cells. The malignant cells have a finely vacuolated cytoplasm, irregular nuclear contours and prominent nucleoli (Papanicolaou stain, 60X).

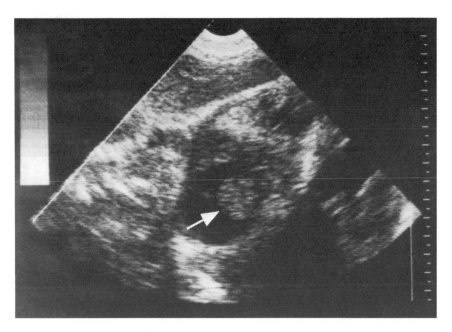

Figure 61. Echocardiogram showing an intracavitary right ventricular mass in a patient with lymphoma (circle and arrow).

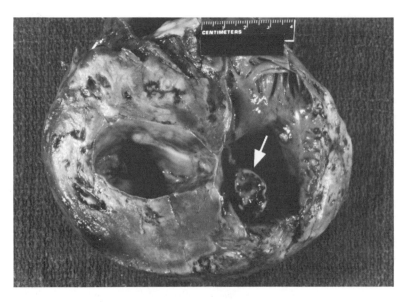

Figure 62. Transverse section of the heart showing an intracavitary right-sided mass (arrow) and patchy involvement of the myocardium by a fleshy, hemorrhagic tumor. The patient had been diagnosed with Non-Hodgkin's lymphoma.

210

Cases # 23, 24 and 25

The following brief clinical vignettes each have one common symptom with 3 completely different, rare, but important etiologies that should be considered in a differential diagnosis. Sometimes the hoof beats really do come from a zebra rather than a horse!

Case # 23

A 25 year old man, bodybuilder, sought medical attention due to several brief episodes of syncope, each lasting less than one minute. His physical exam and ECG were within normal limits. The chest-x-ray was significant for mediastinal fullness, possibly due to enlarged lymph nodes. The patient also complained of malaise, shortness of breath and productive cough with white sputum. He was treated with a course of broad spectrum antibiotics with no improvement. Several weeks later, the patient was found dead in his apartment. The autopsy revealed a 500 g heart with a dilated left ventricle measuring 1.3 cm in thickness. The right ventricular wall measured 0.3 cm. The coronary arteries were clean and patent. The lungs were edematous and weighed 1020 g combined. Microscopic evaluation of the heart showed large areas of the myocardium entirely replaced by non-caseating, confluent granulomas (Figure 63). The granulomas were active for the most part, but old, hyalinizing granulomas and extensive foci of replacement fibrosis mimicking remote myocardial infarcts were also present. Special stains for microorganisms (acid fast bacilli and fungi) were negative.

Case # 24

A 20 year old college student presented with episodes of 'heart racing' and occasional lightheadedness. In addition, she described a brief episode of syncope. An ECG was done revealing normal sinus rhythm. Her treating physician recommended a Holter monitor which showed several intermittent episodes of transient heart block each lasting less than one minute, and a heart rate of 55 pulsations per minute. She was scheduled for electrophysiological examination, but died before the test was done. The autopsy showed a normal-sized heart for her age. The endocardium, myocardium, valves and coronary arteries were all unremarkable. The only significant finding was a 1.0 cm tumor in the area of the atrio-ventricular node. Microscopically, the tumor consisted of multiple cystic spaces lined by several layers of bland, polygonal, mucin-producing cells. No other similar lesions were found in any other organ (Figure 64).

Case # 25

A 32 year old woman came to the hospital complaining of several episodes of syncope occurring within a few weeks period. Some of the episodes lasted several minutes. A computerized tomography (CT) of the brain with contrast revealed a few small resolving cerebral infarcts. The cerebrospinal fluid yielded an increased number of reactive, mature lymphocytes with no evidence of cytologic atypia. The physical exam was significant for the presence of a II/VI diastolic murmur with click. She was scheduled for an echocardiogram, but days prior to the test she developed acute mid-abdominal pain and was admitted with the diagnosis of small bowel obstruction. A nasogastric tube was placed, but provided no relief. The patient underwent a laparotomy with resection of necrotic segments of small intestine. An embolus was found occluding the superior mesenteric artery. Histologically, the embolus was composed of myxoid material, blood vessels and stellate-shaped cells. A post-operative echocardiogram was performed revealing the presence of a left atrial mass. A CT scan of the chest with contrast confirmed a space-occupying lesion in the left atrium.

Analysis

These 3 cases have one clinical manifestation in common: syncope. Syncope is defined as temporary loss of consciousness and postural tone. It differs from fainting in the quality and duration of the event. It usually occurs when the patient is in an upright position and there is a sudden reduction of cerebral blood flow. Additional syncope-triggering circumstances include hypotension with impaired vasoconstrictor mechanisms, hypovolemia, reduced cardiac output, reduction of venous return, arrhythmia and cerebral ischemia. Other causes of syncope are those that affect the metabolism of the brain such as hypoxia, hyperventilation, anemia and hypoglycemia.

Normally, humans maintain an upright posture and sufficient cerebral blood flow, because of a continuous venous return to the heart and pressor reflexes that allow an adequate cardiac output. Since we started this discussion with a brief mention of horses and zebras, you might have wondered why giraffes do not have syncope. The answer is that they have a systolic blood pressure that reaches 350–400 mmmHg, generated by a massively hypertrophied left ventricle. Then you might ask why, when giraffes put their head down to drink water, they do not have a massive stroke as a result of such high blood pressure that is no longer countered by the effects of gravity?. The answer to this riddle is that their carotid arteries enter a sinusoidal network at the base of the skull that dampens the pressure before blood is supplied to the brain. To the best of our knowledge, Lamarck did not know this when he proposed that giraffes developed long necks by reaching to eat leaves from high tree branches.

Not uncommonly, healthy individuals may experience syncope due to increased vagal activity. These episodes of loss of consciousness and generalized muscle weakness are triggered by stress, high temperatures, lack of ventilation, mild blood loss and physical pain, and are preceded by nausea, tachypnea, tachycardia and sweating. Sudden change of posture may also result in syncope. In vasovagal syncope, hypotension occurs, but is not followed by a compensatory increase in cardiac output. Instead, bradycardia and reduced arterial pressure ensue, which exacerbates the patient's condition. Strength is regained by placing the patient in supine posture and elevating the legs to facilitate venous return.

In case # 23, syncope was the result of reduced cardiac output and conduction abnormalities due to severe myocardial damage. The presence of multiple, confluent, non-necrotizing granulomas replacing the myocardium and involving the mediastinal lymph nodes, is diagnostic of sarcoidosis. Sarcoidosis is a systemic disease that commonly affects individuals younger than 40 years of age. It is more common in females. The etiology is unknown, but the manifestations are the result of an exaggerated response of T-helper lymphocytes leading to activation and recruitment of mononuclear phagocytes and granuloma formation. The lymph nodes and lungs are virtually always involved, but the heart is affected in only 5% of the patients. In this case, the involvement was so extensive that it caused cardiac failure. The flu-like symptoms interpreted by the patient and his physician as a viral or possibly a bacterial infection were no more than symptoms of congestive heart failure (CHF), and explain why the empiric treatment with antibiotics failed. CHF was confirmed by the autopsy findings of an enlarged, dilated heart and pulmonary edema. In addition to pump failure, the patient had a component of restrictive heart disease due to the presence of granulomas and extensive areas of replacement and interstitial fibrosis. In this setting, arrhythmogenic events resulting in death are likely to occur. Sarcoidosis in most instances is a diagnosis of exclusion. When a young patient presents with syncope, other heart conditions causing arrhythmia and reduced cardiac output should be considered such as Stokes-Adams-Morgagni syndrome (complete atrio-ventricular block), Wolff-Parkinson-White syndrome, sick sinus syndrome, hypertrophic as well as other types of cardiomyopathy and myocarditis. Massive myocardial infarction must also be excluded.

In case # 24, we are also dealing with a young patient who experienced syncope as well as lightheadedness and tachycardia. However, this case, although interesting, was unlikely to be diagnosed pre-mortem. The characteristics of this patient's tumor (multicystic and multilayered by polygonal cells) are those of a cystic tumor of the atrio-ventricular node (AV node), formerly known as mesothelioma of the AV node. Cystic tumors are located in the atrial septum in the region of the AV node. The cell of origin is unknown. These neoplasms were previously considered mesothelial in nature, but with the advent of immunohistochemical markers, endodermal derivation has been suggested. Although considered a "benign" tumor in terms of its growth rate and potential for metastatic spread, its location is lethal. Cystic tumors of the AV node are rare, and incidentally found in patients that die suddenly of complete heart block or ventricular fibrillation. Clinically, the differential diagnosis in a patient with syncope due to ventricular fibrillation includes long Q-T syndrome, a condition that may be familial and associated with deafness. An important lesson in this case is to think about all the possibilities in a patient that dies of an arrhythmia. Sections of the AV node are not standard in an autopsy. The pathologist has to think about this diagnosis as a possibility in order to take sections of the AV node. The block of tissue for histologic examination should be obtained from the right atrium, near the coronary sinus. The section must include the tricuspid valve leaflet in continuity with the aortic valve leaflet and the atrioventricular septum. The latter contains the AV node immediately beneath the endocardium. Examination of the entire conduction system is not routinely carried out unless structural abnormalities are suspected. Most pathologists are not familiar with the histologic examination of conduction tissues and prefer to refer these cases to cardiovascular pathologists. Nonetheless, it is important to be aware of primary tumors that can potentially cause arrhythmogenic events in addition to cystic tumors of the AV node. These include fibromas, rhabdomyomas, hemangiomas, lymphangiomas and their malignant counterparts fibrosarcoma, rhabdomyosarcoma and angiosarcoma. Other primary tumors of the heart are teratomas and granular cell tumors. These are rare neoplasms and their description is beyond the scope of this discussion. The most primary cardiac tumor of all is illustrated in case # 25.

This young woman presented with episodes of syncope that lasted several minutes and was found to have multiple cerebral lesions that on CT scan were suggestive of infarcts. Weeks later she developed ischemic bowel disease caused by an embolic lesion of the superior mesenteric artery that was histologically consistent with a myxoma. The ischemic infarcts of the brain and small bowel were the result of arterial occlusion by embolic fragments of a left atrial myxoma diagnosed on a post-surgical echocardiogram. Atrial myxomas are benign, pedunculated or sessile tumors composed of a mucopolysaccharide matrix in which polygonal and stellate-shaped cells are embedded (Figures 65 and 66). Occasionally, these cells may have a glandular arrangement and can exhibit tinctorial properties similar to glandular epithelial cells by staining positive for mucin. The majority of these tumors arise in the left atrium (75% of cases) and in middle-aged women. They are often solitary, but a familial, autosomal dominant condition has been

214

described in which the myxomas are multicentric and are associated with endocrine abnormalities and pigmented lesions of the skin (Carney's syndrome).

The clinical presentation of cardiac myxomas depends on the site of origin. In this case, the patient presented with embolic phenomena. Although her cerebral infarcts appeared to have no sequelae, she required surgical intervention to remove a segment of necrotic bowel. Syncope was due to mechanical reduction of venous return, similarly to what occurs when the Valsalva maneuver is applied as the patient strains against a closed glottis. The tumor was pedunculated and acted as a ball valve obstructing the mitral valve outflow. The obstruction was responsible for the diastolic murmur and the click. Both, the diastolic murmur and the click can be mistaken for those of mitral valve stenosis, and in fact, patients with left atrial myxoma were in the past erroneously diagnosed as having rheumatic heart disease. The diastolic murmur caused by atrial myxoma and the diastolic murmur of mitral stenosis can be discriminated on the basis of positional change. The murmur caused by the obstructing tumor diminishes or disappears when the patient changes positions. Similarly, the click (also known as a tumor plop) auscultated in patients with left atrial myxoma can be distinguished from the opening click of mitral stenosis in that the former occurs during ventricular filling when the valve is already open. Right atrial myxomas are less frequent and may be more difficult to diagnose clinically since they can exhibit variable symptomatology. Some of the clinical manifestations include pulmonary emboli, arrhythmias and congestive heart failure. Presumptive diagnosis is made with imaging studies (Figure 67) and the treatment is surgical removal of the tumor. In this case, following the diagnosis, the patient underwent open heart surgery with a curative resection of the tumor.

Suggested Readings

1. Arthur W, Kaye GC. The pathophysiology of common causes of syncope. Postgrad Med J. 2000; 76:750-3.
2. Kapoor WN. Syncope. N Engl J Med. 2000; 343:1856-62.
3. Meyer MD, Handler J. Evaluation of the patient with syncope: an evidence based approach. Emerg Med Clin North Am. 1999; 17:189-201.
4. Shammas RL, Movahed A. Sarcoidosis of the heart. Clin Cardiol. 1993; 16:462-72.
5. Sekiguchi M, Yazaki Y, Isobe M, Hiroe M. Cardiac sarcoidosis: diagnostic, prognostic, and therapeutic considerations. Cardiovasc Drugs Ther. 1996; 10:495-510.
6. Cina SJ, Smialek JE, Burke AP, Virmani R, Hutchins GM. Primary cardiac tumors causing sudden death: a review of the literature. Am J Forensic Med Pathol. 1996; 17:271-81.
7. MsAllister HA Jr. Primary tumors and cysts of the heart and pericardium. In: Current Problems in Cardiology. Harvey WP, ed. Chicago; Year Book; 1979.
8. Shapiro LM. Cardiac tumours: diagnosis and management. Heart. 2001; 85:218-22.
9. Reynen K. Cardiac myxomas. N Engl J Med. 1995; 333:1610-7.
10. Pinede L, Duhaut P, Loire R. Clinical presentation of left atrial cardiac myxoma. A series of 112 consecutive cases. Medicine (Baltimore). 2001; 80:159-72.

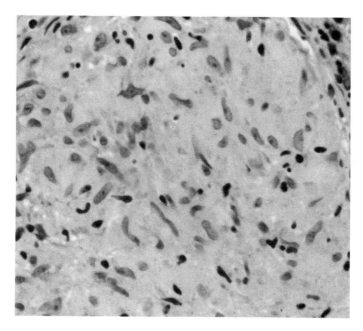

Figure 63. Sarcoidosis, histologic section. Non-necrotizing granuloma (Hematoxylin and Eosin, 20X. Courtesy of Dr. Sui Zee, Albert Einstein College of Medicine).

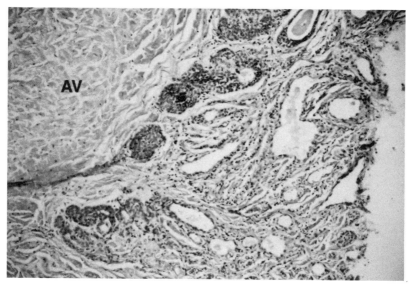

Figure 64. Cystic tumor of the A-V node, histologic section. Nodules and small cysts focally infiltrate the A-V node (Hematoxylin and Eosin, 10X).

217

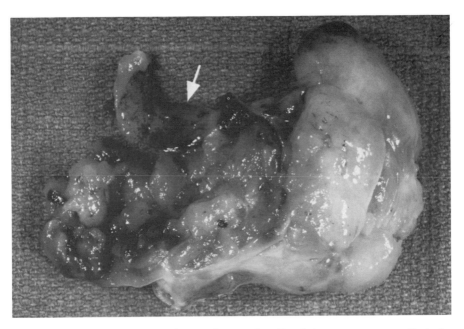

Figure 65. Myxoma. The resected tumor has a polypoid, gelatinous appearance. Foci of hemorrhage are present (arrow).

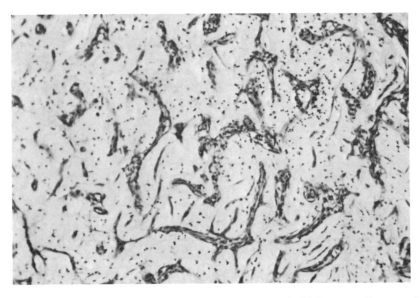

Figure 66. Myxoma, histologic section. The tumor is composed of delicate capillaries and stellate-shaped cells eEmbedded in a myxoid material (Hematoxylin and Eosin, 20X).

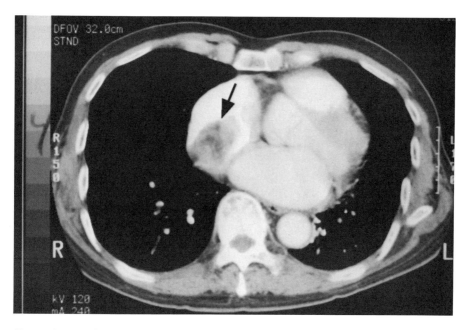

Figure 67. Atrial myxoma. CT scan with contrast reveals a large, lobulated intracavitary mass in the right atrium (arrow). Surgical excision confirmed the diagnosis as myxoma.

Chapter 10

THE PERICARDIUM

Case # 26

Clinical Summary

This 43 year old African American woman, former intravenous drug user with unknown HIV status (spouse was HIV-infected), presented to the emergency room with a 5 month history of weight loss, night sweats, cough with occasional hemoptysis, and 2 weeks of severe pleuritic chest pain and shortness of breath. On initial evaluation in the emergency department she had a normal mental status, but was in significant respiratory distress. There was no jaundice, edema or cyanosis. Head and neck exam was remarkable for oral thrush and no significant lymphadenopathy. The upper extremities had fibrotic areas in the antecubital areas and forearms consistent with old healed scars. Auscultation of the heart revealed S1 and S2, tachycardic, regular rhythm, and a friction rub. No murmurs were reported. There was dullness on percussion at the right lung base, and diffuse crackles over both lungs.

Laboratory data and other tests

Laboratory: WBC 4.6 (S 93, L 4, M 1, E 2), Hb/Hct 7/22, Plt 133; BUN/creat 37/1.4, SGOT 180, protein T/A 7.2/2.2, bilirrubin T/D 2.1/1.5, glucose 124; CK 307, LD 1288. The ECG showed sinus tachycardia at 127 ppm, and low voltage complexes. The chest x ray revealed diffuse interstitial nodular infiltrates with a miliary pattern.

Hospital course: the patient was admitted and started on trimethoprim-sulfamethoxazole (TMP-SMX) for possible Pneumocystis carinii pneumonia and anti-tuberculous drugs (isoniazid, rifampin, ethambutol and pyrazinamide). The following day, she was found without vital signs. Resuscitation efforts were unsuccessful.

Gross Description

The body was that of a thin, well developed African American woman appearing her stated age. It measured 158 cm and weighed 60 kg. The heart weighed 410 g and was of normal shape. However, the pericardial sac was thickened with numerous adhesions. The pericardium and endocardium were diffusely covered by fibrinopurulent exudates and foci of hemorrhage (Figure 68). The myocardium, endocardium and valves were all unremarkable. The coronary arteries were of normal caliber and distribution with no occlusions. The lungs were heavy (combined weight 1700 g, normal is approximately 1% of body weight). The pleural surfaces were diffusely granular. On section, the parenchyma showed multiple white-yellow nodular lesions measuring up to 0.3 cm in diameter present throughout both lungs. The bronchial mucosa was congested. The pulmonary vessels were grossly unremarkable. The mediastinal lymph nodes were diffusely enlarged and had a similar nodular pattern to that noted in the lungs.

Microscopic Description

Sections of the lungs and heart revealed that the nodular areas consisted of caseous necrosis rich in mycobacteria. The inflammatory response was mainly composed of neutrophils, lymphocytes and plasma cells with a few epithelioid histiocytes and Langerhan's giant cells. Well-developed granulomas were not present. Fibrinopurulent material also loaded with acid fast bacilli covered the epicardium and one third of the myocardial wall (Figure 69).

Case Analysis

This woman presented with several months of constitutional and respiratory symptomatology, but recently an acute exacerbation of her respiratory symptoms and pleuritic chest pain had forced her to visit the ER. These complaints primarily indicate a pulmonary and/or pericardial involvement. The clinical hallmarks of pericarditis are pleuritic chest pain and a friction rub, and both were present in this patient. Pericarditis (PC) refers to the inflammation of the pericardium, which covers the heart surface and the proximal part of the great vessels. The pericardium is a 1.0 mm thick membrane of dense collagen lined by a single layer of mesothelial cells. It consists of two layers, the inner or visceral continues with the outer myocardial tissue, and the outer or parietal attaches to the sternum, diaphragm and adventitia of great vessels. Between these two layers there is a virtual space that normally contains about 15 to 50 mL of fluid (filtered plasma), which serves as a lubricant to the heart surfaces. Normally, the pericardial tissue is thin and semitransparent, but with inflammation it reacts by exuding fibrin, fluid, polymorphonuclear leukocytes and/or mononuclear cells. Acute pericarditis may resolve without sequelae. However, if there is proliferation of fibrous tissue, neovascularization and scarring, the end result will be a loss of elasticity (compliance), restriction of heart filling and constrictive pericarditis. The pleuritic pain is classically described as a retrosternal sharp, stabbing, knife-like quality pain, which worsens with inspiration, lying down and swallowing, and improves sitting up and leaning forward. The reasons for the exacerbation and ease of the pain have to do with the position of the heart relative to the rest of the mediastinal structures, which impact on how the pericardium is pulled and stretched, or relaxed. The radiation of the pain relates to the visceral reflections of the pericardium, and is mostly to the shoulder and neck (trapezius muscle). The pain is common in acute infectious pericarditis, whereas insidious accumulation of fluid in the pericardial sac (usually due to non-infectious etiologies) may go unnoticed. The ability of the pericardium to accommodate fluid subacutely or chronically depends on the ratio between production, reabsorption and pericardial distensibility properties. The latter, are a function of the pericardial connective tissue components, which allow for progressive remodeling. With slow accumulation of fluid, or progressive cardiac hypertrophy, the volume of the pericardial sac increases by slippage of the collagen fibers in the parietal layer. With extreme increases of volume, disruption of the collagen fibers can occur. If the increase in pericardial fluid develops too rapidly for the stiff pericardium to respond, tamponade may ensue (see below).

The other critical finding on physical examination was the presence of a friction rub. This variably coarse, scratchy, velcro-like sound, is best heard over the left sternal border, and when the patient is not breathing. It has three components: the atrial systole, the ventricular systole and the rapid ventricular filling. The ventricular systolic component is the loudest and most commonly appreciated. The sound is made when the two roughened and inflamed pericardial layers slide against each other during the cardiac cycle. A disappearing pericardial rub initially heard in a patient who continues to deteriorate clinically, is reason for concern. It implies that the pericardial fluid is increasing and the layers are not in contact at all. The continued accumulation of fluid in the pericardial sac results in interference with heart chamber filling, which leads to increased intracardiac pressures, decreased venous return and eventually a decrease in stroke volume and cardiac output (if untreated, these will eventually lead to death). All these pathophysiological events translate in to the classic Beck's triad of hypotension, jugular venous distension, and low intensity or muffled heart sounds, characteristic of cardiac tamponade. Normally, during inspiration, there is a decrease in intrathoracic pressure, which increases venous return. When the heart pressures are higher, the pulmonary venous blood is prevented from easily entering the left atrium. This causes a decrease in arterial pulse pressure and pulsus paradoxus becomes evident. The latter, is a decrease in systolic blood pressure by more than 10 mm Hg (rarely > 15) during inspiration, because of the decreased venous return. The progressive restriction of ventricular filling triggers a series of compensatory mechanisms similar to those observed in congestive heart failure (CHF). These include an increase in the heart rate, since the stroke volume becomes fixed (there is tachycardia with an abbreviated filling period); peripheral vasoconstriction; and the secretion of humoral or hormonal and renal factors (due to restriction of atrial distensibility there is no significant secretion of the atrial natriuretic factor). In our patient this was evident in the signs and symptoms resembling CHF (e.g. progressive dyspnea, hypoxemia, weakness, passive liver congestion).

Her clinical history had two epidemiologic facts that were extremely important to the overall approach to her illness. First, her immune competence was in question because of the significant risk factors of past intravenous drug use, her spouse being HIV-infected, and the presence of oral thrush. Thus, the index of suspicion for HIV-infection was extremely high as her HIV status was unknown. Secondly, her daughter, who was HIV-infected, had been diagnosed with pulmonary tuberculosis (TB) that did not require hospitalization, and was convalescing in the patient's house. All these elements make our patient a special host, not only because of her possible increased exposure to TB, but also due to a probable dysfunctional immune system which would render her abnormally susceptible to TB (HIV-infection increases both primary TB infection and reactivation). In addition to HIV altering the natural history and epidemiology of TB, there appears to be an equally important influence of TB on the course of HIV-infection. TB can cause CD4 lymphopenia, which reverses after treatment; and TB-related immune activation may increase HIV replication as well. Even more startling is the observation that TB may accelerate the course of HIV disease. Patients dually infected with HIV and TB have worse outcomes (development of opportunistic infections and death) than their counterparts without TB. From a global perspective, TB may be one of the most common HIV-related opportunistic infections.

The cause of death in this patient was a combination of disseminated tuberculous infection, predominantly in the heart (pericardium) and lungs, with a likely underlying acquired immunodeficiency. The pericardial findings demonstrated acute severe fibrino-purulent pericarditis, with adhesions and thickening of the pericardium. The hallmark of her immunodeficiency was the almost complete absence of granuloma formation. This observation suggests that the normal initial mechanisms to contain mycobacterial infection were not in place, and were probably due to cellular immune defects coupled with a lack of immune activation which coordinates the cellular and tissue interaction. The TB pericarditis is rare but a serious complication of tuberculosis. It can lead, in about 30-50% of the cases, to constricitive pericarditis (even if treated), with a particularly higher prevalence in immunosuppressed individuals (especially those with HIV infection). Mycobacterium tuberculosis (MTB) reaches the pericardium via lymphatic or contiguous spread from a lung or a lymph node (peritracheal, peribronchial or mediastinal) focus; or hematogenously from a distant site. Initial stage involves fibrin deposition and multiple granulomas formation with abundant viable MTB. This is followed by a slow accumulation of a serous or sero-sanguineous pericardial effusion, usually without symptoms. Once the effusion is absorbed, further granuloma formation occurs and the pericardium thickens with dense fibrous tissue and collagen deposits. The final stage occurs when the pericardial space is obliterated by dense adhesions, the parietal pericardium thickens and most granulomas are replaced by fibrous tissue and calcification. All these changes result in a markedly constrictive pericardium, where small increments of fluid will produce significant increases in intracardiac pressures, leading to decreased cardiac output. Other causes of pericarditis that must be included in the differential diagnosis are the idiopathic and viral (usually benign, self-limited), purulent pericarditis (fatal if untreated), and the non-infectious group which includes collagen-vascular disease, drugs, post-trauma, malignancies, and uremia.

The laboratory and other diagnostic tests for pericarditis may be non-specific and may reflect the nature of the underlying disease. In general, there may be mild CK-MB elevation (our patient had a modest CK and transaminase increase), which suggests subepicardial myocarditis (contiguous spread). In this case the local invasion to a third of the myocardial thickness reflects the total inability to contain and control the TB infection. Again this is a manifestation of her severely compromised cellular immune response. In addition, abnormal liver function tests may indicate chronic congestion, as seen in cases of CHF. Although, there usually are no systolic abnormalities (except with coexistent myocardial lesions), the constricition of the pericardium resembles the clinical features of CHF (there is diminished functional heart volume, with decreased stroke volume and low cardiac output). The chest x ray may be normal, since only pericardial volumes of above 200-250 mL may present as cardiomegaly. Therefore, a normal cardiac silhouette on CXR does not exclude acute or small pericardial effusions. Although the pericardium does not produce electrical activity, the ECG is abnormal in about 90% of the cases of pericarditis, probably reflecting subepicardial inflammation. The usual changes involve diffuse ST elevation, and after recovery, T wave abnormalities may persist. In addition, the typical low voltage complexes result from the damping of electrical activity due to the pericardial effusion. The echocardiogram may be the most important test to perform in someone suspected of having a pericardial effusion. It not only can accurately detect small volumes, but it can also estimate the pericardial thickness and overall cardiac function. Furthermore, it may even be used to do an ultrasound guided pericardiocentesis both for therapeutic and diagnostic (fluid examination) purposes.

The autopsy findings in this woman were specific for the significant disseminated TB infection, and evident cardiovascular failure. By the time of her presentation, both the TB and her immunodeficiency were at such an advanced stage, that it would have been extremely difficult to reverse the effects of any of them. Her death, under these circumstances was unavoidable.

Suggested Readings

1. Chin DP, Hopewell PC. Mycobacterial complications of HIV infection. Clin Chest Med. N Amer. 1996; 17:697-711.
2. Kardon D, Borczuk AC, Factor SM. Mechanism of pericardial dilatation associated with cardiac hypertrophy and pericardial effusion. Cardiovasc Pathol. 2000; 9:9-15
3. Afzal A, Keohane M, Keeley E, Borzak S, Callender CW, Iannuzzi M. Myocarditis and pericarditis with tamponade associated with disseminated tuberculosis. Can J Cardiol. 2000; 16:519-21.
4. Chen Y, Brennessel D, Walters J, Johnson M, Rosner F, Raza M. Human immunodeficiency virus-associated pericardial effusion: report of 40 cases and review of the literature. Am Heart J. 1999; 137:516-21.
5. Alvarez S, McCabe WR. Extrapulmonary tuberculosis revisited: a review of experience at Boston City and other hospitals. Medicine (Baltimore). 1984; 63:25-55.
6. Myers RB; Spodick DH. Constrictive pericarditis: clinical and pathophysiologic characteristics. Am Heart J. 1999; 138:219-32

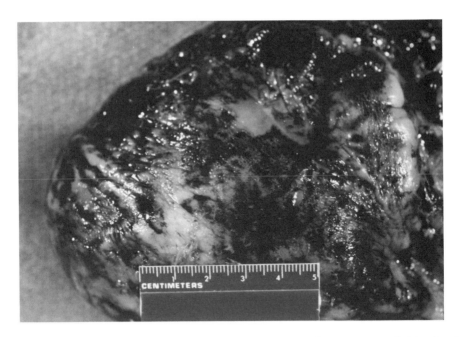

Figure 68. Fibrinous pericarditis. The epicardial surface of the heart is covered by blood and fibrin.

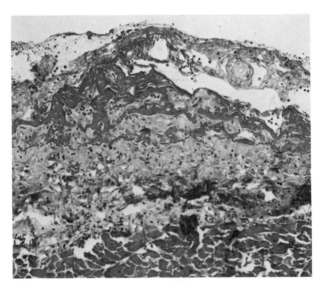

Figure 69. Left ventricle, histologic section, showing fibrinous pericarditis (top) (Hematoxylin and Eosin, 10X).

228

Chapter 11

AORTIC ANEURYSMS

Case # 27

Clinical Summary

This 61 year old hypertensive African American man was brought to the emergency room with severe shortness of breath, pallor, and left abdominal and epigastric pain.

On admission, his vital signs were: BP 188/110, P 138, RR 30 and T 36.8°C. His physical exam was remarkable for a firm pulsatile mass felt in the abdominal lower left quadrant, and decreased femoral pulses. A CT of abdomen and chest revealed an abdominal aortic aneurysm and retroperitoneal blood. In the emergency room, he became bradycardic, apneic and unresponsive, but responded to resuscitation and then was transferred to the operating room. The abdomen was opened and the aorta was clamped above the renal arteries. The retroperitoneum was filled with blood and the margins of the aneurysm were difficult to establish. After five units of blood and 5 liters of crystalloids were given, the patient arrested on the table and was pronounced dead after all resuscitation efforts failed.

Gross Description

The body measured 158 cm in length and weighed 80 kg. The heart weighed 600 g. The pericardium was smooth and shiny. The epicardium had focal petechial hemorrhages on the anterior surface consistent with resuscitation maneuvers. The atria were of normal size without thrombi. The right and left ventricular walls measure 0.6 and 1.6 cm in thickness, respectively. The valve leaflets were pliable and the chordae tendineae were thin. The endocardium had foci of hemorrhage. The myocardium was grossly normal. The coronaries revealed mild atherosclerosis with no occlusions. The aorta showed aneurysmal dilatation extending from the celiac artery to the iliac bifurcation. The aneurysm measured 19 cm in length by 8 cm in diameter and had a large defect with ragged edges measuring up to 15 cm in length. The wall of the aneurysm was very thin and covered with atherosclerotic plaques and areas of necrosis. There was an aneurysmal dilatation of the aortic arch measuring 4 cm in greatest diameter. The brachiocephalic artery was also dilated, and was occluded by a recent thrombus.

Case Analysis

This man presented to the hospital with shortness of breath and severe abdominal pain of acute onset. Although he had tachycardia (138/min) suggesting hypovolemia, he was hypertensive (188/110 mmmHg), most likely due to peripheral vasoconstriction. On physical examination, a pulsatile mass in the left lower quadrant was evident. A CT scan of the abdomen and chest revealed an aortic aneurysm from the thorax to the common iliac arteries associated with retroperitoneal blood clot. He became unresponsive and had a cardiopulmonary arrest, after attempting stabilization he was taken to the operating room with the presumptive diagnosis of a ruptured aneurysm. The surgeons used a combined thoraco-abdominal incision because of the length of the aneurysm. Despite blood and fluid replacement, he had a cardiac arrest on the operating table, and could not be resuscitated.

The mortality rate of a ruptured abdominal aortic aneurysm that leads to emergency surgery can be as high as 90%. The outlook has improved recently, but still the mortality remains greater than 50%. In contrast, elective surgical intervention performed prior to rupture has a completely different result, with greater than 90% *survival*. Therefore, a primary goal in dealing with patients at risk for abdominal aortic aneurysm is the early diagnosis, and appropriate intervention. The issues we will discuss include the risk profile of patients, the etiology, anatomy and pathophysiology of aneurysms with and without rupture, and the complications beyond free rupture and hypovolemic shock.

An aneurysm is an outward 'bulge' of a vascular structure involving the full-thickness of the vascular wall. For instance, one can have an aneurysm of the left ventricle (a muscular vascular tube) following a myocardial infarction, with replacement of the full thickness of ventricular myocardium by scar tissue. Aneurysm development in arteries can involve the entire circumference of the vessel, in which case there is a **diffuse** or **fusiform** (cylindrical) aneurysm (Figures 70 and 71); or a localized bulge of a segment of the vessel known as a **saccular** aneurysm. Either type is susceptible to rupture or the other complications we will discuss. The term aneurysm is often applied to dissection of a vessel, but this is incorrect. A dissection is a partial tear or separation of layers within the vessel wall. It results in a **pseudo-aneurysm**, where there is a localized vascular rupture partially enclosed by surrounding tissue. Pseudo-aneurysm also can develop with a complete rupture of a vascular structure, and the tear site and hematoma are maintained within the surrounding tissues and organs (e.g.

pleura, pericardium, peritoneum). By this definition, there could be a rupture of a true aneurysm of the aorta, with a secondary pseudo-aneurysm, if the rupture site was walled-off by peritoneum, mesentery, or the vertebral column (Figure 72). The other use of the term aneurysm is applied to **mycotic aneurysm** (Figure 73). Mycotic aneurysm is a pseudo-aneurysm secondary to infection of the vascular wall. In general, the rupture site is an abscess with organizing inflammation. Mycotic aneurysm also can develop within a true aneurysm, following secondary infection. Any of these aneurysms, or pseudo-aneurysms has the potential to rupture.

A somewhat subjective aspect of aneurysms is how much dilatation of the vessel wall is required before it is called an aneurysm. With a focal bulge it is relatively straightforward; a saccular outpouching is easy to recognize and discriminate from the remaining vessel wall. In contrast, a diffuse or fusiform aneurysm may involve a segment of the vessel, or it may be a continuation of a generalized dilatation. The latter, known as **ectasia**, is a common phenomenon in elderly patients over the age of 75 years. The aorta dilates diffusely, and may even become tortuous. As a rule, it is preferred to retain the term aneurysm for focal bulges, whether saccular or fusiform, that are more than 25% over the adjacent vessel circumference.

Although aneurysms can occur anywhere in the vascular tree (e.g. intracerebral arteries, thoracic aorta, etc), abdominal aortic aneurysms have the highest incidence, and are the most likely to have a fatal rupture. Even the familiar shorthand term for abdominal aortic aneurysms, AAA or 'triple A', reflects how common it is. The location of the aneurysm, and the profile of the patient often provides significant clues as to the etiology of the condition. AAAs are predominantly the result of severe atherosclerosis of the aorta. Thus, the risk factors for AAA should be the same of those for atherosclerosis. If this is the case, why is it that some individuals with severe atherosclerosis develop coronary or cerebral complications, while others develop aneurysms of the aorta? Are the risk factors for atherosclerosis a sufficient explanation for the development of AAA? Recent information strongly suggests the answer is a resounding no!

Although aneurysms can develop anywhere in the aorta, the ones due to atherosclerosis are far more common in the abdominal aorta, particularly distal to the renal arteries. They may extend into the iliac arteries as a continuous lesion, or there may form separate iliac aneurysms. Atherosclerosis of the abdominal aorta tends to increase in severity from proximal to distal. The explanation for this is uncertain, although it has been suggested that it is a phenomenon of human upright posture and gravity. The increased vascular wall injury develops secondary to the effects of the pressurized column of blood within the aorta (until the time when humans could live permanently in low gravity conditions, this hypothesis will not be tested). However, what is definitely known, is that there is a significant association of AAA with systemic hypertension, smoking, diabetes mellitus and older age (aneurysms are rare before the 6th decade, and are mos common between the 7th and 9th decades). Even though these are all risk factors for atherosclerosis, there is a disproportionate ratio of male gender. and a known familial predisposition. The presence of an AAA in a sibling or parent, significantly increases the risk for that individual. This familial tendency and male predominance strongly suggests that additional unrecognized entities are interacting with the more common and generally modifiable risk factors, which contribute to the development of atherosclerotic AAA.

Molecular defects that impact on the structural integrity of the vessel wall might explain the known link between aneurysms and several relatively rare genetic disorders. Osteogenesis imperfecta, a disease of the skeleton due to a defect in collagen type I (the primary fibrillar component of collagen), is associated with aortic aneurysms. The basis for Ehlers-Danlos type IV syndrome is a defect of collagen type III (the reticular component of collagen), and it presents with skin, connective tissue and cardiovascular system manifestations, including aortic aneurysms. On the other hand, defective collagen resulting from inadequate cross-linking, due to the effects of β-aminoproprionitrile (the active ingredient in sweat-pea that has been associated with a clinical and experimentally-induced condition known as lathyrism), typically leads to aortic dissection in man and laboratory animals. Therefore, although collagen abnormalities may be associated with aneurysms, it is unclear whether genetic, acquired or both types of collagen defects explain the pathogenesis of aortic aneurysms. It is instructive to recall that for more than half a century the etiology of Marfan's syndrome and aortic dissection was thought to be defective collagen, until the defect was identified in a microfibrillar glycoprotein component of *elastic* tissue, called fibrillin.

There are two other pathogenic considerations that have received interest recently, but before we discuss them we should address the pathological changes that occur within aneurysms. The media of the aorta is an elastic structure composed of approximately 40 stacked layers of elastic tissue fibers, smooth muscle cells, and collagen, called lamellae. There are also vessels in the outer third of the tissue (vasa vasorum), that provide blood supply to the inner media (diffusion of oxygen from the lumen through the tissue is insufficient). Atherosclerosis is initially an intimal disease. However, with increasing severity, it extends into the media where it replaces the lamellar structure with plaque, debris, fibrous tissue, calcification, and inflammation. The loss of elastic lamellae leads to a weakening of the tensile strength of the aorta. If there is only localized atherosclerosis, there may be no adverse consequences; but when it becomes diffuse and involves the full aortic wall thickness, there may be aneurysm formation. The disruption of the tissue by plaque, can also affect the vasa vasorum and their ability to supply blood to the media, thereby causing further damage to the wall. The degenerative process resulting from atherosclerosis is the primary cause of aneurysms; but as we have seen, there appear to be other elements that contribute to the breakdown of the media, and the weakening of the aortic wall.

One potential pathogenic mechanism may be related to the activation of lytic enzymes in the aortic atherosclerotic plaque. Similar to the transformation of a stable coronary artery atherosclerotic plaque into an unstable one, with plaque rupture and coronary thrombosis, the atherosclerotic AAA tissue breakdown can be associated with enzyme activity derived from inflammatory cells in the plaque. In particular, collagenases and elastases may play a significant role in media destruction and mural weakening. There appears to be variability in the degree of inflammation in atherosclerosis regardless of site. Some patients seem to have more inflamed plaques than others, making them more susceptible to atherosclerotic complications. Whether this inflammatory activity is genetically determined is unknown. Another potential etiology is related to the possibility that atherosclerotic plaques may become sites of secondary infection. Bacteria can lead to an inflammatory response and a secondary release of collagenases and elastases from inflammatory cells. Furthermore, they can also elaborate their own collagenases with direct degradation of tissue, which may lead to bacterial spread and abscess formation. Gram negative bacteria, and particularly Salmonella species, have a predilection for the debris and surface thrombus associated with atherosclerotic plaques in the aorta (Salmonella have been cultured from surgically repaired aortic aneurysms). Whether, any or all of these potential etiologies is working separately or together to cause aneurysms is unknown. But, since a number of these mechanisms may be prevented or modified by treatment, medical intervention to avoid aneurysm expansion and possible rupture may be feasible in the future.

Size and expansion is the critical issue with abdominal aortic aneurysms. The diameter of the aneurysm is directly proportional to its likelihood of rupture. Also, whether it is stable or progressing over time, determines its rupture potential. Since both of these parameters can be assessed non-invasively with ultrasound, CT scan, or magnetic resonance imaging (MRI), patients can be followed longitudinally to determine when, or if, it is appropriate to intervene therapeutically. What is the critical size? The normal aorta has a diameter of 2.5-3.0 cm. An aneurysm of 4.0-6.0 cm is at a critical size; beyond that, the potential for rupture increases significantly each year. Furthermore, an unstable aneurysm that expands progressively at a rate greater than 0.5 cm per year is at risk for rupture. A 4.0-6.0 cm aneurysm is generally palpable in most individuals; therefore physical examination is an important screening test. The size of the aneurysm and its growth are determined by the mechanisms discussed above. However, there are also physical factors that impact on the likelihood of rupture. As the aneurysm expands, the increased diameter affects the wall stress and potential for rupture. The relationship is explained by LaPlace's law:

$$\text{Wall Stress} = \frac{\text{Pressure X Radius}}{2 \text{ X Wall Thickness}}$$

Thus, the radius or diameter of the aneurysm is directly proportional to the wall stress (a wall that is already weakened by atherosclerotic degeneration). Essentially, the larger the balloon, the more likely it is to burst. It is critically important to intervene before this occurs, for reasons that became evident in this case.

There are complications of aneurysm in addition to fatal rupture. Aneurysms frequently thrombose and the thrombus may fragment and embolize into the distal circulation of the lower extremities leading to acute ischemia. If the aneurysm is fusiform, and the thrombus continues to aggregate, there may be partial or complete obstruction of the lower abdominal aorta. This can cause lower extremity ischemia, intermittent claudication, or gangrene. When there is lower extremity ischemia involving the thigh and below, in association with impotence, the Leriche syndrome (obstruction of the distal aorta) must be considered. In the absence of significant thrombosis, the ulcerative, atheromatous surface of an aneurysm may be the source of cholesterol and plaque emboli. These usually affect smaller vessels in the distal extremities, but may lead to toe and foot gangrene, or the so-called 'trash foot'.

There are several other complications associated with localized rupture. With progressive atherosclerosis, the abdominal aortic aneurysms often develop inflammation and fibrosis of the adventitia. The inflammatory response may induce the aorta to adhere to the surrounding tissues or organs, which include the intestine, vena cava, and vertebral column. The abdominal aorta is a retroperitoneal structure. It lies immediately posterior to the 3rd and 4th portions of the duodenum, proximal to the ligament of Treitz. The duodenum in this location crosses the aorta at the level of the aortic bifurcation into the iliac arteries. Accordingly, this site, which is the most prevalent for atherosclerotic aneurysms, is susceptible to the rupture of an aneurysm into the intestine. This is known as an **aorto-enteric fistula**. It is virtually always fatal, with exsanguinating gastrointestinal hemorrhage. Rarely, it may produce a slow leak, and be a cause of chronic anemia. If the aortic aneurysm becomes adherent along its lateral wall, it can rupture into the vena cava, causing an **arteriovenous fistula**, and high output congestive heart failure. Finally, if the aneurysm extends posteriorly, either with or without rupture, it can lead to vertebral column erosion and severe back pain.

234

Several comments about diagnosis and treatment. As noted above, aneurysms at a critical size (over 5.0 cm) can be palpated with careful examination of the abdomen at the level of the umbilicus. Palpation of a mass, with characteristic lateral pulsations, is strongly supportive of the diagnosis. It also is noteworthy that aneurysms susceptible to rupture often have slow leakage over days to weeks prior to massive rupture. This can lead to inflammation and irritation of nerves in adventitial tissues, thereby causing back or flank pain. When aneurysms do rupture, the blood generally tracks in the retroperitoneal tissues, causing flank ecchymoses, scrotal hematoma, and inguinal hematoma. Most often, patients with these signs will also be in shock. If the aneurysm ruptures anteriorly, it can 'break through' the peritoneal membrane, and cause massive hemoperitoneum. This is rapidly fatal.

Treatment is dependent on the size and the rate of growth of the aneurysm, and the presence of complications such as thrombosis and embolization. The approach for the last 5 decades has been prosthetic graft bypass of the aneurysm with interposition of a woven, artificial vessel between the aorta and the iliac or femoral arteries. The graft material is usually Dacron, and it functions very effectively with minimal risk of thrombosis. Even though it is a prosthetic material, which is potentially thrombogenic, its large diameter, and the ingrowth of the patient's own cells through the porous spaces (a *de novo* endothelial lining) between the weave fibers prevent thrombosis. For many years the aneurysm was actually resected; currently, the aneurysm is opened and the graft is placed over the aneurysm bed. The major complications of surgery are related to the time required to cross-clamp the aorta. Since most aneurysms occur below the renal arteries, the potential for renal ischemia is minimized. Clamping above the renal vessels puts the kidney at risk for ischemic injury. Other rare ischemic complications include spinal cord damage with hemiplegia due to interruption of vessels supplying the cord, and left colon ischemia due to lack of flow in the inferior mesenteric artery. Both are unusual, because of collateral blood supply that efficiently develops over time, triggered by the longstanding atherosclerotic occlusion of the larger vessel. Other standard surgical complications are bleeding and infection. Moreover, a major cause of morbidity and mortality, is related to cardiac and cerebral ischemia, since patients with AAA, invariably have systemic atherosclerosis.

As a final point, it should be mentioned that a new approach to aneurysm 'repair' is becoming prevalent in selected patients. Aneurysms without significant atherosclerotic stenosis of iliac arteries can be treated with endovascular grafting. Tubular, telescoped grafts can be introduced into the aorta from the femoral artery under radiographic control, where they can be extended from the normal aorta superior to the aneurysm to the iliac arteries. They function as a conduit across the aneurysm, thereby eliminating the risk of aneurysm rupture, and any of the surgical complications associated with repair. It is likely that as with the growing use of stents to maintain coronary patency following angioplasty, endovascular aortic grafting will rapidly become a popular approach to dealing with the common, and dangerous AAA.

Suggested Readings

1. Blanchard JF. Epidemiology of abdominal aortic aneurysms. Epidemiol Rev. 1999; 21:207-21.
2. Dietz HC. New insights into the genetic basis of aortic aneurysms. Monogr Pathol. 1995; 37:144-55.
3. Vorp DA, Trachtenberg JD, Webster MW. Arterial hemodynamics and wall mechanics. Semin Vasc Surg. 1998; 11:169-80.
4. Grange JJ, Davis V, Baxter BT. Pathogenesis of abdominal aortic aneurysm: an update and look toward the future. Cardiovasc Surg. 1997; 5:256-65.
5. Wills A, Thompson MM, Crowther M, Sayers RD, Bell PR. Pathogenesis of abdominal aortic aneurysms--cellular and biochemical mechanisms. Eur J Vasc Endovasc Surg. 1996; 12:391-400.
6. Pearce WH, Koch AE. Cellular components and features of immune response in abdominal aortic aneurysms. Ann N Y Acad Sci. 1996; 800:175-85.
7. Thompson RW, Parks WC. Role of matrix metalloproteinases in abdominal aortic aneurysms. Ann N Y Acad Sci. 1996; 800:157-74.
8. Lindsay J Jr. Diagnosis and treatment of diseases of the aorta. Curr Probl Cardiol. 1997; 22:485-542.
9. Fillinger MF. Imaging of the thoracic and thoracoabdominal aorta. Semin Vasc Surg. 2000; 13:247-63.

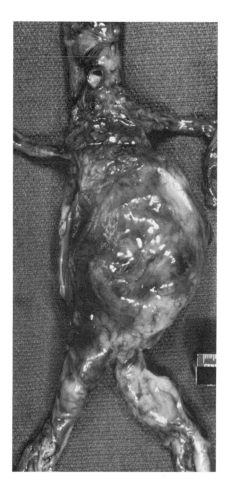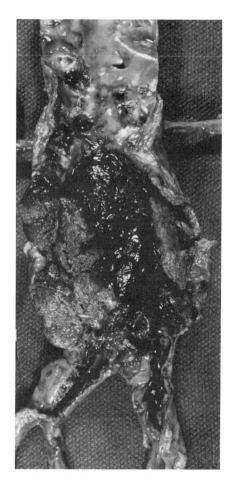

Figure 70 (left). Fusiform aneurysm of abdominal aorta extending from below the renal arteries to the bifurcation of the iliac arteries. There is no evidence of rupture.

Figure 71 (right). Fusiform aneurysm of the abdominal aorta. The aneurysm has been opened to reveal a large thrombus.

238

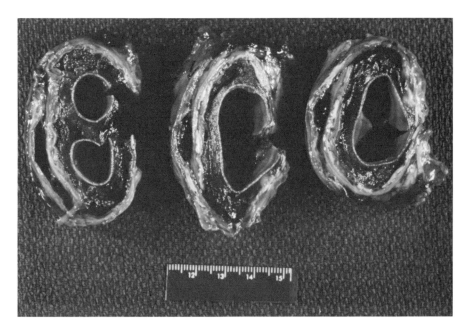

Figure 72. Ruptured aortic aneurysm. Serial transverse sections of an aneurysm of the abdominal aorta revealing a hematoma in the adventitia.

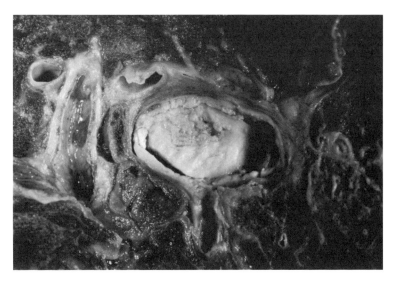

Figure 73. Mycotic aneurysm of the pulmonary artery. The wall of the artery is dilated and the lumen contains a thrombus composed of acute inflammatory cells, fibrin and bacterial organisms.

239

Chapter 12

COLLAGEN VASCULAR DISEASES AND VASCULITIS

Case # 28

Clinical Summary

The patient was a 74-year-old Caucasian man who was admitted to the hospital because of 4-month history of epigastric pain, weight loss of 11 kg and episodes of hematemesis and hemoptysis. The epigastric pain had an insidious onset, was dull, non-radiating, non-exertional, and was not associated with food intake. In addition, he experienced intermittent difficulty in swallowing for which he took antacids with some relief. He also described malaise, hyporexia and nausea. There was a history of hypertension treated with diuretics. The patient also complained about occasional dyspnea on exertion, mild ankle swelling and intermittent claudication. The latter symptoms had developed over a period of a few years, and the patient attributed them to his age. There was no history of rheumatic heart disease, coronary artery disease, gallbladder disease, pancreatitis, hepatitis, change in bowel habits, tuberculosis, bleeding diathesis, or trauma. Surgical history revealed a partial gastrectomy at age 54 for peptic ulcer disease. He drank alcohol socially, and smoked 1-2 PPD for as long as he could remember. He had a chronic productive cough with white sputum, and denied any recent change in the pattern of his cough. He had had multiple sexual partners during his lifetime.

Three months prior to admission, the patient described several episodes of bright red hemoptysis, for which he was admitted to the hospital. He was not certain whether these episodes represented hemoptysis or hematemesis. The physical examination at that time revealed a thin elderly male, appearing chronically ill and somewhat uncomfortable in bed. There was a grade II/VI decrescendo diastolic murmur best heard at the left base. The abdominal examination was unremarkable. There was mild bilateral pitting edema in the lower extremities. The rectal examination revealed no masses and a stool specimen was positive for occult blood. The white blood cell count was normal. The hemoglobin was 8.5 g/dL, and the glucose 136 mg/dL. The transaminases were minimally elevated. The bilirubin and amylase were within normal limits. A urine analysis was unremarkable. The chest-x-ray showed a slightly enlarged heart with a dilated aortic root. The electrocardiogram revealed a pattern compatible with left ventricular hypertrophy. Extensive work-up including GI series, celiac angiogram, and pancreatic scan did not uncover any specific lesion. He was discharged without a definitive diagnosis.

Three days after his release from the hospital, the patient again developed hemoptysis. Meanwhile, his epigastric pain had increased, and he had an overall deterioration of his health with increasing fatigue and anorexia. The temperature was 37°C rectally; pulse 108, respirations 22 and the blood pressure was 140/72 mmHg, without orthostatic changes. The neurologic and HEENT examination was unremarkable. There was no lymphadenopathy. The patient was non-icteric. The carotid pulse was 2+ bilaterally without bruits. The jugular venous pressure was estimated to be within normal limits. The chest was clear to percussion and auscultation. The cardiac examination revealed that the PMI was slightly displaced to the left laterally. Again, there was a grade II/VI diastolic decrescendo murmur that radiated to the left lower sternal border, which was best auscultated at the left base with the patient sitting up and leaning forward. The femoral and popliteal pulses were not palpable bilaterally; however, the pulses of the upper extremities were within normal limits. The abdomen was mildly distended with normal bowel sounds, there was no guarding, rebound tenderness or hepatosplenomegaly. The lower extremities were cool to the touch and had 1+ pitting edema. The rectal examination revealed no masses. A stool sample remained positive for occult blood.

Laboratory data and other tests

Laboratory: WBC 7.0, Hb/Hct 8.4/26, MCV 76, Plt 260 (peripheral blood smear confirmed a microcytic anemia, but was otherwise unremarkable); normal electrolytes, SGOT 48, protein T/A 6.5/3.2, bilirubin T 0.6, LD 378, BUN/creat 28/1.2, glucose 110. The urine analysis was unremarkable. ECG: normal PR and QRS intervals and left ventricular hypertrophy. The CXR showed a moderately enlarged heart with a dilated aortic root. An upright plain film of the abdomen revealed no free air.

While in the hospital, the patient had several more episodes of hemoptysis of about 50 cc each time and one episode of massive bleeding, bringing up an estimate of 1000–1500 cc of bright red blood. Meanwhile, a bronchoscopy failed to reveal any pathology. The bleeding episode recurred and a nasogastric tube was placed revealing fresh blood in the stomach. Irrigation with iced saline, transfusion of 6 units of blood and placement of a Sengstaken-Blakemore tube failed to control the bleeding. The patient was taken to the operating room for a laparotomy and the source of bleeding was located above the stomach. A thoracotomy was performed and a presumptive diagnosis was made. The patient was placed on a partial cardiopulmonary bypass, but had a cardiac arrest and could not be resuscitated.

Gross Description

The body was that of an elderly white male weighing 54 kg. and measuring 167 cm. The heart weighed 400 g, with hypertrophy of the left ventricle. Marked dilatation of the aortic arch was evident. A 10 cm segment of the thoracic aorta below the arch was replaced by prosthesis. Suture lines were intact. The abdominal aorta and iliac vessels showed a moderate degree of atherosclerosis with some calcification. The intimal surface of the aortic root and arch showed changes consistent with a "tree bark" appearance with pearly-grey plaques and sclerosis (Figure 74). The lungs were edematous with centrilobular emphysema. The distal esophagus was adherent to both pleural surfaces and to a massive blood clot associated with fibrous tissue. On opening, a large defect was noted in the esophageal wall approximately 10 cm from the gastric cardia. The defect was consistent with an oval ulcer measuring 3 cm in its greatest dimension that extended through the full thickness of the wall (Figure 75). The edges were sharp, not raised and clearly demarcated. A major portion of the stomach was absent and there was evidence of a Billroth type II anastomosis. The remaining organs showed no significant pathology.

Microscopic Description

The myocardium was essentially normal. There was no evidence of excessive deposition of fibrous tissue. At the site where the aortic root was inserted into the left ventricle there was necrosis of the heart muscle and interstitial hemorrhage. Hemorrhage was also present in the pericardium, the latter finding probably a reaction to the trauma of surgery.

Sections from the aorta showed subintimal sclerosis with deposition of cholesterol and calcium. The adventitia showed a marked perivascular inflammatory cell infiltrate composed primarily of plasma cells. Sections taken from the esophageal ulcer revealed fragments of aortic wall displaying cholesterol and fibrosis, which was adherent to the esophageal wall. These findings were consistent with an aorto-esophageal fistula.

Case Analysis

The two most significant symptoms that this patient experienced were hemoptysis and epigastric pain. The causes of epigastric pain are numerous and include: peptic ulcer disease, pancreatitis, myocardial infarction, aortic aneurysms and malignancies among others. The causes of hemoptysis are primarily of lung in origin, either inflammatory/infectious (bronchiectasis, bronchitis, tuberculosis), neoplastic (carcinoma) or vascular (pulmonary embolism, trauma, pulmonary hypertension and clotting disorders). When it is not possible to determine whether the episodes of bringing up bright red blood represent hemoptysis or hematemesis, aspiration of blood from an upper GI source, or a tracheo-esophageal fistula should be considered. Increased fatigue, tachypnea, tachycardia and anemia were all indicative of ongoing blood loss. A stool specimen positive for occult blood suggested a GI tract origin. Since this patient had a prior history of peptic ulcer disease, a recurrence of an ulcer or a gastric cancer arising in a background of chronic peptic disease, would have explained his symptoms. However, the abdominal exam and an extensive work up that included GI series, endoscopy, celiac angiogram and pancreatic scan failed to reveal any abnormalities. The enzyme values (transaminases, amylase and lipase) eliminated the possible diagnoses of myocardial infarction and pancreatitis. The ECG was only significant for left ventricular hypertrophy and showed normal PR and QRS intervals. The respiratory tract was also unremarkable. The lungs were clear on auscultation and the chest-x-ray as well as a bronchoscopy were negative.

In addition to the epigastric pain and bleeding, the patient experienced symptoms that were important in reaching a diagnosis. Intermittent dysphagia in the setting of a negative endoscopy or GI series, may be explained by the presence of an outside mass compressing the wall of the esophagus. Other symptoms such as dyspnea, dry cough and pain can also be due to a mediastinal mass compressing the airways. The chest-x-ray showed a dilated aortic root, and clinically, he had evidence of aortic regurgitation. This case occurred prior to the use of computerized tomography as a standard ancillary tool, but had it been available, probably a CT scan or even an ultrasound of the thorax, would have confirmed that the lesion represented an aneurysm of the aortic arch.

Aneurysms of the aortic arch are uncommon as compared to the most frequent aneurysms of the abdominal and descending aorta. Nonetheless, when present, the aortic arch aneurysms are often symptomatic due to the compression of adjacent organs. These aneurysms can be either fusiform as in arteriosclerosis or saccular as in syphilis. They are prone to rupture and should be surgically treated despite the fact that the operative risk of death is as high as 50%. The microscopic evaluation of the aorta in our case revealed that the cause of the aneurysm was consistent with syphilitic aortitis. The sections from the aneurysm showed a chronic panarteritis in which the inflammatory infiltrate was composed of plasma cells. The infiltrate is responsible for the destruction of the media and endarteritis of the vasa vasorum in the adventitia (Figure 76). The treponemal organisms bind to the endothelial cells of the vasa vasorum through surface adhesion molecules

244

(Figure 77). A humoral response is triggered with antibody production against spirochete antigens. The humoral response is followed by a cellular immune response, and results in scarring and fibrosis. This leads to a "tree barking" appearance of the aortic arch. Involvement of the aortic valve annulus results in valvular insufficiency and hence, the decrescendo murmur best heard at the left base when the patient was leaning forward. Myocardial ischemia may also occur when there is involvement of the coronary ostia. However, the cause of death is generally the severe congestive heart failure secondary to aortic insufficiency. Dissection of the aortic media is unlikely due to the extensive scarring that obliterates the planes of dissection.

Luetic aortitis is a manifestation of tertiary syphilis that occurs in approximately 10% of the patients. The treponemas appear to have predilection for the proximal aorta due to its rich lymphatic supply. Syphilitic aneurysms are the result of a chronic inflammatory response and damage of the aortic wall. By the time the injury has fully developed, the spirochetes are no longer present within the lesion. Luetic aortitis should be differentiated from mycotic aneurysms due to either bacteria or fungi, and vasculitides that affect the aorta such as giant cell arteritis and Takayasu's arteritis. Infectious aneurysms are often associated with positive blood cultures and elevated white blood count, which this patient did not have. Giant cell and Takayasu's arteritis are characterized by granulomatous inflammation. Giant cell arteritis often involves the temporal artery and the extracranial branches of the carotid artery. It occurs in elderly patients and is associated with polymialgia rheumatica. In contrast, Takayasu's disease usually occurs in patients under 50 years of age. It is often known as the "pulseless disease" because it causes obliteration of the carotid pulses and pulses of the upper extremities when it affects the brachiocephalic trunk and branches. Interestingly, syphilis can also cause symptomatic occlusive disease in the upper extremities when significant arteriosclerosis is superimposed. Our patient experienced intermittent claudication and lack of femoral and popliteal pulses that were most likely the result of peripheral vascular disease and unrelated to his tertiary syphilis. Lastly, syphilis may cause fibrosing mediastinitis similar to that seen in Aspergillus infection, Hodgkin's disease and idiopathic fibrosis of the mediastinum.

In the present case, the patient had a small probability of surviving the operation. By the time the surgical procedure was carried out the patient had bled significantly. Although currently, aortic syphilitic aneurysms are rare, this diagnosis should always be considered, especially in patients with multiple sexual partners and in HIV-infected individuals.

Suggested Readings

1. Dossa CD, Pipinos II, Shepard AD, Ernst CB. Primary aortoenteric fistula: Part I.Ann Vasc Surg. 1994; 8:113-20.
2. Grey TC, Mittleman RE, Wetli CV, Horowitz S. Aortoesophageal fistula and sudden death. A report of two cases and review of the literature. Am J Forensic Med Pathol. 1988; 9:19-22.
3. Coady MA, Rizzo JA, Goldsstein LJ, Elefteriades JA. Natural history, pathogenesis, and etiology of thoracic aortic aneurysms and dissections. Cardiol Clin. 1999; 17:615-635.
4. Amin S. Aortoesophageal fistula: case report and review of the literature. Dig Dis Sci. 1998; 43:1665-1671.

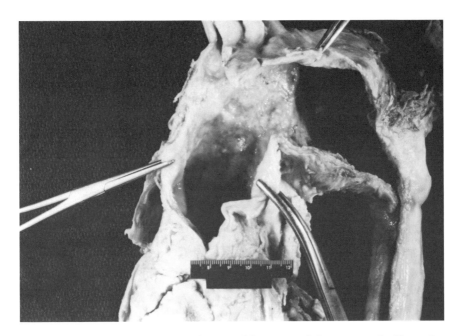

Figure 74. Syphilitic aortitis involving the root of the aorta and the aortic arch. Notice the wrinkling of the intima known as "tree-barking".

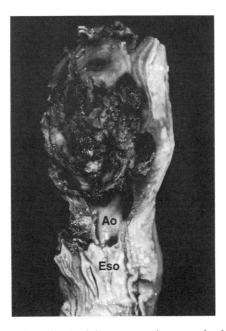

Figure 75. Aorto-esophageal fistula. Syphilitic aortitis that caused a fistulous tract between the aorta (Ao) and the esophagus (Eso). A mass of clotted blood is present at the esophageal lumen

247

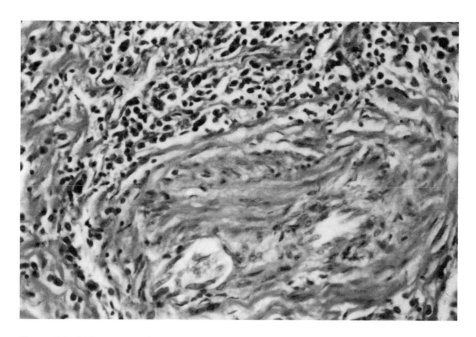

Figure 76. Obliterative endarteritis in syphilis, histologic section. This vessel from the aortic vasa vasorum is rimmed by an inflammatory infiltrate of lymphocytes and plasma cells (Hematoxylin and Eosin, 40X).

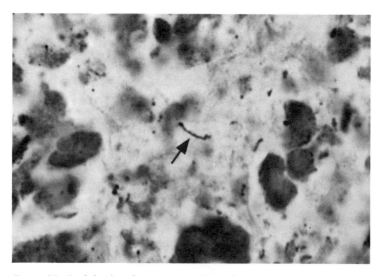

Figure 77. Syphilis, histologic section. Spirochete (arrow) (Steiner stain, 100X).

Case # 29

Clinical Summary

This was a 41 year old woman with a history of scleroderma, who presented with painful ulcers in the fingers and heels. She was diagnosed with scleroderma when she experienced shortness of breath and esophageal dysmotility. Previously, she had been admitted to the hospital with bilateral hand and foot pain, sclerodactyly and Raynaud's syndrome. On that admission, an echocardiogram showed right atrial and ventricular dilatation, and moderate to severe tricuspid regurgitation. Recently, she was unable to ambulate due to bilateral heel ulcers. She had also developed constipation, abdominal pain and mild dysuria. Her social history included smoking 25 packs a year and previous cocaine abuse (for which she received rehabilitation).

Physical examination on admission revealed a patient with moderate distress. Vital signs were: BP 110/82, P 120, R 20, T 37.8°C. Heart: S1, S2 tachycardic, no murmur, evident S3 and S4 gallop. Necrotic ulcers were present on both heels and the tips of all fingers, bilaterally.

Laboratory data and other tests

Laboratory: WBC 14; Hb/Hct 14/42; creatinine 0.9, bilirubin T/D 0.8/0.5, SGOT 63, LD 48, PT 18; CK 112. Pulmonary function tests were consistent with restrictive lung disease. CXR: bilateral ground glass costophrenic angles at bases, and a thick and dilated esophagus.

During her hospital stay, she deteriorated. Her pain became unresponsive to meperidine, and her liver function tests became abnormal. Ten days after admission, the patient was found restless and weak. She became pulseless. Despite resuscitation efforts, she was pronounced dead.

Gross Description

The patient weighed 60 kg and measured 172 cm. On external exam, both hands and feet showed necrotic changes at the tip of all fingers and toes. The heart weighed 450 g. The pericardial surface was rough with fibrous adhesions. Both atria were hypertrophic and dilated with multiple intramural thrombi present. Both ventricles were also hypertrophic and dilated, with right and left ventricular wall thickness measurements of 0.8 cm and 1.8 cm, respectively. The valves measured as follows: tricuspid 13, pulmonic 10, mitral 11 and aortic 9. The leaflets were pliable. There was no significant coronary artery disease. The lungs weighed 1300 g. Fibrous plaques were present on the parietal pleura, more remarkable on the right side. The cut surface of the lung revealed a honeycomb appearance due to severe interstitial fibrosis. In addition, the parenchyma showed multifocal hemorrhage and mild anthracosis. The mediastinal lymph nodes were enlarged. The esophagus was thickened and dilated. The liver weighed 1100 g and had a firm texture

Microscopic Description

Sections from the heart showed marked interstitial and replacement fibrosis, thickening of intramyocardial arterioles and chronic pericarditis. Sections from the lungs showed diffuse interstitial fibrosis. Smooth muscle proliferation was present, along with medial thickening of the vessels, consistent with pulmonary hypertension. Hyaline membranes characteristic of diffuse alveolar damage were also present. Sections from the liver showed periportal fibrosis and thickening of the portal artery wall. Sections from the skin showed dense dermal and subcutaneous fibrosis. There was moderate atrophy of the epidermis and dermal appendages.

Case Analysis

This young woman had many of the classic complications of scleroderma, a disease of unknown etiology, but one generally classified within the group of collagen-vascular disorders. Her clinical presentation was of relatively short duration, and the course of her illness was rapid. This suggests that her disease was either fulminant, or that her symptoms did not become manifest until she had a prolonged period of clinically 'silent' tissue damage. The extent of the organ damage and its histologic chronicity, evidenced by extensive mature tissue fibrosis, suggests that she had a long course of illness.

Her disease represented one of the subsets of scleroderma, known as the CREST syndrome. The latter is a symptom complex that includes Calcinosis, Raynaud's phenomenon, Esophageal dysmotility, Sclerodactyly, and Telangiectasia. Calcinosis is dystrophic calcification in soft tissues; Raynaud's phenomenon is the spasm of distal blood vessels usually in response to cold; esophageal dysmotility results from fibrosis of esophageal muscularis; sclerodactyly occurs secondary to contractures of distal phalangeal skin and bone degeneration secondary to ischemic atrophy; and, telangiectasia is the prominence of dilated small blood vessels visible through the stretched and thinned skin characteristic of the disease. Scleroderma is generally associated with abnormal tissue fibrosis affecting multiple organs, but particularly the skin, lungs, kidneys and heart. The pathogenesis of the systemic fibrosis is at least partially mediated through abnormal reactivity of small blood vessels. This accounts for symptoms such as Raynaud's phenomenon, and for pathological microscopic foci of replacement fibrosis in the myocardium due to reperfusion necrosis mediated by spasm of the intramyocardial small arteries and arterioles. Early in the disease, the microvasculature may be 'leaky', as one of the initial symptoms of the disease is soft tissue edema. The increased microvascular permeability that leads to release of cytokines and proteins into the interstitial space stimulating fibrogenesis, may also be a manifestation of vascular spasm and localized vessel injury. However, there is very little scientific evidence to support this hypothesis, and it still remains an interesting speculation.

Before discussing the pathogenesis of this patient's terminal course, it is worthwhile to mention one confounding variable in her medical history that could account for at least some of her symptoms. She had been a known cocaine user, although allegedly she had been clean for the past 5 years. Cocaine causes a local build-up of norepinephrine (NE) at the neuromuscular junction due to its inhibition of the alpha-2 adrenergic receptor that permits the re-uptake of NE. This results in increased alpha stimulation of the muscle, and subsequent vasospasm. When large vessels such as coronary arteries or cerebral arteries are affected, it can result in myocardial infarction or stroke. However, the effect may be at the microvascular level thereby leading to local tissue necrosis and microscopic scars. Thus, small foci of myocardial and renal fibrosis may develop. Chronic vessel damage may occur, with vascular sclerosis (e.g. fibrosis and smooth muscle hyperplasia) even in the absence of hypertension. Although it is not well recognized clinically, Raynaud's phenomenon and distal tissue damage affecting the extremities may also occur with cocaine abuse. If particularly severe, or in hypersensitive individuals, cocaine-associated vasospasm and ischemia can even lead to gangrene of the upper and/or lower extremities. Thus, at least some of the findings in scleroderma such as peripheral Raynaud's vasospasm and gangrene, cutaneous ulceration, sclerodactyly and myocardial tissue fibrosis could be explained by persistent cocaine use. On the other hand, the delay between this patient's alleged cessation of drug use and her symptoms (five years), her clinical presentation with the CREST syndrome, and her significant pulmonary symptomatology, all strongly support the view that she had scleroderma and not cocaine-induced tissue damage.

As is often the case with many systemic diseases like scleroderma, there are adverse effects on multiple organs that interact to contribute to the patient's death. In this case, she had esophageal dysmotility and esophageal dilatation due to fibrosis of the muscularis propria, which resulted in her inability to swallow properly, and led to chronic aspiration pneumonia. These pneumonias caused additional tissue damage and scarring in the lung beyond that expected from scleroderma alone. In addition, she had acute ischemic bowel disease, partially secondary to decreased cardiac output, but also as a result of local vessel sclerosis in the bowel wall. Bowel ischemia with superficial mucosal necrosis may be an additional risk factor for septicemia, which would place a further stress on an already compromised cardiovascular system.

The primary cause of this woman's death, however, was a result of her chronic scleroderma lung disease and the stress it placed on her damaged heart. She had interstitial pulmonary fibrosis, a recognized complication of severe systemic scleroderma (it should be noted that scleroderma can be localized only to the skin, and this is known as Morphea). The pathogenesis of interstitial pulmonary fibrosis in scleroderma remains unknown. However, there are important implications of the pathologic lung changes. There is 'remodeling' of the pulmonary parenchyma that leads to the development of 'honeycomb' lung. This occurs when there is injury to the alveolar-capillary interface and the alveolar unit. There is airspace enlargement due to interstitial inflammation and damage, and with the scarring process there is a decrease in surface area for gas exchange (e.g. multiple small alveolae have a greater surface area than larger cyst-like spaces). In contrast to alveolae, which generally require magnification to be clearly identified, the cyst-like honeycombs can be recognized on gross examination of the lung. The honeycomb lung may also have bullae, particularly in the periphery, which if ruptured, are associated with spontaneous pneumothorax. As a consequence of interstitial fibrosis and honeycomb lung, patients develop restrictive lung disease due to a loss of the usual elasticity (compliance) of the pulmonary parenchyma. They may be severely dyspneic, often at rest but certainly with exercise; and generally will have some degree of hypoxemia and hypercapnia. Furthermore, due to the damage of the alveolar wall including the alveolar-capillary unit, there is both a loss of capillaries and damage to arterioles and venules. This leads to a decrease in the vascular volume, and an increase in pulmonary vascular resistance. Ultimately, the result is pulmonary hypertension. The latter has chronic effects on the heart, and particularly the right heart, leading to the clinical syndrome of *cor pulmonale*, or right-sided cardiac dysfunction due to chronic lung disease. It was cor pulmonale that led to this patient's death.

This patient had a hypertrophied and dilated right ventricle, with a wall thickness of 0.8 cm (twice normal), mural thrombi in the right atrium and ventricle (Figure 78), dilatation of the tricuspid and pulmonary valve rings, and echocardiographic evidence of tricuspid valve regurgitation. All these, represent characteristic features of cor pulmonale. She most likely had a somewhat compensated right ventricular function, as she did not have evidence of significant pleural effusions or ascites. However, the findings of mural thrombi in the right atrium and ventricle do indicate abnormal contractile function of these chambers, and turbulent blood flow causing endocardial damage with platelet and fibrin aggregation and adherence to the tissue. She also had chronic congestion in the liver, with central venous sclerosis due to transmitted elevated right atrium pressure to the hepatic veins. Chronic congestion accounted for the elevation of her liver function tests during her last admission.

Patients with cor pulmonale are highly susceptible to develop heart failure, as well as sudden death due to cardiac arrhythmia. In this case, she also had damage to her left ventricular myocardium as a result of small vessel disease. This led to microscopic foci of replacement fibrosis. Myocardium around such foci is electrically unstable and may be arrhythmogenic. Furthermore, the basic underlying cause of the replacement fibrosis - vascular hyper-reactivity - can persist, and lead to sudden development of microscopic areas of reperfusion necrosis characterized by contraction bands. Reperfusion necrosis is highly arrhythmogenic, as well.

The terminal event of a sudden cardiac arrest resulted from a combination of cardiac and pulmonary compromise. The major effects were on the right side of the heart, but there was also left ventricular injury. Her disease was progressive, and only partially controlled by steroid therapy. Even if entirely controlled, however, once the pulmonary and cardiac damage develops it is irreversible. When the effects of chronic aspiration pneumonia due to esophageal dysmotility, and bowel necrosis due to local intestinal ischemia are superimposed on the primary lung and heart damage, it is not surprising that she developed a sudden fatal cardiac arrhythmia.

Suggested Readings

1. Gurubhagavatula I; Palevsky HI. Pulmonary hypertension in systemic autoimmune disease. Rheum Dis Clin North Am. 1997; 23:365-94.
2. LeRoy EC. Systemic sclerosis. A vascular perspective. Rheum Dis Clin North Am. 1996; 22:675-94.
3. Rump AF, Theisohn M, Klaus W. The pathophysiology of cocaine cardiotoxicity. Forensic Sci Int. 1995; 71:103-15.
4. Deswal A; Follansbee WP. Cardiac involvement in scleroderma. Rheum Dis Clin North Am. 1996; 22:841-60.
5. Bolster MB; Silver RM. Lung disease in systemic sclerosis (scleroderma). Baillieres Clin Rheumatol. 1993; 7:79-97.

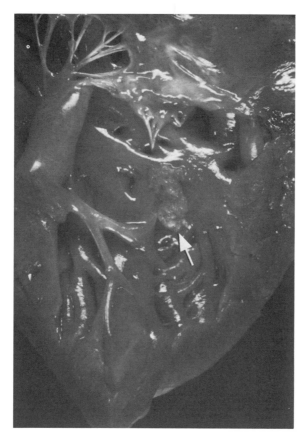

Figure 78. Cor pulmonale. The right ventricle shows severe hypertrophy. A mural thrombus is present (arrow).

Case # 30

Clinical Summary

This 20 year old Caucasian woman, diagnosed at 8 years of age with systemic lupus erythematosus (SLE), presented to the hospital with a one month history of non-traumatic low back pain. She was significantly incapacitated and required crutches for ambulation. The pain had a sudden onset and woke her up from her sleep. There was no history of recent changes in her urinary or gastrointestinal functions. Prior to admission, she had been seen by a physician who prescribed ibuprofen (400 mg q6h), but with no relief. Other medications at the time of admission were prednisolone (60 mg/day) and furosemide (20 mg QD). She had increased her steroid dose on her own because of worsening arthralgias. She had not visited her rheumatologist for a considerable period of time and admitted poor compliance regarding scheduled medical appointments. Her knowledge of her medical condition was limited. The initial presentation during childhood was that of epistaxis secondary to thrombocytopenia. She had primary amenorrhea, with some breast development and minimal growth of axillary and pubic hair. In addition, the patient had a history of avascular necrosis of the hips and she had also developed cataracts.

The physical examination on admission revealed truncal obesity and cushingoid facies. The vital signs were T 37.8°C, P 104/min, R 20/min, BP 120/80 mmHg. She had a dry oral mucosa and supple neck. The lungs were clear. On auscultation she had normal S1 and S2, regular rhythm and no murmurs. The abdomen had striae. No organomegaly was noted. She had large hematomas on both shins. Her sensation and reflexes were intact, but her motor functions could not be explored due to pain.

Laboratory data and other tests

Laboratory: WBC 8.5 (S 96%, L 3%), Hb/Hct 9.6/28, MCV 91, Plt 75, PT/PTT 14/36; Calcium 6.6, SGOT/SGPT 92/30, protein T/A 4.1/2.1, bilirubin T 0.3, BUN/creat 21/1.1, glucose 133. Arterial blood gas: pH 7.38, pCO_2 32, pO_2 80, HCO_3 19, and base excess –4.1. In addition, her serology was positive for anti-double stranded DNA and anti-cardiolipin antibodies. The urine analysis showed trace protein, many bacteria, and amorphous crystals. ECG: sinus tachycardia, otherwise unremarkable. The chest-x ray had evidence for increased pulmonary vascular congestion. An x-ray of the spine demonstrated diffuse demineralization and loss of height of vertebral bodies.

256

The patient was evaluated by a rheumatologist who prescribed pain medication as needed (meperidine 75 mg IM, and acetaminophen/oxycodone 2 tab). In the hospital, prednisone was started at 30 mg/day (during the first 2 days) and then tapered over the following days. Calcium carbonate and vitamin D were also prescribed in view of the severe osteopenia. During the initial hospital days, the patient reported slight symptomatic improvement. A CT scan of the lower thoracic and lumbar spine revealed excessive epidural lipomatosis compressing cauda equina nerve roots. Diffuse osteopenia was again noted, in addition to multiple compressed vertebral bodies.

Several days after admission, the patient developed severe dyspnea in association with tachypnea (44/min) and tachycardia (140/min). Arterial blood gases (ABG) performed at that time revealed severe hypoxemia with respiratory alkalosis. She was intubated, and heparin was initiated (V/Q scan was reported as negative). In view of continuing clinical deterioration with worsening tachypnea (60/min) and tachycardia (150/min), the patient was admitted to the intensive care unit (ICU). Repeat chest-x-ray showed bilateral interstitial infiltrates and was reported consistent with adult respiratory distress syndrome (ARDS). Antibiotics were started to provide coverage for possible opportunistic pathogens. Bronchoalveolar lavage was performed and was reported positive for Pneumocystis carinii. A Swan-Ganz catheter was inserted revealing pressures within the normal range. The remainder of her hospital stay was characterized by a severe decrease in peripheral platelet numbers together with persistent fibrin degradation products (FDP) at > 1:20, falling fibrinogen levels and hem positive stools (signs of disseminated intravascular coagulation or DIC). Purpuric lesions and violaceous plaques developed on the trunk and extremities, with eventual evolution to vesicular lesions on breasts and abdomen. A series of chest-x-rays showed progressive worsening of the bilateral interstitial infiltrates. She became markedly hypotensive with a systolic blood pressure of 60 mmHg and a heart rate of 60 ppm. Shortly thereafter, she went into asystole. In accordance with the expressed wishes of the next-of-kin, no further measures were taken and the patient was pronounced dead.

Gross Description

The body measured 150 cm and weighed 55 kg. External examination revealed truncal obesity, "buffalo hump" on the nape of neck, vesicles on both breasts, and purpuric and violaceous plaques on the trunk and extremities.

The heart weighed 430 g. The pericardium had fibrous adhesions consistent with chronic pericarditis (Figure 79). The epicardium was shiny with a marked increase in subepicardial fat. The atria were normal in size and free of thrombi. The foramen ovale was closed. The right and left ventricular walls measured 0.4 and 1.4 cm in thickness, respectively. The tricuspid valve showed small (up to 1mm) brown, soft vegetations near the line of closure of the leaflets (Figure 80). The mitral valve showed fibrous thickening of the leaflets, more remarkable in the posterior leaflet, with fusion of the commissures and chordae tendineae. The endocardium and myocardium were grossly unremarkable. The coronaries were of normal caliber with no occlusions. Fatty intimal streaks were present in the aorta maximal near the ostia of the celiac and mesenteric vessels.

The lungs weighed 1175 g together and had bilateral patchy areas of consolidation with focal hemorrhage, more prominent in the right middle and lower lobes. The pulmonary artery and its major branches were devoid of occlusions and had a smooth and shiny intima.

Other significant autopsy findings included bilateral adrenal gland atrophy (combined weight 3 g, normal 8 g), small female genital organs, excessive epidural lipomatosis and severe osteopenia of the spine with multiple compression fractures in the thoracic and upper lumbar regions.

Microscopic Description

Sections of the heart showed biventricular hypertrophy, fatty infiltration of the myocardium and mild interstitial fibrosis. Sections of the tricuspid valve confirmed the presence of non-bacterial endocarditis. The mitral valve was fibrotic.

Sections from both lungs revealed vascular congestion, interstitial and intra-alveolar edema and multiple alveolar spaces filled with foamy, proteinaceous material and cell debris. In these areas, silver stain (Grocott-Methenamine-Silver) revealed the presence of numerous organisms consistent with Pneumocystis carinii.

Case Analysis

The clinical history and the autopsy findings illustrate the potential life-threatening complications of long-term high dose steroid use, but also the cardiac manifestations of this patient's underlying disease, SLE.

Systemic Lupus Erythematosus (SLE) is a chronic, systemic disease associated with abnormalities of the immune system. The cause of this disorder is unknown, but its basis is the production of autoantibodies, particularly antibodies against nuclear proteins, DNA, and RNA. The deposition of antigen-antibody complexes in different organs accounts for most of the pathological and clinical manifestations of the disease.

The hallmark of the therapeutic approach to SLE in the past decades has been the use of corticosteroids, and recently adjuvant cytotoxic and antimetabolite drugs have been added successfully. Therefore, the cardiovascular manifestations in patients with SLE are a combination of the inflammatory processes characteristic of the disease itself, and the secondary effects of corticosteroid/immunosuppressive therapy. In the heart, the most affected sites are the pericardium and endocardium. Patients with SLE often present with pericarditis (approximately 80%), and it can be acute (fibrinous pericarditis) or chronic. Recurrent or persistent inflammation of the mesothelial lining of the pericardium may lead to mesothelial hyperplasia and fibrosis with the development of adhesions and subsequent obliteration of the pericardial cavity (fibrous pericarditis). Occasionally, examination of pleural fluid can reveal the presence of lupus erythematosus (LE) cells. These are macrophages or neutrophils that have phagocytized nuclei denatured by circulating antinuclear antibodies (ANA). Similar cells, known as LE or hematoxylin bodies can also be identified in tissue samples (Figure 81). Less commonly, myocarditis with a non-specific mononuclear infiltrate can occur. It is usually subtle, causing spotty myocardial necrosis, and is diagnosed when there is a high level of suspicion leading to an endomyocardial biopsy. The clinical presentation varies from tachycardia to complete heart block. Moreover, inflammation with subsequent scarring may affect the sinus and atrioventricular nodes as well as the bundle of His. Newborns of mothers with SLE and anti-Ro (Sjögren Syndrome A or SS-A) antibodies may develop heart block secondary to transient myocarditis. The latter are anti-nuclear antibodies directed against 52 and 60 kilo-Dalton (kDa) proteins, and are present in approximately 35% of patients with SLE and in patients with Sjögren syndrome. Anti-Ro IgG can cross the placenta and may cause a neonatal lupus-like syndrome. These maternal autoantibodies disappear within a 6-month period; however, long lasting conduction abnormalities in the offspring have been reported.

Valvular endocardial damage was more dramatic in the pre-steroid era. The classic valvular lesion of SLE is known as Libman-Sacks endocarditis (described in a necropsy series by Drs. Libman and Sacks from Mount Sinai Hospital, New York in 1924). It is a non-infective endocarditis manifested by the presence of small verrucous lesions on any valvular surface of the heart. The vegetations are composed of a mixture of immune complexes, inflammatory cells and fibrinoid necrosis. Significant valve dysfunction requiring valvular replacement is rare unless superimposed bacterial infection ensues. Aortic and mitral valvulitis are common in SLE, particularly in patients with antiphospholipid antibodies. The clinical manifestations in patients with the antiphospholipid syndrome (e. g. phospholipid or cardiolipin antibodies), which include venous and arterial thrombosis, recurrent miscarriages and thrombocytopenia, are secondary to a hypercoagulable state, and to the cellular damage caused by the antibodies.

In our patient, the valvular abnormalities were most likely the result of her independent, high-dose steroid abuse rather than her positive anticardiolipin status. Recently, prolonged use of corticosteroids has been linked to the development of a serious form of valvular pathology characterized by rigid and thickened valvular leaflets. The patient had fibrosis of the mitral valve leaflets with fusion of the valve commissure and chordae tendineae similar to that seen in patients with rheumatic heart disease (RHD). Could these changes be the result of chronic rheumatic heart disease? They could, but the clinical history and presence of other elements of cardiac involvement favor SLE and steroid use as etiologic factors for her valvulopathy. The vegetations present on the tricuspid valve were more consistent with non-bacterial thrombotic (marantic) endocarditis than with Libman-Sacks endocarditis. Marantic endocarditis occurs in chronically ill or debilitated patients and is manifested by the presence of small, brown vegetations situated close to the line of closure of the leaflets. Microscopically, they consist of non-infectious and non-inflammatory fibrin aggregates. These small thrombi may detach and embolize causing infarcts in the brain or other organs. They differ from Libman-Sacks vegetations by their location, and absence of inflammation and valvular damage. However, in some cases, they may be indistinguishable from each other.

Other cardiovascular manifestations of SLE include coronary artery disease and acute necrotizing vasculitis. Patients with long-standing SLE, especially those diagnosed at a young age, are prone to develop accelerated coronary atherosclerosis. Risk factors for coronary artery disease and ischemia such as early onset hypertension, glucose intolerance, obesity and hyperlipidemia are strongly associated with long term glucocorticoid treatment (e.g. cushingoid features). Atherosclerosis is also more common in patients taking 10 mg or more of prednisone a day. Our patient had early atherosclerotic changes in the coronary arteries, and in the aorta near the ostia of the celiac and mesenteric vessels. Despite the fact that her cholesterol levels were not elevated, the presence of multiple abdominal lipomas, fatty infiltration of the myocardium and excessive epidural lipomatosis reflected the alterations of this young woman's lipid metabolism. The fat distribution affected by steroid treatment not only involves visceral organs and soft tissues, but bone as well. She had a history of avascular necrosis of the hips probably due to fat emboli involving osseous arterioles, and microvessel occlusion secondary to hypertrophy of bone marrow adipocytes.

Acute necrotizing vasculitis can occur in any tissue and involves small arterioles and capillaries. Histologically, it is characterized by inflammation of the vessel wall and fibrinoid necrosis (Figure 82). Endothelial damage causes extravasation of red blood cells, thrombosis and ischemia. The pathogenesis of vasculitis is complex and not completely understood. Potential causal mechanisms include deposition of immune complexes in the vessel wall as well as direct damage of the endothelium by antiendothelial cell antibodies.

In this case, the cause of death as well as the clinical signs and symptoms were the result of her dependence on corticosteroids. The cushingoid facies, cataracts, centripetal obesity, bilateral adrenal atrophy, myopathy and severe osteopenia were all adverse effects of steroid therapy. Corticosteroids cause osteopenia by inhibiting osteoblastic function and intestinal calcium absorption, and by increasing bone turnover and parathyroid activity. Steroid therapy is effective in suppressing the acute inflammatory manifestations of SLE, but carries a significant risk since it inhibits the host's response to infections. Infectious complications in an immunocompromised host, like this patient, can be due to the usual organisms affecting the normal general population. However, what makes these hosts unique is their susceptibility to infections caused by opportunistic pathogens (e.g. Pneumocystis carinii, Cryptococcus neoformans). The latter group of agents can be difficult to diagnose, since they would not normally pose a threat to the normal host. Therefore, the medical personnel taking care of immunosuppressed individuals must have a high index of suspicion when approaching acute, subacute or chronic infections in these patients. This woman died as a result of overwhelming infection with Pneumocystis carinii leading to adult respiratory distress syndrome, disseminated intravascular coagulation and fibrino lysis. Unfortunately, she attributed her back pain to her underlying disease when in fact it was caused by her self-prescribed treatment. Even though steroids and other immunosuppressive agents have proven to be very effective in controlling autoimmune diseases, the patients have to be carefully monitored to prevent or closely follow any significant deleterious effects that may arise as a consequence of these medications use or abuse.

Suggested Readings

1. Roberts WC, High ST. The heart in systemic lupus erythematosus. Curr Probl Cardiol. 1999; 24:1-56.
2. Nesher G, Ilany J, Rosenmann D, Abraham AS. Valvular dysfunction in antiphospholipid syndrome: prevalence, clinical features, and treatment. Semin Arthritis Rheum. 1997; 27:27-35.
3. Moroni G, La Marchesina U, Banfi G, Nador F, Vigano E, Marconi M, Lotto A, Ponticelli C. Cardiologic abnormalities in patients with long-term lupus nephritis. Clin Nephrol. 1995; 43:20-8.
4. Ben-Chetrit E. The molecular basis of the SSA/Ro antigens and the clinical significance of their autoantibodies. Br J Rheumatol. 1993; 32:396-402.
5. Bruce IN; Gladman DD; Urowitz MB. Premature atherosclerosis in systemic lupus erythematosus. Rheum Dis Clin North Am. 2000; 26:257-78.
6. Cunnane G; Lane NE. Steroid-induced osteoporosis in systemic lupus erythematosus. Rheum Dis Clin North Am. 2000; 26:311-29.
7. Stuck A, Minder C, Frey F. Risk of infectious complications in patients taking glucocorticoids. Rev Infect Dis. 1989; 11:954-963.

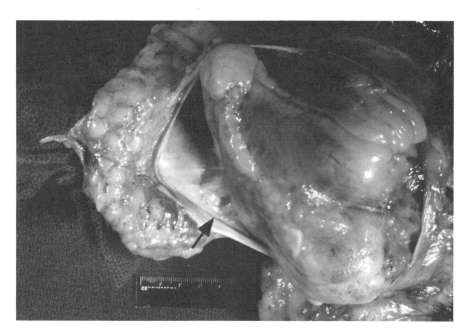

Figure 79. Chronic pericarditis. Fibrous adhesions are present between the epicardial surface and the pericardial sac (arrow).

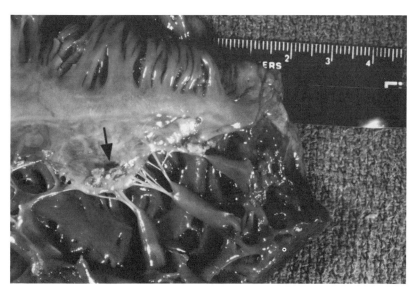

Figure 80. Libman-Sacks endocarditis. Small, friable vegetations are present on the tricuspid valve (arrow).

263

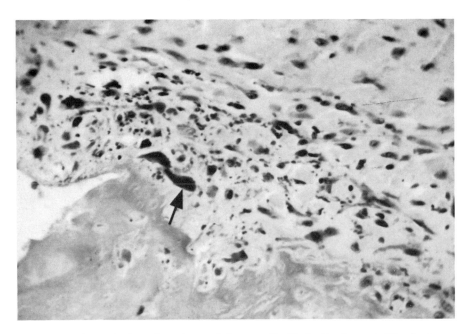

Figure 81. Libman-Sacks endocarditis with hematoxylin-like bodies (arrow) (Histologic section, Hematoxylin and Eosin stain, 40X).

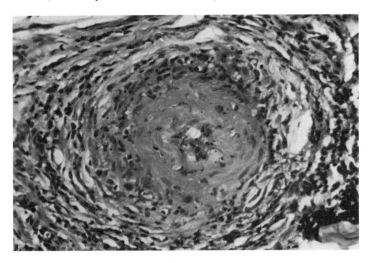

Figure 82. Systemic lupus erythematosus (SLE). This small-sized vessel of the dermis shows fibrinoid necrosis of the wall with infiltration of polymorphonuclear leukocytes and extravasation of red blood cells. In addition, there is fragmentation of the nuclei of the neutrophils (karyorrhexis). These changes are consistent with necrotizing (leukocytoclastic vasculitis) (Histologic section, Hematoxylin and Eosin, 40X).

264

Case # 31

Clinical Summary

A 35 year old Hispanic woman was brought to the ER because of acute chest pain and shortness of breath. Her medical history included hyperthyroidism treated for 4 years with PTU (propylthiouracil), tonsillectomy at 15 years of age, and cigarette smoking for the past 20 years. The patient described non-progressive dyspnea on exertion, and occasional episodes of chest pain and abdominal pain after each meal. She had not taken any medications recently. Upon arrival, her pulse was 120 ppm with diminished carotid and lower extremity pulses and absent pulses in the upper extremities. Her BP was 97/68 mmHg. There was central cyanosis. An ECG showed RBBB and ST elevation in the anterolateral leads. An arterial blood gas showed hypoxemia. The chest x ray was unremarkable (no cardiomegaly). Blood chemistries revealed slightly low albumin (normal total protein), calcium and uric acid; slightly elevated LDH, SGPT, CK, alkaline phosphatase and creatinine, and normal bilirubin and SGOT. The differential diagnoses included pulmonary embolism and myocardial ischemia. The patient suffered a cardiorespiratory arrest and despite prolonged resuscitative efforts was pronounced dead 3 hours after admission.

Gross Description

The body measured 158 cm in length and weighed 52 kg. The heart weighed 300 g and was of normal shape. The heart measurements were: LV 1.2 cm, RV 0.4 cm, TV 10 cm, PV 6 cm, MV 9 cm and AV 6 cm. The cardiac cavities were of normal size and the foramen ovale was closed. The endocardium was smooth and the valve leaflets and chordae tendineae were normal. The myocardium of the septum and free wall of the left ventricle had a brown, dull appearance compatible with acute myocardial infarction (6-12 hours). The epicardium was normal. The coronary arteries were distributed normally. The right coronary ostium was severely narrowed and the left mildly narrowed. The aortic root was abnormal; it was thickened with superficial intimal plaques and scarring. The changes extended with diminishing severity through the aortic arch. The proximal right coronary artery showed intimal focal sclerosis with 50–60% occlusion; distally, it had focal but less marked sclerosis. The proximal left anterior descending (LAD), and left circumflex (LCX) coronary arteries showed similar sclerosis, but with 95% and 50-75% occlusion, respectively. The descending aorta was less involved by this process. However, just above the aortic bifurcation there was a segment of approximately 3 cm in length, which was narrowed to a diameter

265

of about 1.5 cm, and was completely occluded by laminated white firm material (Figure 83). The portion of aorta distal to this segment appeared to branch normally into the common iliac arteries, and these were unremarkable except for patchy superficial intimal plaques. The celiac trunk branched into the splenic and common hepatic arteries. The superior mesenteric artery was larger in caliber than usual. The inferior mesenteric artery was unremarkable. There were 2 renal arteries on the left side, the smaller supplied the upper part of the left kidney and was patent. The larger artery supplied the lower 2/3 of the left kidney, and an ulcerated plaque occluded the ostium of this vessel. The right renal artery had a single origin from the aorta, but branched approximately 3 cm proximal to the holus of the kidney. This vessel was patent throughout its course. The right kidney weighed 130 g and showed multiple healed infarcts. The left kidney was approximately one half the size of the right and weighed 80 g. The lower 2/3 of the left kidney corresponded to the occluded lower left renal artery and showed severe ischemic atrophy. The liver and lungs were congested, but otherwise unremarkable. The pulmonary vessels, however, showed similar changes to those seen in the aorta and its branches.

Microscopic Description

Multiple sections of the heart, coronary arteries and aorta were examined. The myocardium showed focal contraction bands, hyper-eosinophilia and margination of neutrophils, some of which were interstitial. These changes were seen in the left ventricular free wall, left ventricular papillary muscle and septum, and were consistent with an acute, focal myocardial infarction of 6–12 hours duration. The mitral valve showed fibromyxomatous degeneration. The right ventricle and tricuspid valve were unremarkable. The coronary arteries revealed prominent focal subintimal fibrous thickening associated with scattered collections of lymphocytes and occasional neutrophils. There was also thickening of the adventitia, which showed a more prominent mixed inflammatory infiltrate, with more neutrophils, lymphocytes, and plasma cells. No significant changes were noted in the vasa vasorum. There were foci of calcification between the intima and media. The media itself was focally thinned or absent and elastic stains showed focal destruction of the internal and/or external elastic laminae. In the proximal LAD, there was a recent thrombus superimposed on these changes with virtual occlusion of the lumen. The proximal RCA was approximately 85% occluded by the subintimal fibrosis, although there was no plaque hemorrhage or thrombus. The left circumflex showed 50–75% occlusion. The overall findings were consistent with end-stage coronary arteritis.

The aortic root and the occluded segment of the abdominal aorta showed extensive subintimal fibrous thickening with foci of cholesterol clefts. Scattered collections of acute and chronic inflammatory cells were present in the subintimal areas (Figure 84). Within the media, which was focally destroyed, there were similar collections of neutrophils, lymphocytes and plasma cells. The adventitia was markedly thickened by fibrous tissue and calcifications, and its vessels showed intimal fibrosis, and in some areas, perivascular inflammation. Similar changes, but to a lesser extent, were noted in sections from aortic arch, descending aorta, iliac arteries and left lower renal artery.

Case Analysis

The cause of death in this patient was an acute antero-septal myocardial infarction, which was evident by the chest pain, elevated enzymes (LDH, CK and SGPT) and ECG changes. However, the most significant findings were related to the aorta and coronary arteries. The gross and microscopic changes in combination with the clinical history and distribution of lesions (e.g. large caliber vessels and branches), are in keeping with the diagnosis of aortitis and coronary arteritis. Although many of the findings described, such as intimal fibrosis, cholesterol clefts and focal calcification, are by themselves indicative of atherosclerosis and non-specific, their occurrence in a young woman, especially in association with focal inflammation of the vessel wall, support this diagnosis. Furthermore, atherosclerosis may be superimposed upon a vessel damaged by vasculitis.

The forms of vasculitis that affect large vessels include: Giant cell arteritis and Takayasu's arteritis. Giant cell arteritis occurs in patients over 50 years and commonly involves small muscular arteries such as the temporal and carotid arteries. Two histologic variants have been described: 1) granulomatous with giant cells and mononuclear cells infiltrating the inner half of the media; and, 2) non-specific panarteritis that comprises a mixed inflammatory infiltrate. Although giant cell arteritis has a female preponderance and carotid involvement, our patient was young and did not have evidence of temporal arteritis.

Takayasu's arteritis (TA) is a disease of younger individuals, particularly females and it is the most likely diagnosis in this case. It is characterized by a panarteritis that may affect any segment of the aorta and its branches. It is presumably an autoimmune disorder that in early phases presents with non-specific symptoms but later evolves into a more severe disease. The symptoms are related to the portion of aorta that becomes involved. In this patient, symptoms such as chest pain, dyspnea and shortness of breath associated with hypoxemia, were due to acute pulmonary edema

267

secondary to myocardial infarction caused by the inflammation and subsequent thrombotic occlusion of the coronary vessels. This last event was preceded by episodes of angina pectoris and angina intestinalis (the post-pyramidal abdominal pain was related to mesenteric involvement). She was hypotensive due to decreased peripheral vascular resistance. However, it is significant that there was no history of hypertension, which is a common symptom in TA as it is related to renal artery stenosis. The patient had no involvement of the right renal artery, and in the left side, one of the two vessels was patent and maintained the function of the upper 1/3 of the left kidney; therefore, sparing her of renovascular hypertension. The left pulmonary artery showed intimal proliferation and thickened adventitial vessels with perivascular infiltrates. These changes were focal with no significant occlusion; thus, the absence of pulmonary hypertension and right ventricular hypertrophy. It is worth mentioning that TA may present with a distinct pulmonary arteriopathy that consists of outer media defects with capillary ingrowth in this layer and in the thickened and fibrosed intima.

The occlusion of the subclavian and iliac arteries was responsible for the diminished or absent peripheral pulses. The asymmetry as well as the absence of the peripheral pulses is quite characteristic of this entity, hence the term "pulseless" disease. TA is not a common disorder; therefore, other causes of reduced peripheral pulses should be considered such as arteriosclerotic occlusive disease, coarctation of the aorta, syphilis and neoplasias.

Coarctation of the aorta is more common in males and in patients with gonadal dysgenesis. It is also associated with other congenital cardiac abnormalities in approximately 10% of cases. It presents in early childhood unless the coarctation is distal to the ductus arteriosus, in which case the onset of symptoms occurs much later in life. This could have been a consideration in this case, because coarctation of the aorta can present with diminished pulses in the lower extremities. Additionally, it is associated with cardiomegaly, hypertension in the arms and engorged collateral vessels in the intercostal and subscapular areas. Both the clinical history and autopsy did not reveal any of these findings in our patient. Coarctation of the aorta has a characteristic chest X ray with a "3" sign made by the stenotic area and the 2 adjacent dilated segments. The ECG and echocardiogram invariably show left ventricular hypertrophy, but other findings depend on the location of the coarctation and presence of other heart anomalies.

Syphilis is another form of arteritis that might be considered in this case, but it is usually seen in older patients and most often spares the abdominal aorta. The characteristics features of syphilitic arteritis were not present in our patient. Although there was perivascular inflammation involving the vasa vasorum of the adventitia, it was not prominent and the infiltrate did not consist predominantly of plasma cells.

TA is suspected to be an autoimmune disorder, but the etiology and pathogenesis are not known. HLA typing studies have shown some correlation with the markers HLA-A10, B5 Bw52, DR2, DR4, and MB1. In addition, TA has been associated with other diseases. One of these, is ulcerative colitis, a gastro-intestinal inflammatory disease in which HLA DR2 expression has also been described. Another important association is the one between TA and ankylosing spondylitis, despite the lack of association between TA and the expression of HLA-B27, which is frequently present in ankylosing spondylitis. Some authors have proposed that TA may be the result of an abnormal immune response elicited by certain infectious organisms (e.g. acid fast bacilli). As in other forms of vasculitis, sensitized T cells have been considered to play an important role in the manifestation of the disease. Abnormal endocrine manifestations have also been reported, which may be an interesting observation, since our patient had a history of hyperthyroidism of unclear etiology.

Suggested Readings

1. Kerr G. Takayasu's arteritis. Curr Opin Rheumatol. 1994; 6: 32-8.
2. Matsubara O; Kuwata T; Nemoto T; Kasuga T; Numano F. Coronary artery lesions in Takayasu arteritis: pathological considerations. Heart Vessels Suppl. 1992; 7:26-31.
3. Hall S; Buchbinder R. Takayasu's arteritis. Rheum Dis Clin North Am. 1990; 16:411-22.
4. Rizzi R, Bruno S, Stellacci C, Dammacco R. Takayasu's arteritis: a cell-mediated large-vessel vasculitis. Int J Clin Lab Res. 1999; 29:8-13.
5. Morita Y, Yamamura M, Suwaki K, Mima A, Ishizu T, Hirohata M, Kashihara N, Makino H, Ota Z. Takayasu's arteritis associated with ulcerative colitis; genetic factors in this association. Intern Med. 1996; 35:574-8.

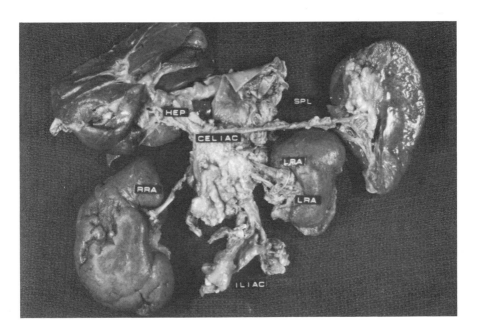

Figure 83. Takayasu's arteritis. Segment of aorta narrowed before the bifurcation into the common iliac arteries (RRA = right renal artery, LRA = left renal artery, Hep = hepatic artery, Spl = splenic artery).

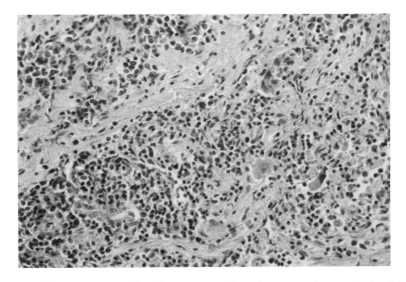

Figure 84. Takayasu's arteritis, histologic section. Granulomatous inflammation involving the adventitia of the aorta. The infiltrate consists of lymphocytes, hystiocytes and giant cells (Hematoxylin and Eosin, 20X).

271

Case # 32

Clinical Summary

This is the case of a 31 month old girl who was admitted to the hospital because of increasing respiratory distress and wheezing. She was a full-term baby after an uncomplicated pregnancy, vaginal delivery and post-natal period. Past medical history was remarkable for: 1) mild intermittent asthma diagnosed at 8 m of age; 2) hospitalization at 20 m of age for an episode of intussusception which resolved uneventfully with medical treatment; 3) since her 2nd birthday she complained of intermittent arthralgias (mostly lower extremities) to the point of sometimes refusing to walk. At 30 m she was given a tentative diagnosis of juvenile rheumatoid arthritis because of these arthralgias and a new onset conjunctival injection that was diagnosed as uveitis (of note is that all her clinical work-up was unremarkable, except for mild hypergammaglobulinemia). She was given naproxen PO twice a day and a steroid based ophthalmic solution for her eyes, which significantly improved her symptoms. The day of her admission, she had a 2-day history of worsening respiratory distress and wheezing with minimal response after the usual home treatments with nebulized albuterol. She was admitted with an acute asthma exacerbation and probable pneumonia. Over the first hours she remained stable, her physical exam was remarkable for Temp 38.2 °C, HR 174, RR 42, and pulse oxymetry on room air 97 %. She seemed alert and interactive with moderate respiratory distress (increased expiratory phase, mild nasal flaring, mild to moderate intercostals, and subcostal retractions). The lungs had decreased air movement with diffuse wheezing; there was tachycardia with a regular rhythm and no reported heart murmur. There was hepatomegaly (10 cm liver span) and no splenomegaly or abdominal masses. The laboratory results (CBC and chemistries) were unremarkable. The chest x-ray showed diffuse infiltrates bilaterally. The respiratory signs progressed and she turned restless, agitated and developed perioral cyanosis. Concomitantly, her blood gasses deteriorated. As her cyanosis progressed, she became lethargic and was intubated and transferred to the pediatric intensive care unit. There she had a cardiopulmonary arrest with good response to resuscitative maneuvers, and was stabilized. Two hours later, despite vasopressors, her blood pressure dropped, and again she became pulseless. This time there was no response and she was pronounced dead about 20 hours after admission.

Gross Description

The body was described of an average built and weight for the stated age of 31 months. External examination was unremarkable. The heart was enlarged (weight. 100 g, normal heart weight between 24 months and 3 years of age 58–72 g). There was an aneurysmal dilatation of the left descending coronary artery which measured 2 cm in length and 1 cm in diameter. It was occluded with thrombi (Figures 85 and 86). Extensive areas of scarring consistent with remote myocardial infarctions were present in the left anterior ventricular wall. There was hepatomegaly and generalized lymphadenopathy.

Microscopic Description

Microscopic examination of the heart revealed focal areas of scarring consistent with remote infarctions (Figure 87). Coronary artery sections showed a chronic inflammatory infiltrate and marked dilatation of lumen with thickened tunica media and intima. The lumen was occluded with organizing thrombi. Some sections revealed chronic fibromuscular intimal hyperplasia with recent thrombosis (Figure 88). There were signs of multifocal recent and remote myocytolysis and fibrosis. There were changes of diffuse alveolar damage and bronchopneumonia in both lungs, and some of the larger pulmonary vessels showed intimal thickening consistent with pulmonary hypertension. The liver showed central vein dilatation and sclerosis, large intralobular xanthogranulomatous nodules with lymphocytes, foamy histiocytes and multinucleated giant cells.

Case Analysis

This is an important case because it demonstrates potential pitfalls in the approach of acutely ill febrile children, and underscores the implications of a well documented past medical history.

Let us start with the presenting symptom: a known asthmatic 31m old girl complaining of increasing respiratory distress. This initial scenario may not be particularly concerning because of its frequency and usual uncomplicated resolution. Very commonly asthmatic children will have intermittent asthma exacerbations, which will respond rapidly to the usual home and occasionally office or hospital therapy. The usual asthma triggers are: upper respiratory infections (common colds), allergies, drugs and exercise. In this case, the child had some fever and did not improve her respiratory symptoms with home and office therapy. She was then admitted for further management. Despite optimizing her asthma treatments and adding an antibiotic for a probable lower respiratory infection, over the

273

following hours the child failed to improve. At this point, one must consider several possibilities: 1) that there is a severe bronchospasm which will be difficult and may take some time to control; 2) that the infectious component may be more significant than initially suspected, and this too will take longer to control; 3) that this child may have an underlying condition that was not diagnosed earlier, which could potentially complicate even more her treatment; and 4) a combination of the aforementioned factors. For all these situations, respiratory support has to be readily available.

In this case, a probabilistic approach to the presenting clinical complaint would mainly include an acute asthma exacerbation followed by an infectious problem; but given the lack of improvement, it is of particular importance that one explores the possibility of a cardiac co-morbidity, mostly pericardial and/or myocardial disease. In general, even with a history of chronic pulmonary disease, cardiac dysfunction, e.g. heart failure, can present clinically as persistent and progressive respiratory distress. Once the contributing heart pathology is identified, the addition of cardiovascular drugs may be followed by an improvement in the clinical course. The documentation from this admission did not alert to any arrhythmias or any significant cardiac finding, and what may have confused or complicated the situation even more was that the chest x-rays did not suggest a cardiac problem.

Another crucial part of the history is that for several months before her death this girl had been complaining of intermittent arthralgias (there were never signs of inflammation), which occasionally would prevent her from walking. These symptoms, together with the new ophthalmologic findings of uveitis, introduced a new diagnosis of Juvenile Rheumatoid Arthritis. Briefly, this is a systemic vasculitis syndrome that typically presents at this age with joint manifestations, both peripheral and axial, and systemic organ involvement. Frequently, it is only diagnosed on the basis of clinical signs. Because of this presumptive diagnosis, chronic therapy with a potent non-steroidal anti-inflammatory drug was started, which seemed to have controlled her symptoms.

As the course of the acute illness evolved, the child became hemodynamically unstable and went into cardiorespiratory arrest. Once stabilized, she required vasopressors and ventilatory support. These facts indicate progressive cardiopulmonary compromise, which essentially occurs due to overall cardiac dysfunction often triggered either by intrinsic heart conditions (e.g. myocarditis), pericardial disease (e.g. pericardial effusion, restrictive pericarditis) and/or worsening pulmonary insufficiency (e.g. adult respiratory distress syndrome or ARDS, Pneumocystis carinii pneumonia). The crucial observation in this case was that there were no clinical features that pointed to a particular etiology and her rapid deterioration was completely unexpected as were the pathology findings.

The autopsy showed a heart with signs of significant coronary artery disease. The left descending coronary artery had marked aneurismal dilatation with organizing thrombus and diffuse damage to the vessel wall. There was evidence of extensive remote subendocardial and transmural myocardial infarctions, and multifocal recent and organizing myocytolysis. Except for the heart (coronary arteries) there was no evidence of vasculitis in other organs. In addition, lung sections revealed features of ARDS and focal pneumonia. The cardiac findings were classic for Kawasaki's disease (KD). The latter is an acute febrile illness of young infants and children of unknown etiology, which is associated with systemic vasculitis of the extraparenchymal portions of medium and large size arteries, with a predilection for coronary arteries. It is thought to be a superantigen mediated illness, with activated T and B lymphocytes and increased production of cytokines. The clinical criteria for the diagnosis of KD include fever of more than 5 days, and four of the following signs: bilateral conjunctival injection, mucous membrane changes, edema/erythema of the extremities or generalized/peripheral desquamation, rash and cervical lymphadenopathy (Figure 89). Because of the usual skin and mucous membrane involvement this syndrome is also known as Mucocutaneous Lymph Node Syndrome. The initial management of these children is a full pediatric and cardiologic evaluation, including an initial and several follow-up echocardiograms to assess the coronary arteries and cardiac function. Prognostic factors that correlate significantly with coronary involvement are: age less than one year, male gender, Japanese origin, prolonged or recurrent fever, low albumin and hemoglobin levels, and cardiac manifestations (e.g. arrhythmias, pericardial effusion). The mainstay of therapy is intravenous immune globulin (IVIG) within 10 days of the onset of the fever, and anti-thrombotic medication (aspirin). It has been shown that if children are treated early in the course of the illness the coronary changes are prevented. Recently, clinicians are more inclined to diagnose atypical cases of KD since not always all the criteria are present. The basis for this over-conservative approach is that in untreated children with KD, coronary artery ameurysm or ectasia can develop in up to 15–25% of the cases. The implications are tremendous since the coronary injury may lead to myocardial infarction and sudden death as occurred in this case (reported mortality rate oscillates around 0.1%). Furthermore, in the United States, KD is the most common cause of acquired heart disease, surpassing rheumatic heart disease.

In retrospect, this girl had a very unusual presentation of KD, probably affected by the use of NSAID. It was about one month before her death when she had conjunctival injection, interpreted at the time as uveitis. Bulbar conjunctivitis (one of the diagnostic criteria) and uveitis can be signs of KD, but since there was no fever, rash, or other mucocutaneous manifestations, the diagnosis was not considered. With the autopsy findings, the differential diagnoses are those syndromes affecting medium and small

275

arteries. The main one is Polyarteritis Nodosa (PAN). The onset of PAN is insidious and frequently presents with constitutional symptoms, fever and weight loss. In contrast with this case, PAN usually affects not only the cardiac, but also the renal and nervous systems (peripheral and central). There is significant organ involvement and abnormal laboratory findings are the rule (CBC, ESR, UA, serum immunoglobulins). Pathologically, the two conditions may be undistinguishable. Other important conditions that were excluded clinically or based on the autopsy findings were streptococcal and staphylococcal-related syndromes (toxin-mediated), drug toxicity and hypersensitivity reactions.

In summary, given the severe coronary involvement found in this girl, and the fact that it went undetected for a long period of time, it is highly unlikely that she would have survived. It is possible that the use of NSAID prevented the expression of the full inflammatory syndrome, and thus the diagnosis of KD was never considered.

Suggested Readings

1. Rowley AH, Shulman ST. Kawasaki syndrome. Pediatr Clin North Am. 1999; 46:313-29.
2. Laupland KB, Dele Davies H. Epidemiology, etiology, and management of Kawasaki disease: state of the art. Pediatr Cardiol. 1999; 20:177-83.
3. Burns JC, Kushner HI, Bastian JF, Shike H, Shimizu C, Matsubara T, Turner CL. Kawasaki disease: A brief history. Pediatrics. 2000; 106:E27.
4. Meissner HC, Leung DY. Superantigens, conventional antigens and the etiology of Kawasaki syndrome. Pediatr Infect Dis J. 2000; 19:91-4.
5. Suzuki A, Miyagawa-Tomita S, Nakazawa M, Yutani C. Remodeling of coronary artery lesions due to Kawasaki disease: comparison of arteriographic and immunohistochemical findings. Jpn Heart J. 2000; 41:245-56.
6. Reich JD, Campbell R. Myocardial infarction in children. Am J Emerg Med. 1998; 16: 296-303.
7. Brenner JL, Jadavji T, Pinto A, Trevenen C, Patton D. Severe Kawasaki disease in infants: two fatal cases. Can J Cardiol. 2000; 16:1017-23.

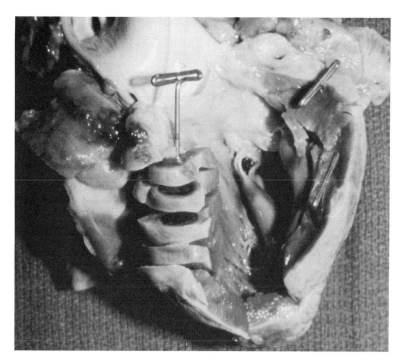

Figure 85. Kawasaki's disease. The heart has been opened and a probe has been inserted in the lumen of the left anterior descending coronary artery (LAD). The wall of the vessel is markedly dilated and the lumen is entirely occluded by an organizing thrombus.

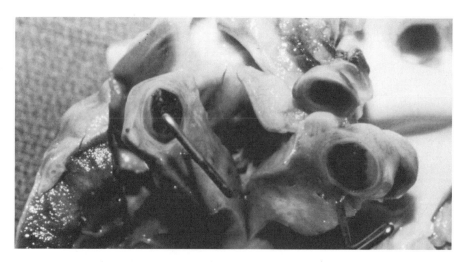

Figure 86. Kawasaki's disease. Close up of different segments of the LAD coronary artery showing complete thrombotic occlusion of the lumen and significant aneurysmal dilatation of the vessel wall.

278

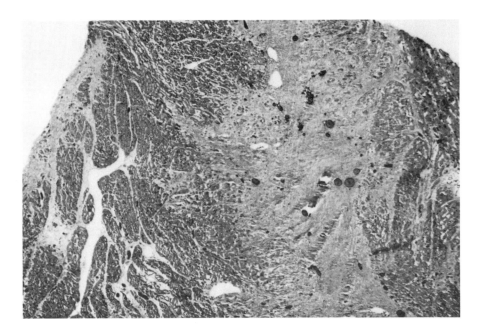

Figure 87. Kawasaki's disease, left ventricle, histologic section. Extensive area of scarring consistent with remote myocardial infarction (Hematoxylin and Eosin, 20X)

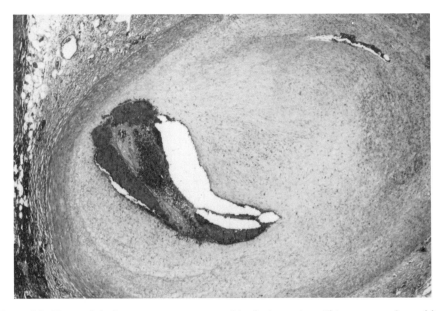

Figure 88. Kawasaki's disease, coronary artery, histologic section. This segment of vessel has chronic fibromuscular hyperplasia secondary to prior inflammatory damage occluding 95% of the lumen. There is an acute thrombus in the residual lumen (Hematoxylin and Eosin, 10X)

279

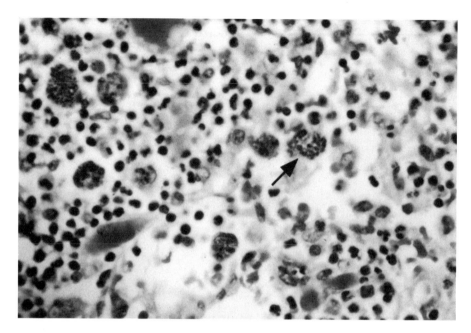

Figure 89. Kawasaki's disease. Histologic section of a cervical lymph node showing numerous neutrophils and histiocytes engulfing nuclear debris (arrow). The lymph nodes in KD demonstrate patchy foci of necrosis and fibrin thrombi occluding capillary vessels (Hematoxylin and Eosin, 40X)

Chapter 13

MEDICINE, LAW AND THE HEART

Cardiovascular Disease in the Medico-Legal Era: An Introduction

The United States is a litigious society, far more so than other regions of the world with sophisticated healthcare systems and economies comparable to ours, such as Canada, Western Europe and Great Britain, and Japan. A major focus of this litigation deals with medical malpractice, with patients or survivors suing healthcare providers for either a real or claimed injury. Cardiovascular disease represents a disproportionate number of these cases, along with failure or delay in the diagnosis of cancer, or complications following surgery. The defense of these cardiovascular law suits often requires knowledge of complex medicine, and a correlation with cardiac pathology and pathophysiology. Similarly, the plaintiff must be aware of mechanisms of cardiovascular disease and the actual pathology in order to make an effective argument to a jury.

Other types of litigation such as personal injury (e.g. automobile accident), or product liability (e.g. adverse drug affects, or claims that cars or tires were defective leading to an accident) often also require knowledge of cardiovascular disease. For instance, an automobile accident may apparently lead to the death of the driver as a result of trauma; however, if the driver actually had an arrhythmic cardiac arrest prior to the accident (e.g. coronary artery ischemia or cardiomyopathy) and then crashed, this would mitigate if not eliminate the liability of insurers or the automobile manufacturer. In another instance, a so-called drug adverse effect may represent the natural consequences of the underlying disease for which the drug was prescribed, rather than a complication of the drug. An example of this phenomenon is sudden cardiac death during sexual activity of an individual with diabetic cardiomyopathy, who is taking Viagra® for erectile dysfunction secondary to diabetic neuropathy. Association is not the equivalent of causation; however, unless one is aware of diabetic cardiomyopathy as an entity, and its potential for causing sudden cardiac arrhythmias, a law suit against the manufacturer of the drug, or the prescribing doctor, might be successful.

Different types of cardiovascular disease, many of them discussed in this book, present with atypical complaints (or no complaints at all, such as 'silent ischemia'). These are conditions that affect the heart and blood vessels, and are often the source of medico-legal suits. Two frequent sources of suits are those dealing with ischemic heart disease (IHD), and infectious endocarditis (IE). Failure to or delay in the diagnosis of IHD may lead to a myocardial infarction or death; and in the cases of IE, this may result in failure to perform a valve replacement or death. Typical scenarios are those of subtle electrocardiographic changes such as non-specific ST-T wave abnormalities, or atypical chest pain misconstrued as chest wall pain or dysphagia, which then result in death or a myocardial infarction. Another common situation is a patient who presents with low-grade fever and malaise diagnosed as an upper respiratory infection, and the diagnosis of IE is overlooked. Thus, it becomes crucial to be aware of these cardiovascular conditions, and to recognize the pathological changes that may have important implications for the plaintiff or the defense. For instance, the timing or dating of a coronary thrombus or plaque rupture, may help in determining whether the symptoms or signs ascribed by one party to IHD, in fact were present at or around the time of the abnormal ECG or the atypical chest pain. Similarly, not only is the dating of the valvular endocarditis important to assess how long it had been active, but it is important to determine how much valve destruction had taken place. If the valve was sufficiently damaged, or if there were other conditions such as an annular abscess that would require surgical intervention, a delay in diagnosis might have no bearing on whether the valve could have been salvaged with an earlier diagnosis. This is known as a **proximate cause defense**. In other words, the failure in timely diagnosis had no bearing on the ultimate outcome.

The following 2 cases were selected because they represent unusual cardiovascular complications that led to a medico-legal suit. In one instance, the complication resulted from application of an organo-phosphate insecticide; thus, this was a product liability case. In the other instance, the complications followed coronary artery intervention with atherectomy and angioplasty; and therefore, a medical malpractice case. It is not entirely surprising that often medico-legal suits result from rare or unexpected complications, or unusual disease manifestations. The usual and common presentations of disease are generally diagnosed with facility; it is the atypical presentation that leads to medical puzzlement, patient dissatisfaction, or adverse outcome.

Case # 33

Clinical Summary

This is the case of a 47 year old man who presented to the emergency room two weeks after a pesticide application in his home, with complaints of itchy eyes, blurred vision, "foggy" sensorium, dizziness and headache. His vital signs were unremarkable, although his diastolic pressure of 96 mmHg was higher than it had been five months ago (86 mmHg). He was treated with diphenhydramine. The symptoms persisted. A laboratory test demonstrated a red blood cell cholinesterase of 5.6 u/mL (normal range 3.8-8.0 u/mL).

Two weeks later he presented again to the emergency room with acute complaints of stabbing chest pain for two days radiating to the back. He had a new murmur of aortic insufficiency, acute anuria, cyanosis of the right lower extremity, and unstable blood pressure readings of 190/110 to 130/80 mmHg. The diagnosis of aortic dissection was made. He was found to have a type I dissection with extension into the abdominal aorta, and with absent filling of the superior mesenteric, celiac and right common iliac arteries. He was immediately taken to the operating room and placed on cardiopulmonary bypass. The intraoperative findings included a non-ruptured aorta with a dissection beginning 1.5 cm above the aortic valve. An intimal flap extended from above the valve to near the origin of the brachiocephalic artery. The aortic valve was thick with fibrosis, and was bicuspid. The valve was replaced by a mechanical St. Jude prosthesis, and the ascending aorta was repaired with a graft. The patient tolerated the procedure well and was stable. He was immediately taken to angiography to assess the abdominal vessels. While the angiogram was being performed, he developed sudden bradycardia and hypotension, and he arrested with ventricular fibrillation. Resuscitation efforts were unsuccessful.

Past medical history

The patient was 18 years old when a coarctation of the aorta was diagnosed by catheterization. This finding was confirmed by echocardiography 16 years later. He also had a mild aortic regurgitation murmur of II/VI. In addition, he had mild hypertension for 3 years for which he was given antihypertensive medication. Subsequently, and until the acute episode of dissection, he did not have any recorded blood pressures in the hypertensive range nor was he taking any medication for blood pressure control. Other pertinent findings included a chest-X-ray that demonstrated an ectatic and prominent ascending aorta. He was also noted to have a mid-systolic click murmur compatible with a mitral valve prolapse syndrome. His habitus was average (180 cm, 95 kg) and he was not Marfanoid in appearance. An ECG suggested the presence of multiple old myocardial infarctions of indeterminate age. He was also a 2 pack per day cigarette smoker.

Gross Description

Upon exam, the surgical anastomoses were intact, and the aorta had not ruptured. Infarction of the small intestine and liver were noted. The dissection extended into both common iliac vessels. There was minimal atherosclerosis of the aorta and coronary arteries. The heart weighed 335 g (normal), but the left ventricular wall was concentrically hypertrophied at 2.2 cm. No abnormality of the mitral valve was seen. The lungs were significantly heavy (2360 g, normal 685-1050 g) with pulmonary edema. Post-mortem pseudocholinesterase levels of 1151 u/mL (approximately 50% of normal) were measured.

Microscopic Description

Examination of the autopsy slides confirmed that the dissection was acute, with the histological changes of no more than 24–48 hours in duration. The dissection occurred in the outer segment of the aortic media; and was associated with a fresh fibrin coagulum in the false channel along with focal neutrophils in the adventitia and media. The latter inflammatory cells may represent a cellular response to the acute injury, and/or a reaction to surgical manipulation occurring during the attempted repair of the lesion. There was no hemosiderin (iron) pigment in the adventitia, thus further confirming that the dissection was acute and had not caused any blood leakage from the false channel greater than 48 hours before death. In the aortic wall there was insignificant intimal atherosclerosis. More importantly, in the media there were focal areas of elastic lamella and smooth muscle degeneration with concomitant increase of basophilic mucoppolysaccharide. These are the types of change commonly associated with aortic dissection. However, the medial degeneration did not appear as severe as is often seen in those cases associated with known connective tissue disease (e.g. Marfan's syndrome) or hypertension.

Case Analysis

Two cardiovascular aspects should be addressed in this case:
1) The chronic underlying disease
2) The acute dissection with the potential role played by the organophosphate toxicity

This patient appeared to have two distinct and probably unrelated conditions: coarctation of the aorta associated with a bicuspid aortic valve, and chronic stable aortic degeneration suggestive of a connective tissue abnormality. The coarctation of the aorta and bicuspid aortic valve are well-recognized and relatively common congenital abnormalities that often occur together. The aortic constriction present at or just distal to the left subclavian artery and the ductus arteriosus varies in severity. It ranges from completely asymptomatic and clinically silent to marked obstruction of the aortic flow and severe hypertension. The aortic valve disease may also be asymptomatic, or may be associated with clinically significant aortic insufficiency or stenosis. In this case, the coarctation and the aortic valve disease were apparently mild. It is noteworthy that he was found to be hypertensive for only 3 years; however, by the time his aorta was noted to be prominent on chest-X-ray, he no longer required antihypertensive medication, and with no therapy, he remained normotensive. This is an unusual and atypical pattern for hypertension associated with coarctation. This suggests that he "healed" or compensated for his coarctation by mildly dilating his aorta due to an underlying tissue disorder. The aortic valvular disease was not particularly severe, as judged by the murmur and the lack of physical limitations (e.g. absence of symptoms referable to congestive heart failure). The valve degeneration, rather than the hypertension, is most likely the explanation for the concentric left ventricular hypertrophy. However, it should be noted, that hypertension occurring several years previously, still could have contributed to chronic damage to the aortic media, thereby increasing its susceptibility to dissection with the appropriate stimulus.

The suggestion that the patient had an underlying connective tissue disorder is based on several findings:
1) The dilatation of the aorta as noted on the chest X ray in the absence of atherosclerosis (confirmed by the autopsy).
2) The dissection as a terminal event
3) The findings of elastic tissue degeneration associated with increased mucopolysaccharide material in the aortic media
4) The clinical findings strongly consistent with mitral valve prolapse

Although this patient did not have the habitus of a patient with Marfan syndrome, it is known that patients can have similar aortic pathology with dilatation and a susceptibility to dissection. In the absence of specific genetic or biochemical studies of the glycoprotein abnormality in Marfan's syndrome (e.g. fibrillin), or of the collagen and elastin that provide the tensile strength of the aorta, it cannot be established with certainty if any connective tissue abnormality existed in this patient.

In regard to the issue of organophosphate poisoning and its role in inducing aortic dissection, there are several pertinent observations:

Aortic dissection virtually never occurs in the presence of an anatomically and microscopically normal aorta. In young individuals (2nd though 4th decades) with overt Marfan's syndrome or other recognized heritable connective tissue disorders, it may occur spontaneously with no associated hypertension. In older individuals without Marfan's syndrome, it is strongly associated with hypertension (generally greater than 75% of those affected). In both situations, cardiac and blood vessel contractility is thought to play a major pathogenic role. Increased cardiac contractility places abnormal stress on the ascending aorta (the commonest site for initiating dissection); whereas increased smooth muscle contractility may be important in generating local damage in the aortic wall, and may cause tears with hemorrhage in the vasa vasorum that supply the media along the plane in the aortic wall where dissection typically occurs (e.g. outer 2/3 of the media where the vasa vasorum branch parallel to the intimal surface, thereby providing a potential anatomic cleavage plane). Damage to the vasa vasorum may lead to focal hemorrhage that dissects through the tissue until it eventuates in an intimal tear, with subsequent distal propagation of the dissection. It also has been shown that agents that cause relaxation of smooth muscle and vasodilatation can be injurious to the media. Dysfunction or necrosis of smooth muscle is a correlate of the focal lesions that occur as a predisposition to dissection. The smooth muscle cell not only serves as a contractile modulator of the aortic tone, but it is also critical in the synthesis of the connective tissue components of the media. Smooth muscle damage, occurring either as a consequence of increased constriction (e.g. spasm) or increased relaxation, may be deleterious to medial integrity. This is of particular relevance in the present case because of the known effects of undegraded acetylcholine (Ach) at the neuromuscular junction that causes vasodilatation in certain vascular beds, and vasoconstriction in vessels with chronic pathological damage (e.g. atherosclerosis or endothelial injury). Underlying damage to previous episodes of hypertension, increased turbulence secondary to the coarctation in the proximal descending aorta, as well as in the ascending aorta due to bicuspid valvular dysfunction, is highly likely to have made the patient's aorta susceptible to the dilating and/or constricting effects of ACh. As noted previously, there was focal chronic damage of smooth muscle cells and elastic tissue in the aortic media at a distance from the acute dissection. These are pathological changes that could increase the susceptibility of the aortic media to the hemodynamic effects of ACh as a vasodilating or vasoconstricting agent.

There is an obvious temporal relationship between the onset of organophosphate poisoning and the development of the aortic dissection in someone who was entirely stable and asymptomatic, approximately one month before. It is known that organophosphates, as inhibitors of acetylcholinesterase (AChE) can lead to unrestrained effects of ACh at neuromuscular junctions and in the central nervous system. ACh can act as a smooth muscle relaxing agent in normal blood vessels, but it is known to act as a constrictor in pathological vessels. It is impossible to predict which effects it might have had in this patient's aorta; but in addition to potential medial smooth muscle injury, either effect could have led to abnormal motility of the vessel or of the vasa vasorum causing damage. ACh inhibitors typically cause bradycardia, but under certain circumstances they may lead to

286

tachycardia, presumably as a result of central nervous system actions. In addition, there may be a reduction in peripheral vascular resistance (due to the vasodilating effects of ACh) that can cause increased systemic catecholamine secretion leading to enhanced cardiac contractility, a major cause of aortic dissection in the setting of an abnormal vessel. It has been shown that prophylactic treatment of patients with Marfan's syndrome by using beta adrenergic blockers or calcium channel blocking drugs to decrease heart rate and cardiac contractility, can prevent or significantly delay the development of aortic dissection. Similarly, although AChE inhibitors are generally associated with hypotension, their central nervous system activity may lead to hypertension, specifically through the stimulation of the locus ceruleus, which is involved in peripheral sympathetic tone control. Thus, the potential cardiovascular effects of ACh inhibition by an organophosphate agent with increased ACh activity are complex and difficult to predict; however, they are clearly consistent with the development of vascular and cardiac instability that in the appropriate setting of underlying aortic disease could directly lead to dissection.

The effects of AChE inhibition with a build-up of ACh at the neuromuscular junction and in the central nervous system (CNS), are comparable in many ways to the effects of cocaine, crack, and methamphetamines at the neuromuscular junction and in the CNS. However, the latter agents exert their effect through different receptors than AChE inhibition. Specifically, cocaine, crack and methamphetamines act to block a receptor on the nerve ending, the alpha-2 adrenergic receptor. This receptor is involved in the re-uptake of norepinephrine (NE) at the neuromuscular junction. Receptor blockade leads to an increase of catecholamines at the junction, thereby causing unrestrained stimulation of smooth muscle. This is comparable to the build-up of ACh at the junction following AChE inhibition by organophosphate agents, which can cause either relaxation or stimulation of the smooth muscle cell. With catecholamines, the vascular smooth muscle is constricted. This hypercontractile effect can then lead to muscle cell necrosis, overlying endothelial damage with the development of vascular thrombosis and eventual atherosclerosis, intensifying the immediate effects of tissue injury (e.g. myocardial infarction or stroke). These agents have also been associated with aortic dissection. If the effects of organophosphate poisons, which produce irreversible inhibition of the AchE, are not counteracted rapidly, they lead to a prolonged build-up of ACh at the neuromuscular junction. In contrast, the cocaine class of drugs does not irreversibly bind to the neuromuscular receptor, and they can be rapidly reversed by alpha or beta adrenergic receptor antagonists, or by other drugs that act as smooth muscle relaxants (e.g. calcium channel blockers or drugs that act by releasing nitric oxide).

287

In regard to the patient's terminal event, it is noticeable that he survived the surgery in apparent good condition and the decompensated suddenly during the post-surgical angiogram. Although he still had significant abdominal cardiovascular compromise that would have required further immediate revascularization, the pattern of collapse is in keeping with an abrupt cardiovascular event possibly related to the autonomic dysfunction secondary to the organophosphate poisoning. Specifically, if he had cardiovascular collapse secondary to the infarcted bowel, it would be anticipated that he might become hypotensive with tachycardia; yet his initial rhythm was bradycardia. It is very likely that he had an atypical reaction to the angiographic agent due to persistently dysfunctional autonomic neuromuscular junctions. Unless AChE inhibitors are reversed with a specific antidote such as pralidoxime within the first 48 hours of exposure, the binding to the junction becomes irreversible and requires de novo synthesis of AChE that can take one to three months to be completed. Therefore, when the patient was undergoing surgery, he still was in a state of relative AChE inhibition that could have made him overly sensitive to the normally hypotensive effects of the angiographic dye. With the release of toxins from the necrotic small intestine, the AChE inhibition may also have contributed to furthering its vasodilating effects. This combination of the angiographic dye and the septic shock may have caused a loss of peripheral vascular resistance in a vascular bed blocked from normal constriction. The resulting hypotension then could have led to heart failure and arrhythmia as terminal events.

Suggested Readings

1. Marrs TC. Organophosphate poisoning. Pharmacol Ther. 1993; 58:51-66.
2. Ward C. Clinical significance of the bicuspid aortic valve. Heart. 2000; 83:81-5.

Case # 34

The death of this middle-aged man several weeks after an interventional catheterization and coronary artery procedure resulted in a suit against the treating cardiologist. The claim against the physicians is based on the performance of an unjustified procedure in lieu of recognized interventions with high clinical success and low morbidity or mortality, such as undertaking a coronary artery bypass or a balloon angioplasty with stenting. It is also suggested that the failure to adequately follow the patient after the procedure contributed to his death. The further claim was that the unjustified procedure not only did not improve the coronary stenosis, but actually directly contributed to his death through unexpected complications. The first claim may be countered by establishing that the decision to carry out the procedure is a matter of medical judgment and not negligence, and the lack of follow-up may have been the result of patient uncooperation. However, it would be very difficult to argue that the improper procedure did not negligently cause this patient's death, as will be established below.

This 51 year-old man, with a strong family history of coronary artery disease, complained of new onset chest pain. He had undergone a relatively recent screening procedure, **ultrafast CT scanning**, which revealed significant calcium scores in his coronary arteries. This test has received much hype in the medical community over the last 5 years, as a non-invasive test to determine the presence of coronary disease. It has yet to be established prospectively that the claims for the test's sensitivity or specificity are scientifically justified. There is evidence that coronary atherosclerosis (particularly vulnerable plaques with high susceptibility to rupture, associated with unstable angina or myocardial infarction) may have minimal or no calcification; and calcification is not necessarily an indication of luminal occlusion or narrowing. Obviously, a positive test that then leads to a positive confirmatory finding is valuable; however, a negative test may not rule out the potential for a serious coronary lesion. Ultimately, it will have to be determined that the benefit of the test justifies its cost.

Regardless, in this symptomatic patient the test was positive, and it led to coronary catheterization that demonstrated severe complex stenoses of the proximal left anterior descending coronary artery (LAD), and high grade stenosis of the mid-right coronary artery (RCA). The left circumflex artery (LCX) was apparently had minimal involvement. With two-vessel disease, particularly with involvement of the proximal LAD, it would have been prudent to recommend coronary artery bypass grafting (CABG). The LAD could have been bypassed with an internal mammary artery with a very high guarantee of long-term success, since the internal mammary artery is minimally susceptible to atherosclerotic stenosis. The RCA would have required either a vein-graft, or a free arterial graft with a radial artery. This procedure, particularly in a young man with no prior cardiac damage, could have been performed with very low morbidity, and a mortality rate of at most 1-2%. The survival of the grafts could be estimated in the range of 15-20 years, or more.

A considerably riskier approach would be to perform a balloon angioplasty with stenting. This is potentially dangerous with proximal lesions, particularly when there are multiple sites within the same vessel, along with high-grade disease in another major vessel. The placement of stents would function to maintain vessel patency post-angioplasty. Angioplasty, however, does have the significant potential of re-stenosis, with a rate of 30-40% in the first 3-4 months after the procedure, and a slowly progressive increase thereafter. Although somewhat ameliorated with the use of stents, re-stenosis can occur, and occasionally even at an accelerated rate. Moreover, with multiple sites of stenosis in the LAD, the vessel would have required multiple stents. Although technically feasible, this may prolong the procedure and make the left ventricle susceptible to ischemia or infarction.

The procedure that was employed known as atherectomy, is rarely used today, since it was supplanted clinically by angioplasty and stenting in the mid 1990's. Atherectomy uses a variety of cutting catheters, including sharp blades or rotating blades (and experimentally, lasers), to excise plaque material from the vessel wall and re-establish an adequate lumen. The plaque material is then suctioned through the coronary catheter, and removed from the patient. Atherectomies became valuable source of research tissue in a number of centers investigating atherosclerosis and re-stenosis, since it was the only methodology that provided fresh atheroma for biochemical, histochemical, or molecular studies. The tissue fragments were composed of all of the elements of atherosclerotic plaque including fibrofatty tissue, lipid core, calcium, and inflammatory cells. Not infrequently, segments of medial smooth muscle were included; yet, there was only a rare case of actual coronary artery rupture that required surgical intervention. Complications other than vessel rupture include vessel collapse or spasm, coronary dissection, and lumen thrombosis. These complications are prevented by stenting, which can be used with atherectomy. In this case, stenting or removal of plaque debris was not performed. There has been some concern about this approach over the years, but there are few clinical data to demonstrate a potential adverse affect of allowing fragments of plaque (even microscopic) to embolize downstream in the coronary circulation.

This patient had an apparently successful procedure carried out in the LAD and RCA on separate days. He allegedly had good coronary flow with widely patent vessels and no residual stenosis. He did have bleeding complications at his arteriotomy site, but this is not unusual. He also had minor elevations of creatine kinase (CK), with a significant increase of his

MB iso-enzyme after the LAD procedure. He was maintained on aspirin prophylactically. Approximately 3 weeks after the procedure, he returned to his executive position overseas. On the following day, he collapsed suddenly and died. The autopsy was carried out in a well-recognized academic center with sophisticated knowledge of cardiovascular disease.

Before actually turning to the specific autopsy findings and discussing them in detail, it might be worthwhile to address this patient's death from a clinical perspective. What are the likely cause(s) of his sudden cardiac arrest? Although some unrelated event only indirectly related to the coronary artery procedure could have occurred (e.g. stroke), the temporal proximity to the cardiac catheterization and intervention, strongly suggests an association. Acute coronary occlusion is a likely cause, with several etiologies possible. Neo-intima proliferation, thrombosis, and vessel trauma should be considered. As a general rule, neo-intimal proliferation leading to re-stenosis requires months to develop sufficiently to cause coronary artery ischemia; although the process may have begun over 3 weeks, it is not likely to cause sufficient occlusion to lead to ischemia and arrhythmia. There could have been an acute thrombus developing at an atherectomy site with sudden myocardial ischemia or infarction. Thrombus, however, is much more likely to develop shortly after the procedure, not weeks later. There could have been a 'silent' complication of the atherectomy and balloon angioplasty such as a delayed rupture of a pseudo-aneurysm (e.g. disruption of the vessel during the procedure leading to a localized hematoma that then ruptured weeks later with pericardial tamponade). There also could have been a dissection of the coronary artery with a delayed rupture. If any of these complications had actually been the cause of death, then the medico-legal aspects of this case would have focused on the utilization of the atherectomy procedure rather than coronary artery bypass grafting.

What did happen? In fact, 3 things occurred that together contributed to his death:
1. Persistence of high-grade coronary stenosis
2. Focal coronary artery dissection that contributed to the stenosis
3. Multi-focal myocardial necrosis secondary to embolization of plaque debris and other foreign material

We will address each of these processes.

High-grade Coronary Artery Stenosis: Despite the clinical impression that following the atherectomy and balloon angioplasty there was wide patency of all coronary arteries, the autopsy showed otherwise. The left main coronary artery (LM) was narrowed 50-75%, the LAD and RCA were 90% occluded focally, and the LCX was 75% occluded. Although it is possible that there was a complete mis-reading or inaccurate reporting of the actual degree of coronary artery patency, it is more likely that other related phenomena can explain this significant discrepancy. There often is an angiographic underestimation of coronary lumen narrowing. This almost certainly accounts for the presence of high-grade stenoses in the LM and LCX, since these vessels were not manipulated, and it cannot be assumed that they developed severe atherosclerotic disease in 3 weeks. If a vessel has an eccentric lumen, the angiographic dye may fill a flattened oval or slit-like lumen; if viewed perpendicular to its wide axis, the vessel may appear to have a larger lumen (since the dye is only visualized in 2 dimensions). Ordinarily, by rotating the angle of view, this effect should be minimized or eliminated, but it is not unusual to find a lack of close correlation between angiographic and post-mortem estimates of coronary patency.

The vessels that were instrumented with the atherectomy device and the angioplasty balloon, may have undergone post-procedure **remodeling**. In other words, because of medial smooth muscle stretching immediately following the intervention, the vessel lumens may have appeared larger than they actually were. Subsequently, the media may have recovered its tone, and elastically rebounded to a smaller diameter. This effect is prevented by the placement of a metallic stent, which maintains a fixed lumen diameter.

At the time of autopsy, the third contributor to significantly smaller caliber vessels was the development of coronary artery spasm. Although often occurring at the time of the procedure, spasm of multiple coronary vessels may occur at the time of cardiac arrest. Sometimes, when localized, it may be the actual cause of the arrest; whereas, when generalized it is more likely associated with a high output of catecholamines and other stress hormones. The vascular spasm may be prevented with intra-coronary stenting, but if persistent post-mortem, it may affect the estimation of the lumen diameter.

In this case, it appears most likely that the marked discrepancy between the coronary artery lumens post-intervention, and the findings at autopsy, were due to mis-interpretation of the angiograms, and the effects of re-modeling of the vessels with subsequent recovery.

Focal Coronary Artery Dissection: The autopsy also demonstrated a dissection of the LAD outer media (Figure 90), which was a direct unrecognized complication of the procedure. The occurrence of this event could be dated with certainty to the time of the atherectomy and angioplasty, since the dissected false lumen had maturing granulation tissue within an organizing thrombus that was approximately 3 weeks in age. It probably resulted from the balloon angioplasty, since in the intima overlying the dissected channel, there was a thin layer of loose connective tissue consistent with an early neo-intima, within which fibromyoblasts were proliferating. The association of coronary dissection and angioplasty is common; in the present case it contributed to a focal area of LAD stenosis. Moreover, dissection can also be prevented or minimized with the use of intra-coronary stents.

Multi-focal Myocardial Necrosis: Throughout the left ventricle and in a few areas of the right ventricle, there were multiple foci of sharply demarcated, small areas of myocardial necrosis, known as **myocytolysis**. These foci were generally in the range of 200-500 microns, with infiltration by mononuclear inflammatory cells (lymphocytes and monocytes), and histiocytes. The histiocytes had phagocytized myocyte cell debris, including lipofuscin. Within the foci, myocytes were generally completely destroyed with empty 'ghosts' maintaining myocyte shape and size; hence the term myocytolysis. Some organization, with in-growth of connective tissue was present, consistent with a process that was about 2-3 weeks old.

Most significantly, in many small intra-myocardial arteries in the general vicinity of the foci of myocytolysis, there was tissue debris within the vessel lumens. Some of the debris was calcified, and some was clearly recognizable as atherosclerotic plaque material. In one somewhat larger intra-myocardial artery, there was foreign (non-biological) material, consistent with some type of fiber (possibly cotton) (Figure 91) and/or plaque debris, which elicited a local giant cell reaction. The plaque emboli were predominantly subepicardial and mid-wall vessels, although occasionally they were seen in the subendocardium.

Clearly, this embolic biologic and foreign material was secondary to the two atherectomy procedures. The dating of the focal myocytolysis associated with the emboli, provides a temporal relationship to the coronary intervention occurring 3 weeks before death. It is noteworthy, that at the time of the atherectomy, the patient developed an abnormally elevated creatine kinase, with a positive MB fraction. This was not considered to be significant clinically. Yet, in retrospect, the elevated CK enzyme was due to multi-focal small areas of reperfusion myocardial necrosis secondary to coronary micro-emboli. Whether it was the multiple areas of healing necrosis with surrounding viable but ischemic myocardium, or whether it was the severe high-grade coronary disease with ischemia that elicited a sudden fatal arrhythmia, cannot be determined; however, either could have done so. Both entities represent significant complications of the original procedure; neither would have occurred if this patient had been treated with CABG, or even angioplasty with stenting.

A final point relates to the pathogenesis of myocytolysis, and the potential role of coronary micro-emboli. Myocytolysis is a type of reperfusion necrosis associated with an abnormal microcirculation. As described elsewhere in this book, the coronary microcirculation is an end-vessel network; thus, distal arterioles supplying capillaries and small volumes of myocardium, do not anastomose with other arterioles. If those arterioles or more proximal small intra-myocardial arteries develop spasm, the myocardium supplied by those vessels may develop a type of reperfusion necrosis (e.g. there is initially ischemia, followed by blood flow). This causes free radical damage to the myocyte, with rupture of the sarcolemma and an influx of calcium into the cell causing an 'explosive' type of necrosis (hence, lysis). Most often, there are concurrent high-catecholamine states such as shock; however, other vasoactive substances can cause microvascular vasospasm. Myocytolysis is a very common finding in cardiomyopathies of many etiologies, myocarditis, and ischemic heart disease.

Although it is logical to assume that micro-embolization would cause localized myocyte necrosis due to obstruction of the vessels, in fact, the morphology of the microscopic necrosis with areas of contraction bands (a reperfusion lesion that precedes myocytolysis) or myocytolysis, suggests a reperfusion process. Experimentally, embolization of 25 and 50 micron-sized microspheres into the coronary circulation of animals led to identical areas of microscopic necrosis as seen in this case. Interestingly, treatment of the animals with drugs that prevent coronary artery or microvascular spasm (calcium channel blocking drugs, or alpha-adrenergic blocking drugs), significantly prevented the necrosis even with the microspheres in the circulation. Thus, it is not obstruction, but spasm that leads to myocytolysis. The plaque emboli caused multiple areas of microvascular spasm and myocyte necrosis in this patient. It is not known where the foreign fiber material came from, but it is likely to have been a contaminant of one of the coronary catheters. Since the sections of myocardium that demonstrated these changes were randomly sampled (e.g. the pathologist performing the autopsy did not see any grossly visible areas in the myocardium to sample specifically), then the plaque emboli, and probably the foreign material, were probably a generalized and widespread phenomenon throughout the heart.

In summary, this case has many interesting clinical and pathological features, but it also clearly indicates why it led to a negligence suit against the cardiologists performing the coronary interventional procedure. The wrong treatment, and its subsequent complications, was medical negligence that unfortunately caused the death of this treatable patient.

Suggested Readings

1. Carroza JP Jr, Braim DS. Complications of directional coronary atherectomy: incidence, causes, and management. Am J Cardiol. 1993; 72: 47E-54E.
2. Hinohara T, Robertson GC, Selmon MR, Vetter JW, McAuley BJ, Sheehan DJ, Simpson JB. Directional coronary atherectomy complications and management. Cather Cardiovasc Diagn. 1993; Suppl 1:61-71.
3. Kaufmann UP, Meyer BJ. Atherectomy (directional, rotational, extractional) and its role in percutaneous revascularization. Curr Opon Cardiol. 1995; 10:412-9.
4. Corcos T, Zimarino M, Tamburino C, Favereau X. Randomized trials of direccional atherectomy: implications for clinical practice and future investigation. J Am Coll Cardiol. 1994; 24:431-9.

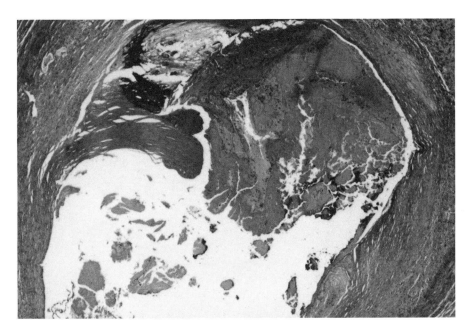

Figure 90. Coronary artery several weeks following balloon angioplasty. There is distortion and disruption of the atherosclerotic plaque and granulation tissue in a medial dissection (arrow) (Hematoxylin and Eosin, 10X).

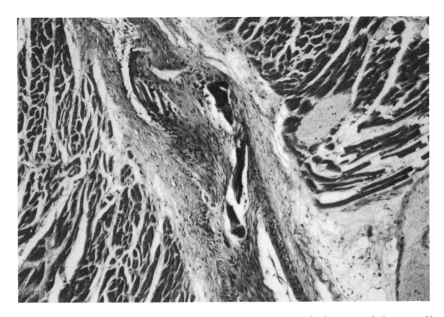

Figure 91. Intramyocardial small artery occluded by foreign body material (? cotton fiber) with an intimal granulomatous and fibrous reaction occluding the vessel (Hematoxylin and Eosin, 20X).

297

Appendix I. Heart Measurements in Adultts (modified from Sunderman FW, Boerner F: Normal values in clinical medicine. Philadelphia. W.B. Saunders Company, 1949).

	Mean (cm)	Range (cm)
Thickness, left ventricular muscle	1.5	
Thickness, right ventricular muscle	0.5	
Thickness, atrial muscle	0.2	
Circumference, mitral valve	10	8-10.5
Circumference, aortic valve	7.5	6-7.5
Circumference, pulmonary valve	8.5	7-9
Circumference, tricuspid valve	12	10-12.5

Appendix II. Normal adult laboratory values

BUN mg/dL	3-25	Uric Acid mg/dL	3.5–7.2
Na mEq/L	135-145	T Prot g/dL	5.3-8.0
K mEq/L	3.5 – 5.0	Albumin g/dL	3.3-5.8
Cl mEq/L	98-108	T Bili mg/dL	0.1-1.0
CO2 mEq/L	20-28	D Bili mg/dL	0.2-0.5
Glucose mg/dL	60-100	Alk Phos U/L	50-375
Ca mg/dL	9.0-10.7	SGOT (AST) U/L	1-40
Creat mg/dL	0.1-1.0	SGPT (ALT) U/L	1-45
Lactate nmol/L	0.3-1.3	LD U/L	100-210
Osmolality mOsm/kg	285-295	CK U/L	5-225
Ion Ca mmol/L	1.12 –1.23	CK-MB/CK	<2.5%
Mg mg/dL	1.6-2.6	Chol mg/dL	< 197
Phos mg/dL	2.7–4.5	PT sec	9.0-11.5
PTT sec	23.0-34.0		

WBC /nL	4.5-13.0	% Gr	40.0-61.5
RBC /pL	4.5-5.3	% Ly	26.7-40.0
Hgb g/dL	13.0-16.0	% Mo	1.0-10.0
Hct vol %	37-49	% Eo	0-3
MCV fL	78-98	% Ba	< 2
MCH pg	25-35		
Plt n/L	150-440		

Appendix III. Abbreviations.

AAA	abdominal aortic aneurysm
ABE	acute bacterial endocarditis
ABG	arterial blood gases
ACh	acetylcholine
AChE	acetylcholinesterase
AIDS	acquired immunodeficiency syndrome
ANA	antinuclear antibodies
ARDS	adult respiratory distress syndrome
ASA	aspirin
ASD	atrial septal defect
ATP	adenosin triphosphate
AV	atrioventricular
BMI	body mass index
BP	blood pressure
CABG	coronary artery bypass graft
CAD	coronary artery disease
CCU	coronary care unit
CEA	carcinoembryonic antigen
CHF	congestive heart failure
CK	creatin kinase
CM	cardiomyopathy
CMV	cytomegalovirus
CNS	central nervous system
CO	cardiac output
COPD	chronic obstructive pulmonary disease
CPR	cardiopulmonary resuscitation
CREST	calcinosis, Raynaud's phenomenom, esophageal dysmotility, sclerodactyly and telangiectasia
CSF	cerebrospinal fluid
CT	computarized tomography
CVA	cerebrovascular accident
CXR	chest x ray
DCM	dilated cardiomyopathy
DIC	disseminated intravascular coagulation
DM	diaebtes mellitus
ECG	electrocardiogram
ECHO	enteric cytopathogenic human orphan viruses
EMD	electro-mechanical dissociation
ER	emergency room
ESR	erythrocyte sedimentation rate

FDP	fibrin degradation products
FHC	familial hypertrophic cardiomyopathy
GI	gastrointestinal
H&E	hematoxylin and eosin
HAART	highly active antiretroviral therapy
Hb	hemoglobin
HCM	hypertrophic cardiomyopathy
Hct	hematocrit
HDL	high density lipoproteins
HIV	human immunodeficiency virus
HSV	herpes simplex virus
HTN	hypertension
ICU	intensive care unit
IE	infectious endocarditis
IHD	ischemic heart disease
IM	intramuscular
JVD	jugular venous distension
LA	left atrium
LAD	left anterior descending coronary artery
LAH	left atrium hypertrophy
LCX	left circumflex coronary artery
LDH	lactate deshydrogenase
LDL	low density lipoproteins
LM	left circumflex artery
LV	left ventricle
LVH	left ventricular hypertrophy
MHC	myosin heavy chain
MI	myocardial infarction
MRI	magnetic resonance imaging
MVP	mitral valve prolapse
NE	norepinephrine
NSAID	non-steroidal anti-inflammatory drug
NSR	normal sinus rhythm
PCR	polymerase chain reaction
PCWP	pulmonary capillary wedge pressure
PDA	patent ductus arteriosus
PDA	patent ductus arteriosus
PDGF	platelet-derived growth factor
PPC	peri-partum cardiomyopathy
PPH	plexogenic pulmonary hypertension
PRBC	packed red blood cells
PT	prothrombin time

PTCA	percutaneous transluminal angioplasty
PTT	partial thromboplastin time
PTU	propylthiouracil
PVD	peripheral vascular disease
RA	right atrium
RAH	right atrium hypertrophy
RBBB	right bundle branch block
RCA	right coronary artery
REM	rapid eye movements
RHD	rheumatic heart disease
ROMI	rule out myocardial infarction
RV	right ventricle
RVH	right ventricular hypertrophy
SAM	systolic anterior motion of the mitral valve
SBE	subacute bacterial endocarditis
SCD	sudden cardiac death
SEMI	subendocardial myocardial infarction
SMA	superior mesenteric artery
SVT	supraventricular tachycardia
TA	Takayasu's arteritis
TB	tuberculosis
TEE	transesophageal echocardiogram
TIA	transient ischemic attack
TMMI	transmural myocardial infarction
TMPs	tissue metalloproteinases
TOF	tetralogy of Fallot
TPA	tissue plasminogen activator
TXa	thromboxane
VF	ventricular fibrilation
VSD	ventricular septal defect
WBC	white blood cell count
WPW	Wolf-Parkinson-White

Index.

basophilic degeneration, 87, 100, 152, 158

Beck's triad, 223

beer-drinkers cardiomyopathy, 103

beri-beri heart disease, 102

bicuspid aortic valve, 153, 155, 284

Blalock-Taussig operation, 141

bulbus cordis, 2, 10, 140

bundle of His, 3, 4, 6, 10, 259

CABG, 29, 32, 35, 290, 294

calcific aortic stenosis, 154, 155

calcific aortic stenosis of the elderly, 123, 155

capillary loops, 4, 49, 70

cardiac metastases, 205

cardiac myxoma, 216

cardiac output, 85, 94, 95, 99, 106, 114, 133, 191, 212, 213, 223, 225, 252

cardiac tamponade, 54, 132, 133, 205, 206, 223

cardiogenic shock, 39, 106

cardiomyopathy, 10, 14, 16, 25, 30, 34, 63, 70, 71, 72, 74, 75, 79, 81, 82, 83, 85, 86, 87, 90, 94, 95, 96, 98, 101, 102, 103, 104, 105, 106, 107, 108, 109, 111, 113, 114, 115, 117, 130, 142, 144, 151, 152, 167, 182, 193, 195, 205, 213, 281

Carney's syndrome, 215

Chaga's disease, 193

changing murmur, 174, 184

chest pain, 19, 20, 21, 36, 37, 52, 53, 54, 57, 58, 64, 79, 99, 119, 132, 152, 161, 193, 221, 222, 265, 267, 282, 283, 290

chordae tendineae, 5, 11, 13, 16, 76, 100, 105, 123, 130, 131, 135, 138, 150, 162, 171, 176, 184, 186, 204, 229, 258, 260, 265

chronic alcoholic cardiomyopathy, 103

chronic obstructive pulmonary disease, 52, 161, 162, 171, 205

clubbing, 52, 57, 84, 137, 138, 143, 144, 162, 164

CO, 85

coagulative necrosis, 40, 46, 101

coarctation of the aorta, 153, 154, 159, 268, 283, 284

cobalt, 103

cocaine, 25, 59, 61, 64, 113, 114, 182, 249, 251, 254, 287

coeur en sabot, 143

collagen vascular disease, 61

collateral circulation, 45, 141, 142, 143

commissure, 5, 154, 260

concentric, 17, 29, 75, 76, 105, 108, 116, 285

concentric hypertrophy, 76, 149

Concentric left ventricular hypertrophy, 122

conduction system, 1, 6, 106, 192, 193, 206, 214

congenital heart disease, 4, 146, 199

congestive heart failure, 13, 17, 25, 67, 70, 76, 99, 101, 102, 103, 106, 119, 120, 122, 137, 142, 150, 151, 155, 175, 180, 192, 198, 205, 213, 215, 224, 234, 245, 285

connective tissue, 1, 2, 3, 5, 6, 7, 11, 12, 13, 14, 16, 32, 38, 43, 48, 62, 69, 103, 105, 131, 135, 143, 154, 164, 173, 175, 223, 232, 284, 285, 294

connective tissue disorders, 62, 85

connective tissue matrix, 12, 13, 78, 85, 95

constricitive pericarditis, 224

contraction band necrosis, 17, 45, 46

cor pulmonale, 161, 163, 164, 165, 252, 253

coronary arteries, 3, 4, 7, 13, 20, 29, 36, 53, 60, 62, 63, 68, 69, 92, 105, 110, 138, 150, 151, 162, 171, 183, 197, 204, 211, 222, 251, 260, 265, 266, 267, 275, 284, 290, 292

coronary artery ameurysm, 275

coronary artery bypass graft, 29

coronary artery disease, 7, 24, 29, 30, 31, 34, 48, 57, 59, 60, 71, 86, 101, 120, 151, 241, 250, 260, 275, 290

coronary artery dissection, 63, 64, 96, 292

Coronary artery dissection, 62, 65

coronary artery spasm, 23, 59, 60, 61, 63, 293

coronary artery vasculitis, 61

coronary ostia, 3, 245

Corrigan's pulse, 183

Coxsackie, 193, 199

creatine kinase, 21, 291, 294

Crohn's disease, 102

cyanosis, 52, 57, 84, 137, 142, 143, 144, 162, 164, 221, 265, 272, 283

cystic tumor of the atrio-ventricular node, 213

Cytomegalovirus, 194

DCM, 76, 78, 85, 86, 87, 113

degenerative valve disease, 123

diabetes mellitus, 14, 19, 20, 21, 22, 24, 48, 57, 59, 60, 67, 68, 69, 149, 155, 174, 232

diabetic cardiomyopathy, 151, 281

diabetic neuropathy, 43, 69, 281

diabetic vascular injury, 69

diastolic dysfunction, 7, 25, 71, 78, 114

dilated cardiomyopathy, 76, 85, 105, 113

dilated congestive cardiomyopathy, 163

dissection, 32, 37, 38, 39, 54, 59, 63, 64, 230, 232, 245, 283, 284, 285, 287, 291, 292, 293, 297

Dressler's syndrome, 132

ductus arteriosus, 8, 138, 140, 141, 142, 144, 166, 167, 168, 268, 284

Duroziez's sign, 183

dyskinesia, 1

eccentric, 17, 293

ECHO, 193, 200

ectasia, 231, 275

Ehlers-Danlos syndrome, 16, 62

Eisenmenger's syndrome, 164

electrocardiogram, 29, 94, 143, 191, 206, 242

electro-mechanical dissociation, 30

endarteritis, 244, 248

endocardial cushion defects, 11, 130

endocarditis, 2, 4, 5, 8, 11, 16, 59, 111, 112, 130, 132, 144, 172, 175, 176, 177, 178, 180, 181, 182, 183, 184, 186, 188, 189, 258, 259, 260, 263, 264, 282

endocardium, 2, 4, 8, 14, 16, 36, 45, 46, 47, 62, 63, 76, 77, 84, 86, 92, 105, 110, 111, 138, 173, 181, 198, 204, 206, 211, 214, 222, 229, 258, 259, 265

Endomyocardial biopsies, 194

endothelin-1, 32

endovascular grafting, 235

eosinophilic vasculitis, 63

myocyte whorls, 78
myocytolysis, 43, 103, 110, 111,
    112, 120, 150, 151, 197, 273,
    275, 294, 295
myofibrils, 15
myosin heavy chain, 79
necrotizing glomerulonephritis,
    174
necrotizing vasculitis, 166, 174,
    260
neo-intima, 32, 293
non-bacterial thrombotic
    vegetation, 100
non-Q-wave MI, 45
non-steroidal anti-inflammatory
    drug, 274
obesity, 14, 161, 162, 163, 164,
    165, 256, 257, 260, 261
Osler's nodes, 174
ostium, 7, 11, 39, 62, 265
papillary fibroelastoma, 10
papillary muscle, 4, 5, 13, 36, 37,
    39, 41, 42, 74, 130, 131, 266
patent ductus arteriosus, 162, 163
pathologic hypertrophy, 31
Pentalogy of Fallot, 141
percutaneous transluminal
    coronary angioplasty, 29, 34
perforin, 193
pericardial effusion, 19, 54, 92,
    110, 111, 132, 152, 161, 191,
    205, 206, 225, 274, 275
pericardial friction rub, 132, 180,
    185
pericardial tamponade, 13, 39,
    186, 292
pericardiocentesis, 185, 205, 225
pericarditis, 58, 59, 75, 129, 132,
    185, 186, 192, 222, 225, 228,
    250, 257, 259, 263, 274
pericardium, 13, 19, 29, 36, 52,
    54, 62, 84, 92, 100, 110, 119,
    123, 129, 132, 138, 161, 171,
181, 185, 186, 198, 204, 205,
    216, 221, 222, 224, 225, 229,
    231, 243, 257, 259
peripartum cardiomyopathy, 63
peri-partum cardiomyopathy, 93
peri-partum cardiomyopathy, 95
peripheral vascular disease, 19, 43,
    245
physiologic hypertrophy, 31
Pickwickian syndrome, 163
platelet-derived growth factor, 32
pleuritic pain, 223
plexogenic pulmonary
    hypertension, 164
pneumococcal endocarditis, 184
Pneumocystis carinii pneumonia,
    221, 274
polyarteritis nodosa, 60
Polyarteritis Nodosa, 276
polycythemia, 143, 144, 162
post-cardiotomy syndrome, 132,
    133
posterior leaflet, 11, 76, 77, 78,
    123, 129, 131, 258
Potts anastomosis, 141
PPC, 93, 94
primary tumors, 204, 214
pseudo-aneurysm, 176, 181, 186,
    230, 292
pseudovalve, 120, 121
pseudoxanthoma elasticum, 62
PTCA, 29
pulmonary adenocarcinoma, 206
pulmonary hypertension, 53, 162,
    163, 268
pulmonary valve, 14, 121, 138,
    141, 252
pulmonic valve, 2, 5, 15, 92, 141,
    186, 204
pulsus paradoxus, 132, 223
Purkinje cells, 46
Purkinje fibers, 6
Quincke's pulse, 183

remodeling, 6, 7, 14, 17, 47, 85, 95, 105, 122, 130, 152, 153, 155, 163, 182, 196, 252, 293
reperfusion infarction, 22, 24
reperfusion injury, 17, 45, 51, 116
re-stenosis, 29, 32, 34, 291, 292
restrictive heart disease, 114, 213
retroperitoneal hematoma, 53
RHD, 120, 123, 260
rheumatic heart disease, 5, 11, 76, 105, 120, 121, 124, 125, 130, 183, 215, 241, 260, 275
rheumatic mitral valve, 123
rheumatoid arthritis, 3, 193, 272
right ventricle, 4, 9, 12, 13, 14, 17, 19, 29, 36, 75, 100, 116, 119, 129, 133, 138, 141, 143, 149, 151, 163, 197, 252, 255, 266, 294
rule out myocardial infarction, 59
ruptured papillary muscle, 39
ruptured plaque, 20, 25
SAM, 75, 77, 78
sarcoidosis, 21, 85, 213, 216
sarcolemma, 15, 17, 45, 111, 295
sarcomere, 15, 17, 79
sarcomeric cardiomyopathy, 79
sarcoplasmic reticulum, 15
SEMI, 43, 44, 45, 46, 47, 48
septum secundum, 8
shock, 37, 39, 99, 106, 110, 114, 191, 230, 235, 288, 295
sick sinus syndrome, 213
sinoatrial node, 14
sinus of Valsalva, 3, 7, 154
sinuses of Valsalva, 14, 123, 154, 160, 186
small vessel disease, 24, 70, 105, 253
splinter hemorrhages, 174
Stokes-Adams-Morgagni syndrome, 213
streptokinase, 22

stunned myocardium, 21
subacute bacterial endocarditis, 172
subendocardial infarction, 23, 44
subendocardial myocardial infarction, 43
sudden cardiac death, 7, 14, 24, 37, 85, 281
Sudden death, 79, 80
superior mesenteric artery, 67, 68, 69, 212, 214, 266
Swan-Ganz catheter, 92, 99, 257
syncope, 58, 61, 94, 143, 208, 211, 212, 213, 214, 216
syphilis, 2, 244, 245, 248, 268
Syphilitic aneurysms, 245
syphilitic aortitis, 38, 244
systemic lupus erythematosus, 61, 256, 262
systolic anterior motion of the mitral valve, 75, 77
Takayasu's arteritis, 2, 62, 245, 267, 271
Takayasu's disease, 245
TB pericarditis, 205, 224
TEE, 9
tetralogy of Fallot, 14, 146
Tetralogy of Fallot, 139, 147
The Dallas Classification, 194
thrombolytic therapy, 21, 26, 52, 53
thromboxane, 32
tissue metalloproteinase, 25
tissue plasminogen activator, 19, 43, 52
TMMI, 46, 47, 48
TPA, 19, 22, 23, 24, 25, 43, 45, 47, 48, 52, 53, 54
trans-esophageal echocardiography, 9
transient cerebral ischemic attack, 149, 150
transmural extension, 44, 47, 197

311